Case-Based Clinical Cardiology

Majid Maleki • Azin Alizadehasl
Editors

Case-Based Clinical Cardiology

Springer

Editors
Majid Maleki
Rajaie Cardiovascular Medical and Research Center
Iran University of Medical Sciences
Tehran
Iran

Azin Alizadehasl
Head of Cardio-Oncology Department and Research Center, Rajaie Cardiovascular Medical and Research Center
Iran University of Medical Sciences
Tehran
Iran

ISBN 978-1-4471-7495-0 ISBN 978-1-4471-7496-7 (eBook)
https://doi.org/10.1007/978-1-4471-7496-7

This Springer imprint is published by the registered company Springer-Verlag London Ltd. part of Springer Nature.
The registered company address is: The Campus, 4 Crinan Street, London, N1 9XW, United Kingdom

Preface

There are many good books on case-based cardiovascular disorders but what distinguishes case-based clinical cardiology from the rest is a strong emphasis on its practical points. All the chapters deal with a specific group of cardiovascular problem and several diagnostic tools. The particular problem depends on the clinical presentation, and once a diagnosis is made, there will be an issue of determining different aspects of the disorder by different diagnostic tools and respective practical points. Almost all of the figures are not simply a single good illustration, but rather they are a sequence of images prepared and gathered from our patients with the problem being demonstrated showing the necessary features for the diagnosis and its severity and how to manage it.

The target group of this book is both those who are new to the field of cardiology and those who are experienced in different areas of this field. This is not intended to be a textbook, but it is a practical guide to all medical students, cardiology residents, and fellows in different aspects of cardiology such as electrocardiography, echocardiography, electrophysiology, interventional cardiology, congenital heart diseases, peripheral disease, and even experienced cardiologists and cardiac surgeons.

Any work has a number of contributors both direct and indirect. Most of the images used in this book were collected by the authors of different chapters to whom we owe a great debt. Expert secretarial help was provided by Sara Tayebi and Arefeh Ghorbani.

Our thanks go to all our families and children who understand the importance of the time spent for preparing and writing this book.

Special appreciation and thanks to Springer and Grant Weston and Anand Shanmugam for their editorial assistance in the preparation of the content of the book.

Tehran, Iran

Majid Maleki
Azin Alizadehasl
Feridoun Noohi
Ata Firouzi
Bahram Mohebbi
Zahra Khajali
Mohammad Javad Alemzadeh-Ansari
Md. Sedigheh Saedi
Zahra Hosseini

Contents

Chapter 1
Electrocardiography Cases

Majid Maleki

Abstract The electrocardiogram (ECG) is one of the most important and one or first tool for diagnosis and management of cardiovascular and sometimes systemic disorders.

Abbreviations

BAA	Biatrial abnormality
Bpm	Beat per minute
DOE	Dyspnea on exertion
Dx	Diagnosis
LAA	Left atrial abnormality
LAD	Left axis deviation
LVH	Left ventricular hypertrophy
MI	Myocardial infarction
NPJT	Non-paroxysmal junctional tachycardia
NSR	Normal sinus rhythm
PRWP	Poor R wave progression
RAA	Right atrial abnormality
RVH	Right ventricular hypertrophy

M. Maleki (✉)
Rajaie Cardiovascular Medical and Research Center, Iran University of Medical Sciences, Tehran, Iran

M. Maleki, A. Alizadehasl (eds.), *Case-Based Clinical Cardiology*,
https://doi.org/10.1007/978-1-4471-7496-7_1

Introduction

The electrocardiogram (ECG) is one of the most important and one or first tool for diagnosis and management of cardiovascular and sometimes systemic disorders.

Also, it can help to diagnose some abnormalities such as electrolyte abnormalities thyroid disease, hypothermia, drug effects, and systemic disease effects on the heart.

Our goal in *this* chapter is just focusing on ECG interpretation in both simple and complex cases with some comments on final diagnosis and if necessary differential diagnosis.

Electrocardiography has its greatest role in diagnosis, treatment, and follow-up the cardiac and noncardiac patients. Not only the diagnosis of abnormality is essential but it is also important to know that ECG may mimic heart disease falsely and can lead to unnecessary medical actions. The presentation and form of this chapter are directed primarily at the clinicians such as cardiologist, internist, and different cardiology fellows in echocardiography, electrophysiology, interventional cardiology, and so on.

The text consists of the case summary, illustrative case studies, interpretation of electrocardiogram, and some important point as a take-home massage.

This chapter is not a detailed presentation of the electrocardiographic manifestation and mechanism of the various ECG abnormalities. But it is intended to be familiar with common ECG abnormalities and their clinical points.

The chapter is rather aimed to be familiar with the genesis, and clinical significance of certain comment electrocardiographic and arrhythmia with focusing on their diagnosis and management.

In summary, the analysis of abnormal rhythm includes three basic steps:

1. Identification and analysis of P wave in ECG
2. Finding out the P.QRS relation
3. The QRS complex analysis

If a bipolar chest leads is used for heart rhythm monitoring, then the modified CL1 (MCL1) lead is a more useful MCL1 lead that has the advantages of not interfering with cardiac physical examination and probable administration of precordial electric shock.

Case 1

Thirty years old man with a history of mitral stenosis

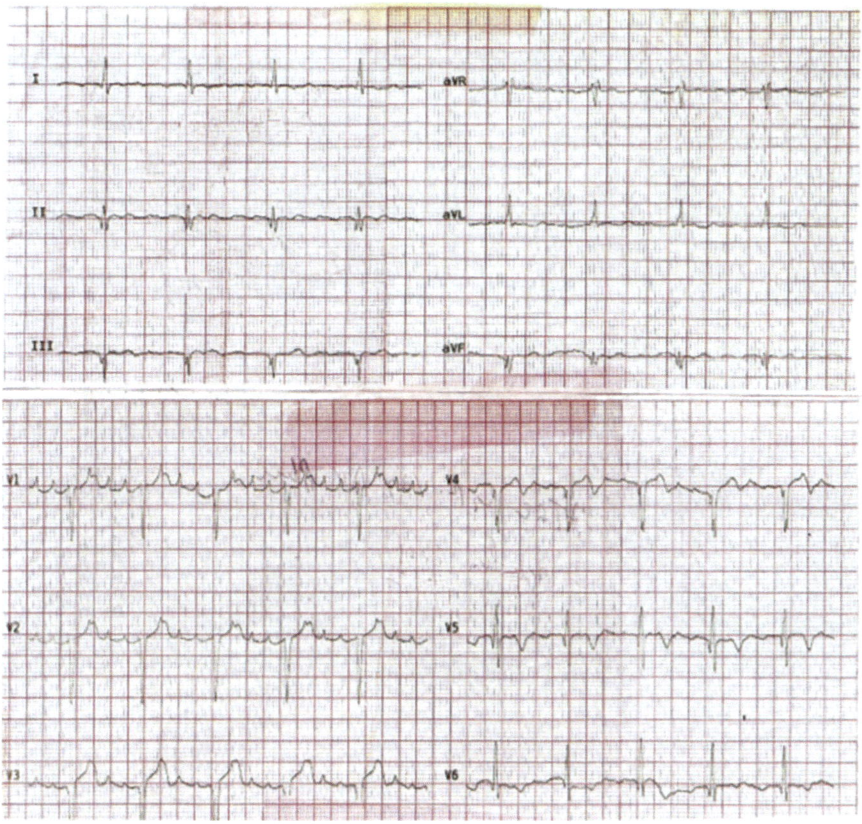

- ECG: atrial flutter with 4:1 conduction
- LAD
- Atrial rate: 300 bpm
- Ventricular rate: 75 bpm
- PRwp
- Diagnosis: atrial flutter with 4:1 conduction

Case 2

Thirty years old man with history of frequent palpitation

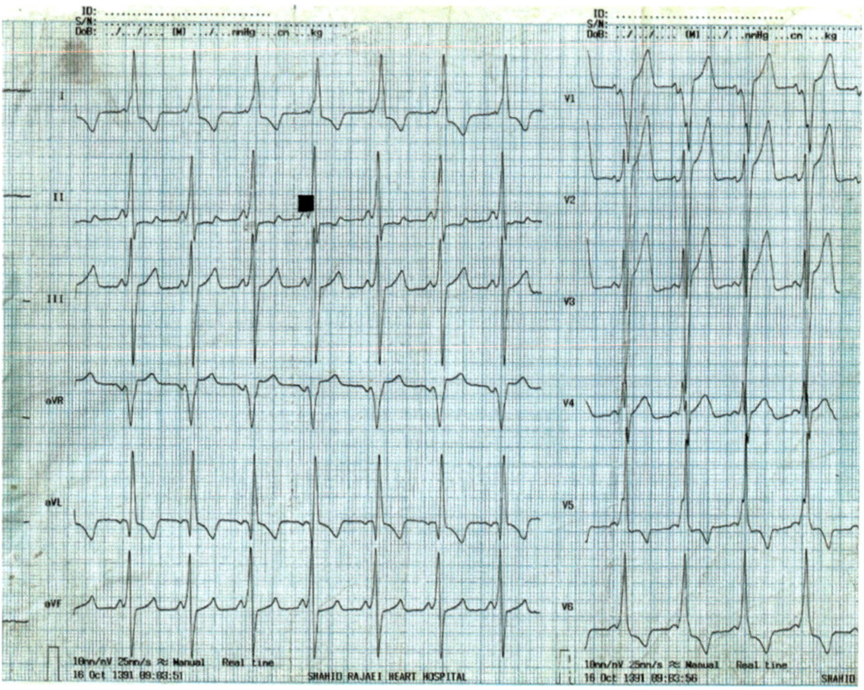

- ECG: NSR
- Normal axis
- 90 bpm
- Short PR interval
- Delta wave presence
- Secondary ST T changes
- Diagnosis: pre-excitation syndrome with accessory pathway probably from RV free wall [1]

Case 3

Thirty-five years old man with history of dilated cardiomyopathy since 1 year age

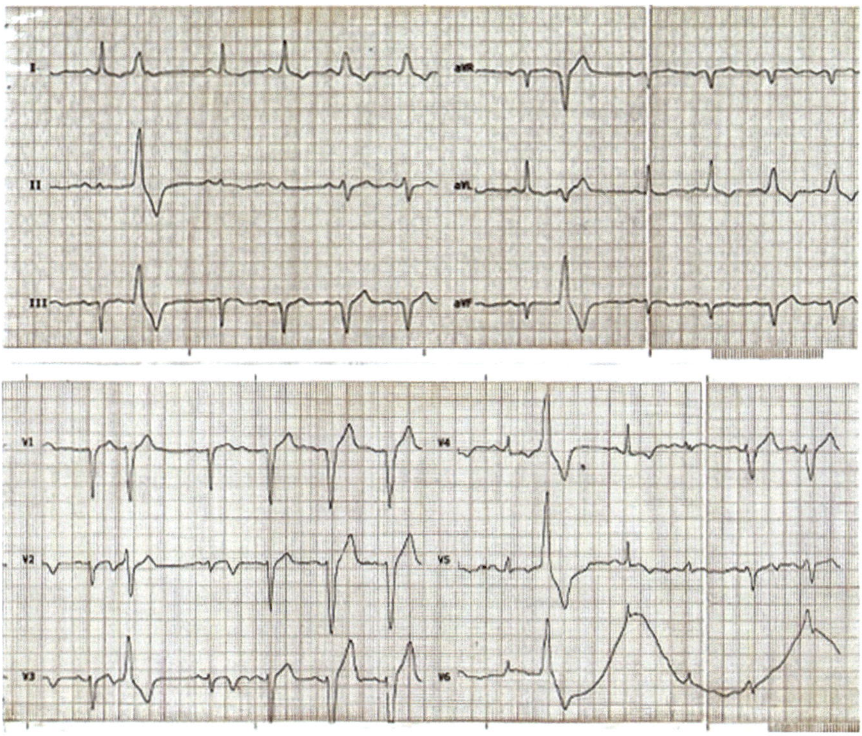

- ECG: NSR
- LAD
- Variable rate between 75 and 77
- Occasional PVC
- Rate-dependent LBBB with fusion beat
- Dx: occasional PVC with tachycardia dependent LBBB pattern [1]

Case 4

Twenty-five years healthy man with atypical chest pain

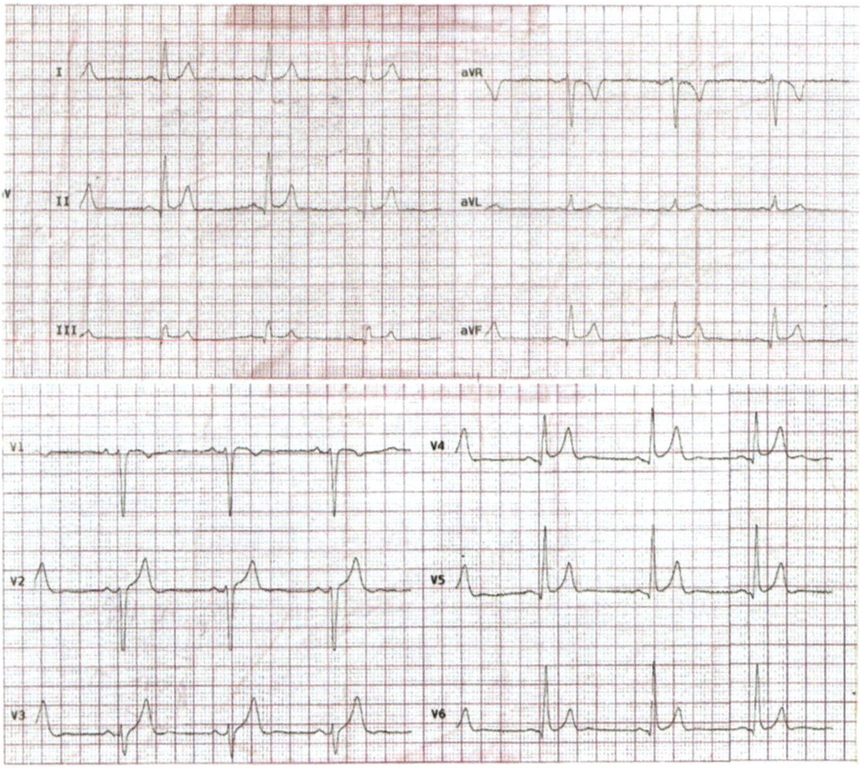

- ECG: Sinus bradycardia
- Normal axis
- Concave st elevation in inferolateral leads
- Dx: early repolarization [2]

Case 5

Seventy years old man with vertigo since 1 month age

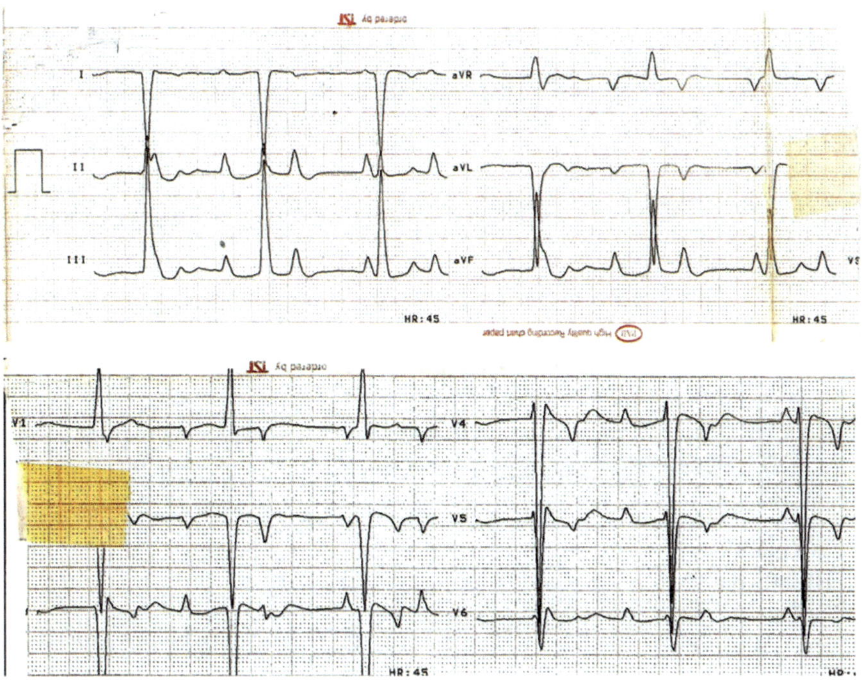

- ECG: Sinus rhythm
- Atrial rate 90 bpm
- Ventricular rate 43 bpm
- AV dissociation
- Dx: complete heart block

Case 6

Sixteen years old girl with clubbing fingers since birth.

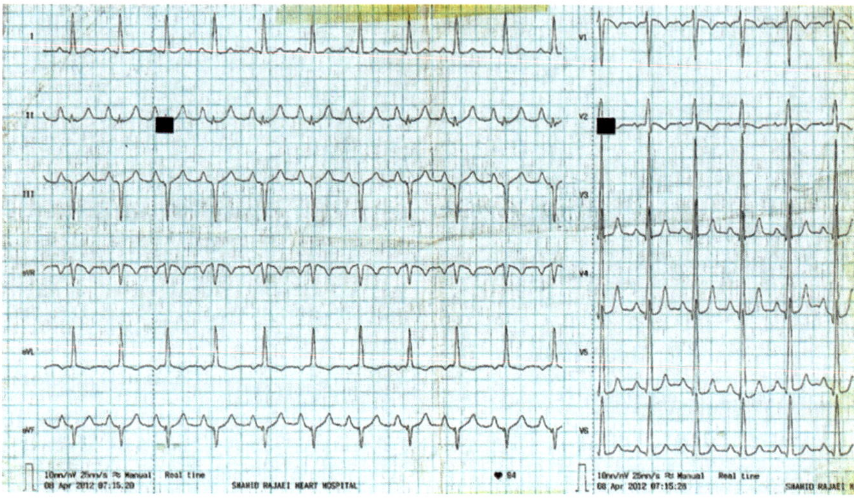

- ECG: NSR.
- HR 80 bpm.
- LAD.
- RAA.
- LVH.
- Dx: NSR, RAA, LVH.
- NOTE: LVH and RAA in a young cyanotic patient are strongly suggestive of Tricuspid Atresia [2].

Case 7

Thirty years old man with history of frequent palpitation since many years ago

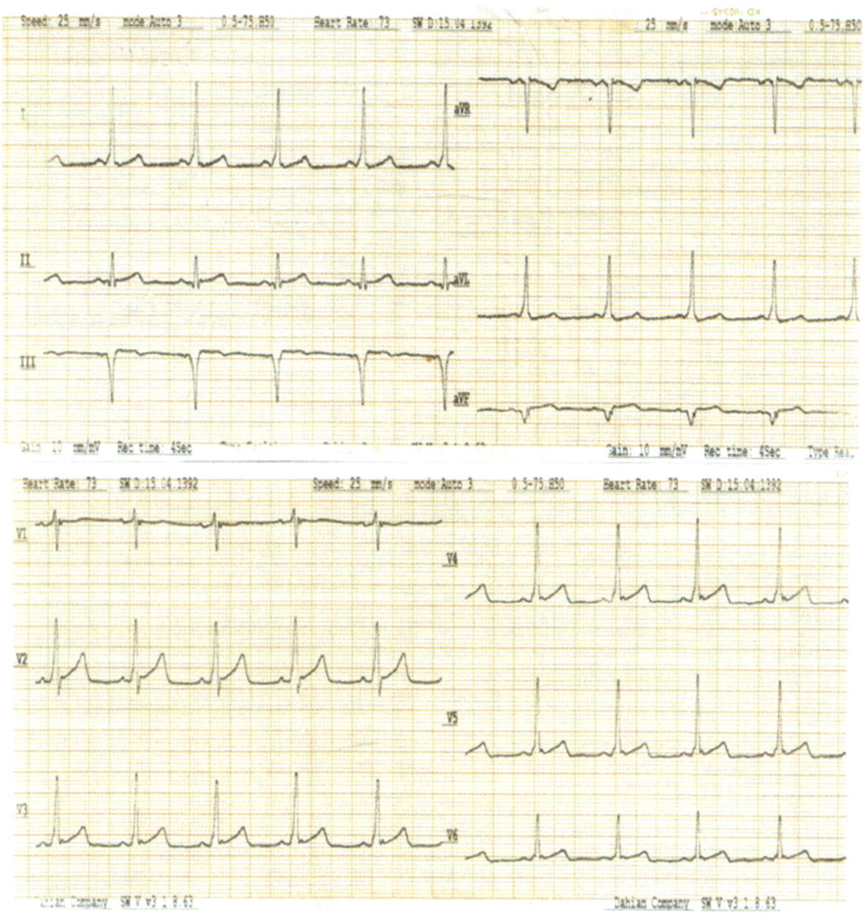

- ECG: NSR
- LAD
- 75 bpm
- Short PR interval
- Delta wave
- Dx: pre-excitation syndrome with accessory pathway originated from mid-septal [3]

Case 8

Fifty years old man with history of valvular heart disease

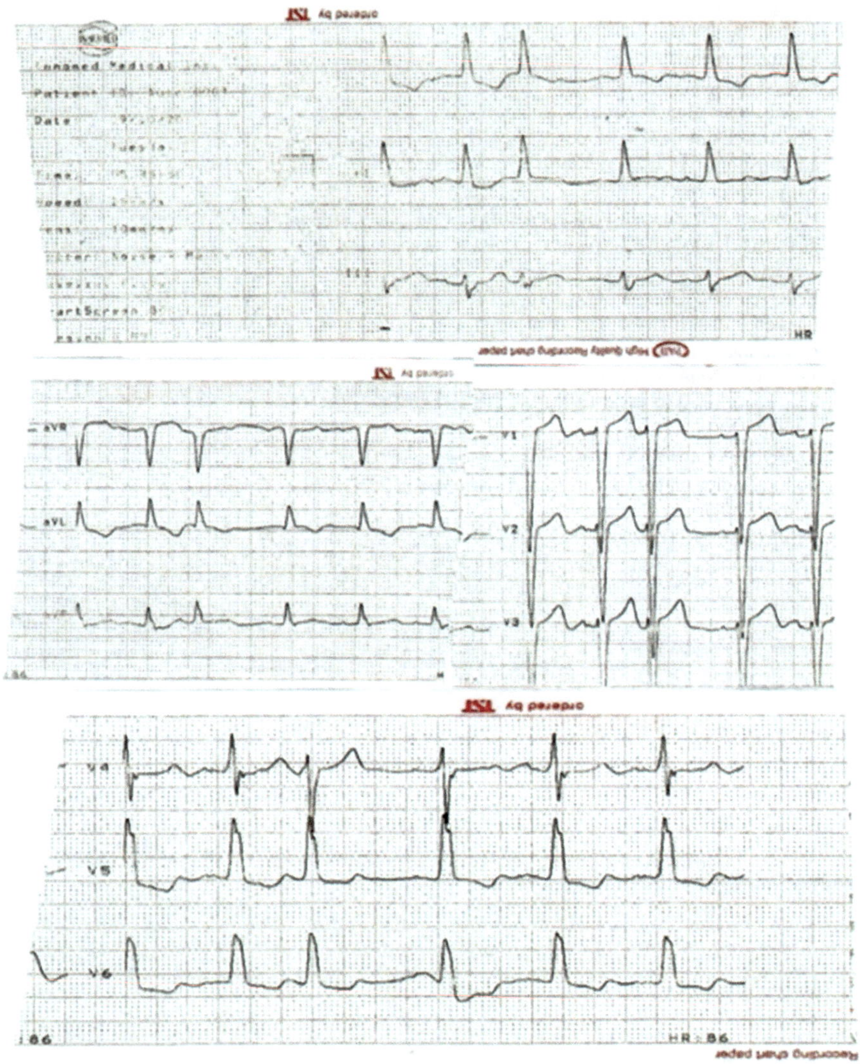

- ECG: NSR
- Normal axis
- 75 bpm
- LBBB pattern with secondary st. T changes occasional PAC.

Case 9

Sixty years old man with history of valvular heart disease.

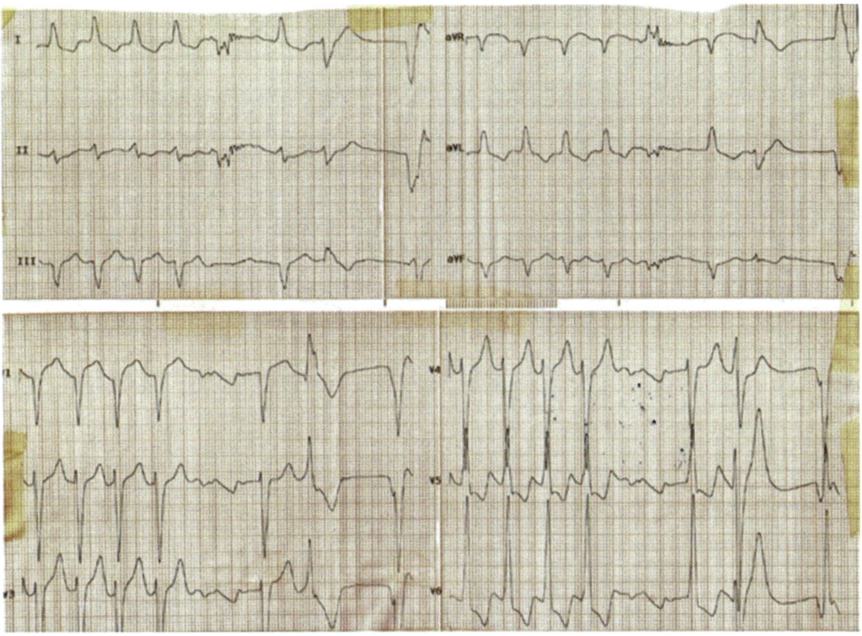

- ECG.
- AF with rapid ventricular response.
- LAD.
- Long pause, short pause with RBBB pattern (Ashman phenomenon).
- Dx: AF, LBBB pattern, with Ashman phenomenon.
- NOTE: sometimes it is difficult to distinguish PVC with RBBB pattern from aberrancy (Ashman phenomenon) in atrial fibrillation with rapid ventricular response. PVC usually has its coupling interval and compensatory and Ashman phenomenon is distinguished in AF with preceding long pause short pause with RBBB pattern [2].

Case 10

Sixty years old man with history of CABGS 1 week ago.

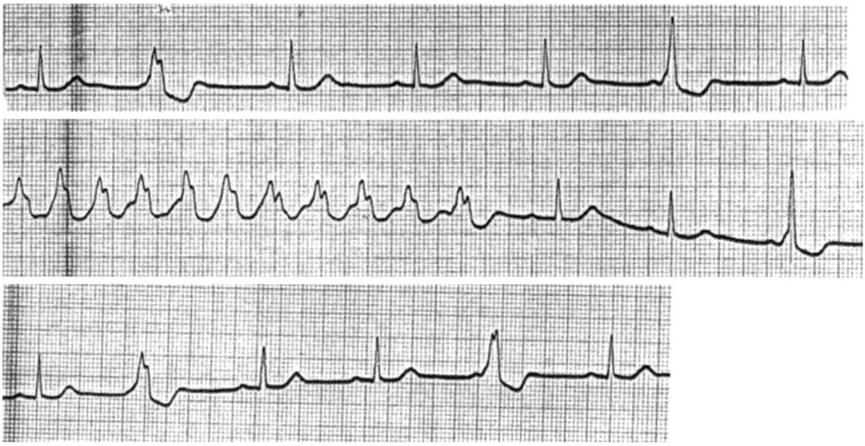

- ECG: Lead II.
- Sinus rhythm.
- PVC (second beat in the first row).
- Fusion beat (sixth beat in the first row).
- Short run of ventricular tachycardia with concealed conduction to AV node and subsequent prolonged PR interval after VT [3].

Case 11

Thirty-eight years old lady with history of Rheumatic heart disease.

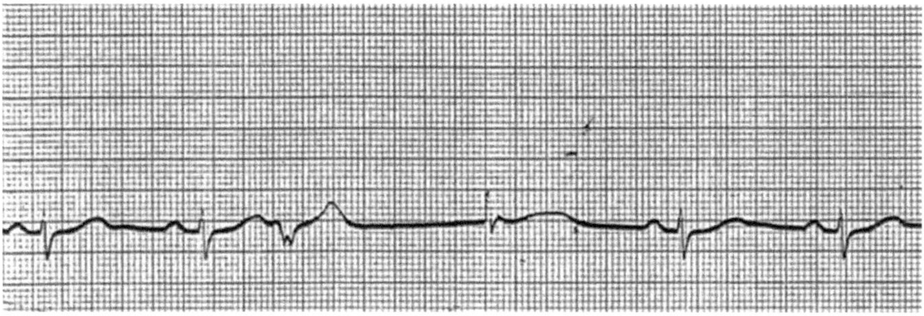

- ECG: Sinus rhythm.
- PVC with compensatory pause junctional escape beat after PVC.
- NOTE: sinus node in patient with sick sinus syndrome may not recover after a compensatory pause with pvc and unusual recovery of the sinus node is suggestive of sinus node disease.

Case 12

Sixteen years old asymptomatic boy with III/VI murmur at lower left sternal border and sail sound due to Ebstein anomaly.

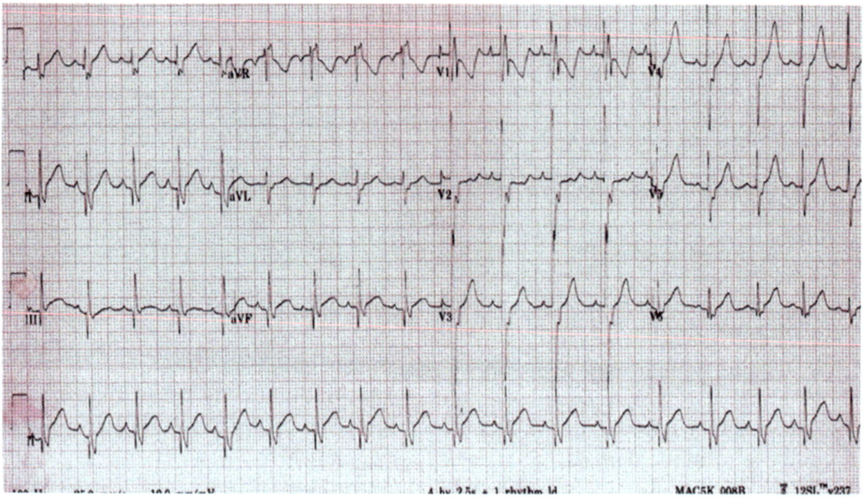

- ECG.
- NSR.
- RAD.
- HR: 100/min.
- RAA.
- RBBB, rsr'.
- Fragmented QRS in V.
- Note: This ECG pattern and Fragmented QRS may be due to atrialization of parts of the right ventricle. Fragmented QRS in right precordial leads may be due to abnormal depolarization of residual right ventricle [2].

Case 13

Thirty years old man with chest pain aggravation by respiration since 1 week ago. He had history of influenza 20 weeks ago.

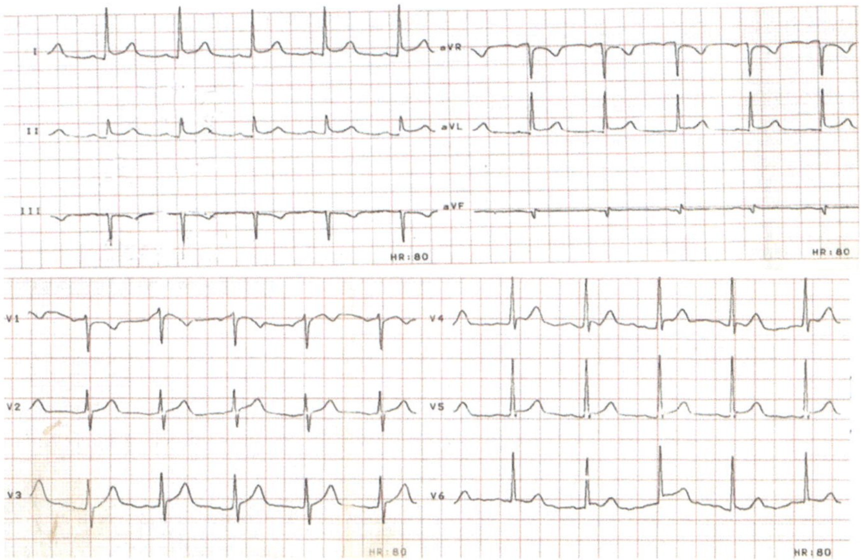

- ECG.
- NSR.
- HR: 80/min.
- LAD.
- ST. elevation in all leads except AVR and V1.
- ST Depression in AVR and V1.
- Note concave st. Elevation in all except AVR and V1 which in characteristics for pericarditis [2].

Case 14

Twenty-three years old man with history of frequent palpitation

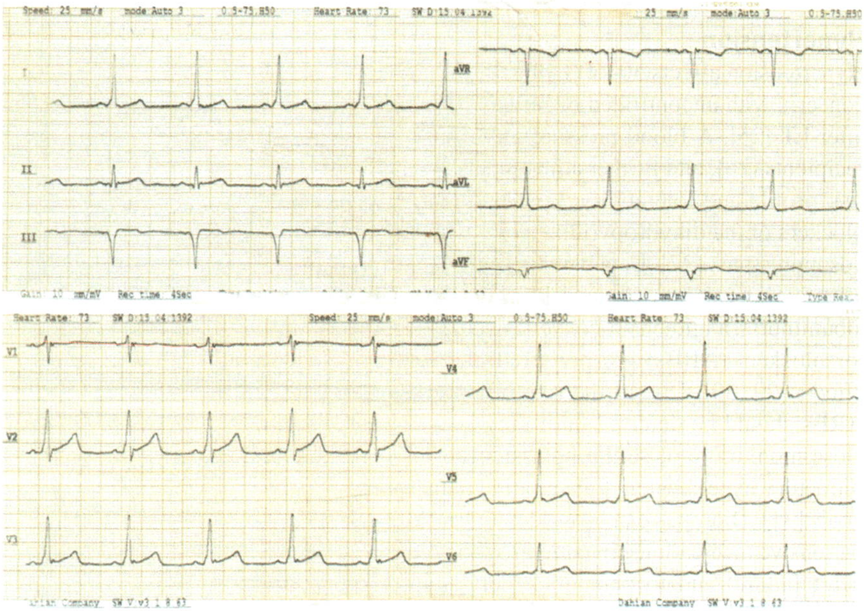

- ECG: NSR
- 75/min
- LAD
- Short PR
- Delta wave
- Tall R in V1-V2
- Diagnosis pre-excitation syndrome (WPV)

Case 15

Fifty years old man with history of myocardial infarction and congestive heart failure. Echocardiography showed enlarged cardiac chambers and reduced Ejection fraction.

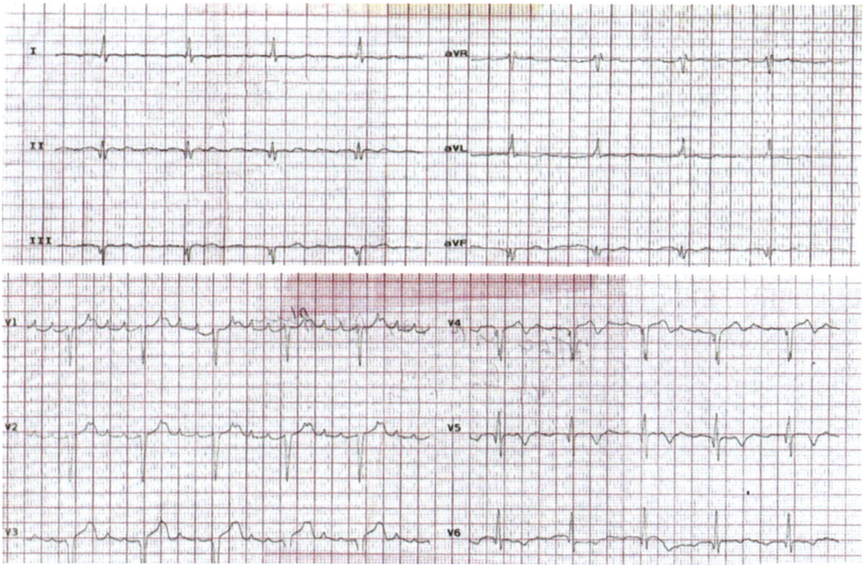

- ECG: Narrow QRS regular rhythm.
- 75/min.
- Q wave in II, III, AVF.
- ST.t change in, AVL, v4-v6.
- QS pattern in precordial leads with inverted T wave in v4-v6.
- Atrial rate 300/min.
- Ventricular rate 75/min.
- Diagnosis, Atrial flutter with 4:1 conduction, old inferior myocardial infarction [4].

Case 16

Twenty years old cyanotic man with dyspnea on exertion (Fc, II, III) since childhood.

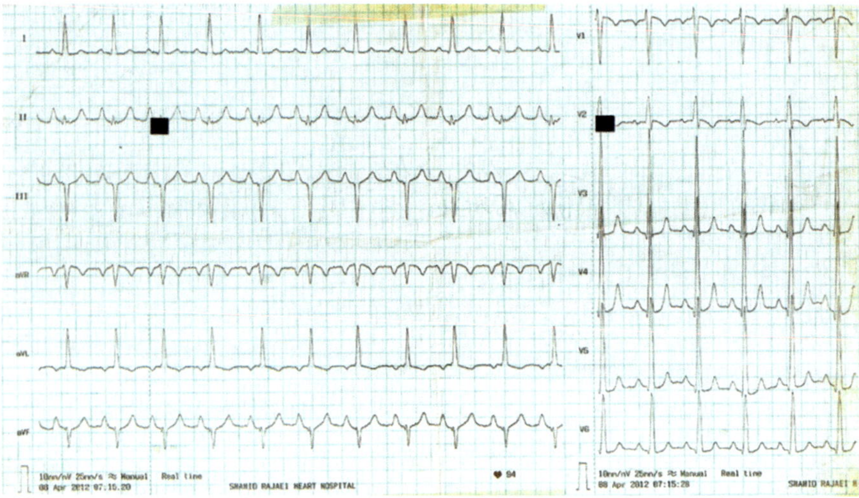

- ECG.
- NSR.
- HR: 100/min.
- LAD.
- RAA.
- High voltage QRS in the precordial lead.
- Diagnosis, RAA, LVH most probably due to Tricuspid Atresia.
- Sometimes thin pattern is seen in a single ventricle too [2].

Case 17

Seventy years old woman with vertigo since last week.

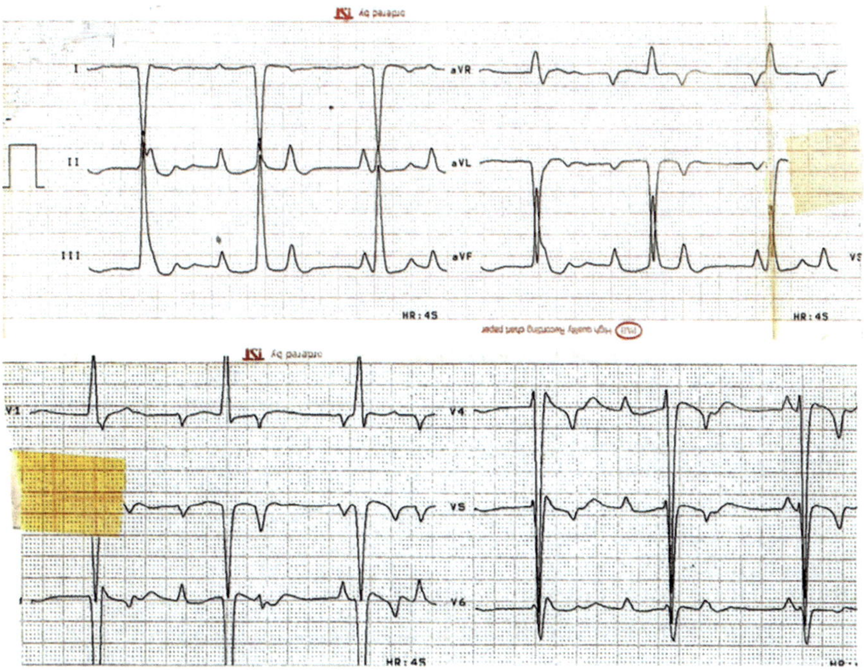

- ECG: Atrial rate 75/min.
- Ventricular rate 48/min.
- AV Dissociation.
- Complete heart block.
- Note: complete heart block usually is Av dissociation too but AV dissociation in not always complete heart block such as ventricular tachycardia.

Case 18

Forty-five years old man with history of dyslipidemia and heavy smoking has been referred to ER due to severe chest pain.

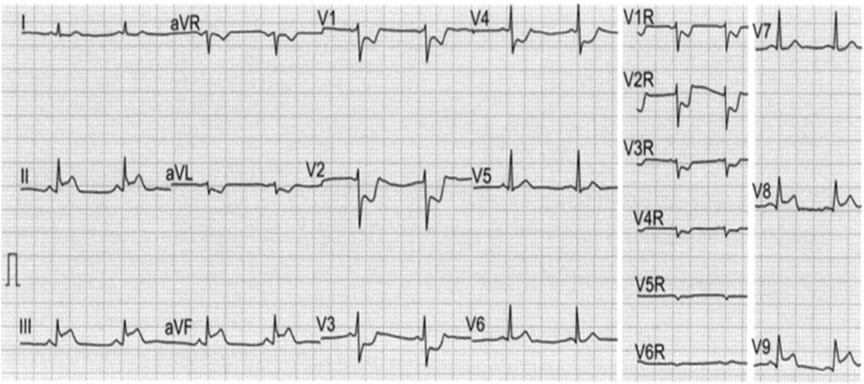

- ECG: sinus Rhythm.
- 115/min.
- St-Segment elevation in inferior leads (II > III and posterior leads).
- Prominent R wave in v1.
- ST depression and T wave inversion in V2-V4.
- ST-segment depression in V4R.
- Diagnosis: acute inferior posterior STEMI most probably due to LCX occlusion [1].

Case 19

Forty years old man with typical chest pain and sweating since 1 day ago.

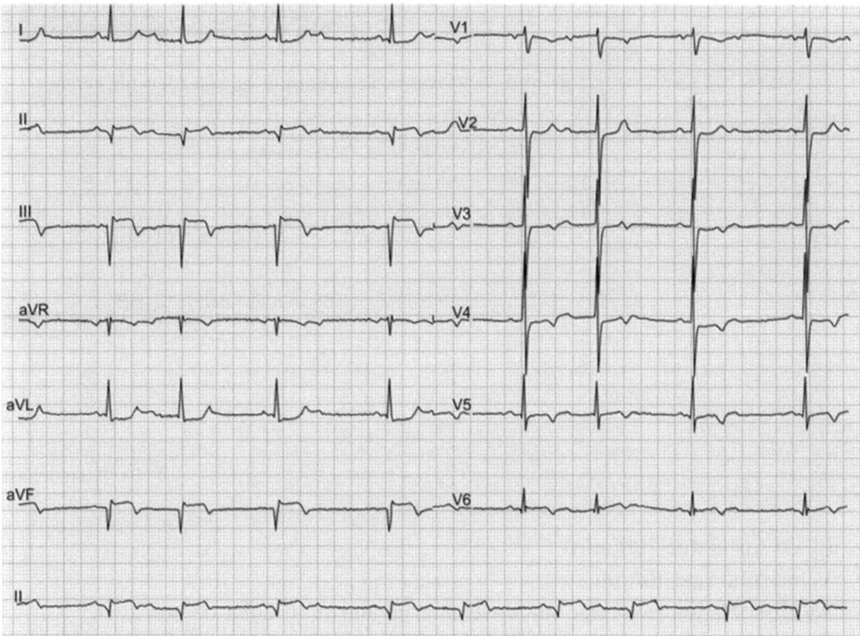

- ECG: sinus Rhythm.
- Q waves in inferior leads.
- ST. elevation in leads II, III, AVF.
- Progressive prolongation of PR interval.
- Diagnosis: type I second-degree AV block (Mobitz type I) due to inferior ST elevation myocardial infarction (STEMI) [5].

Case 20

Fifty years old man with typical chest pain, nausea, vomiting, and vertigo.

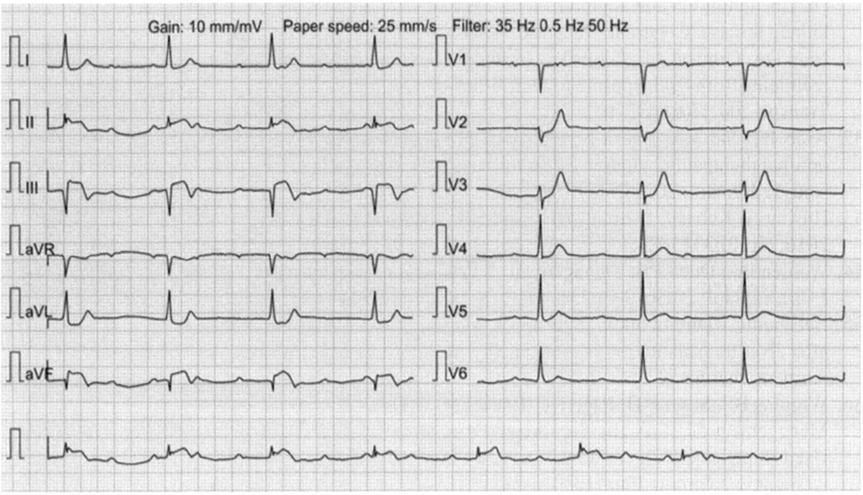

- ECG: Atrial rate 100/min.
- Ventricular rate 40/min.
- AV dissociation (No relation between atrial and ventricular complexes).
- Q wave and ST elevation in inferior leads.
- Diagnosis: complete AV nodal block due to inferior ST elevation MI [5].

Case 21

Twenty years old unconscious man who has been admitted to the ER he had history of severe weight reduction in recent month. (lead v1).

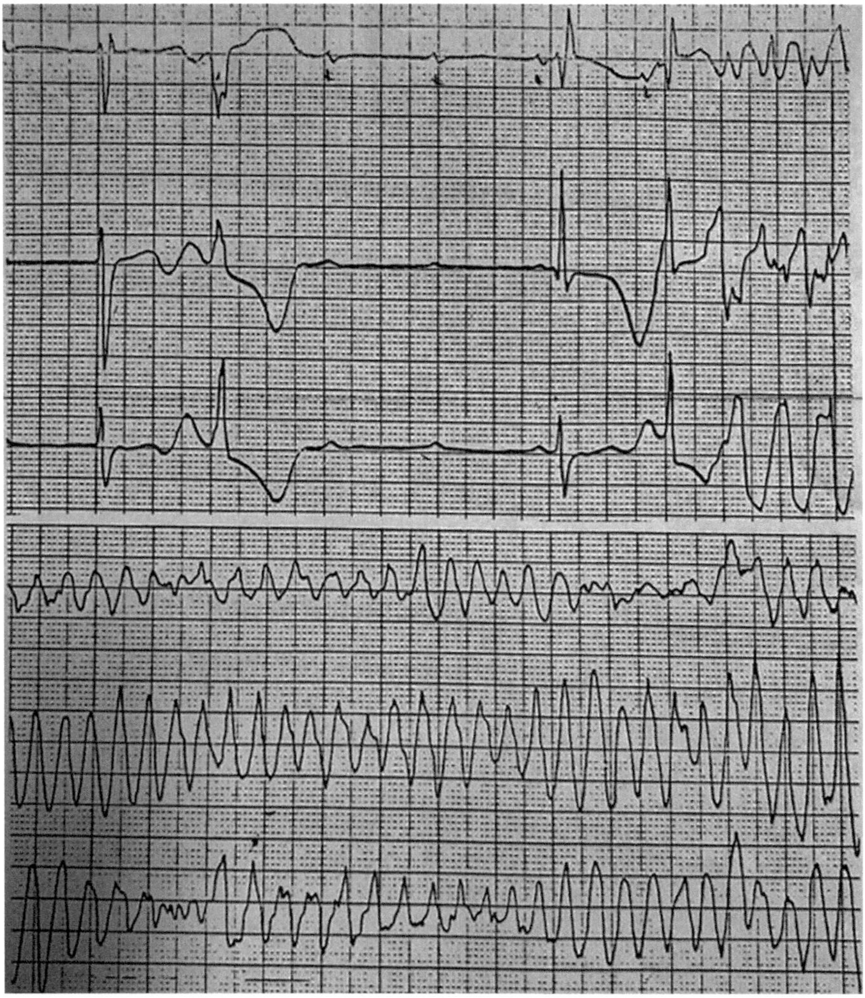

- ECG: Sinus rhythm.
- High degree Av block. Occasional sinus capture beat and PVC.
- QRS rotation about the baseline.
- DX: Episode of torsade de pointe.
- Most probably due to prolonged QT secondary to weight reduction and may be hypokalemia [6].

Case 22

Fifteen years old asymptomatic boy with incidental ECG finding.

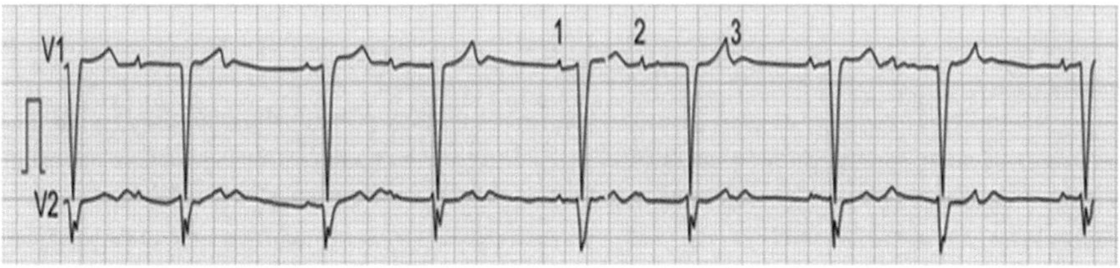

- ECG: sinus rhythm.
- PR interval progressively lengthen (first and second p wave) before the dropped beat (third p wave).
- R-R interval shortening suggestive of second-degree type 1 Av block (Mobitz type I).

Case 23

Twenty years old apparently healthy woman with history of frequent palpitation since last year.

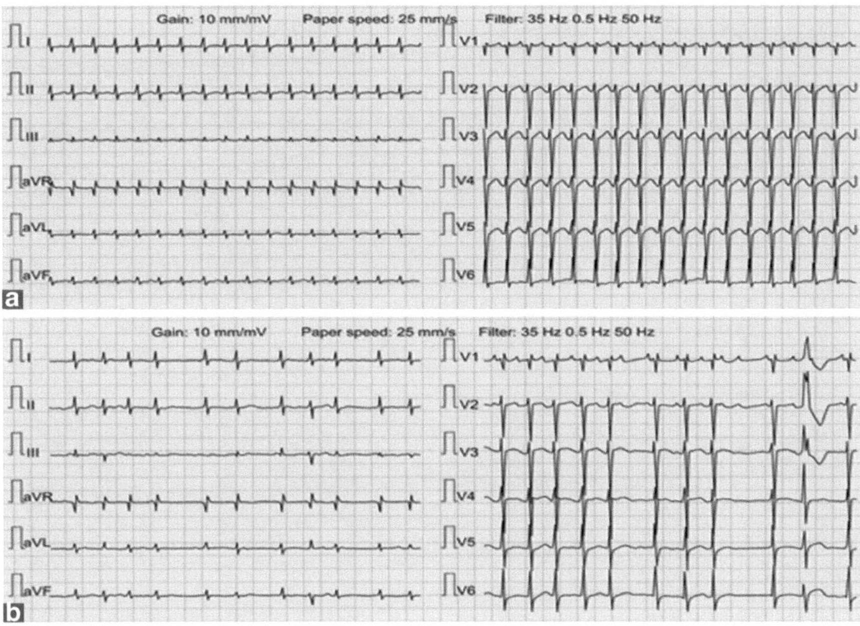

- ECG A: narrow QRS tachycardia.
- HR: 160/min.
- Normal axis.
- 1:1 Av association.
- DX: Atrial tachycardia with one to one atrioventricular conduction.
- ECG B: after rate control.
- Irregular narrow QRS tachycardia.
- With varied Av conduction and Ashman phenomenon before the last beat.
- Note: Ashman phenomenon usually is seen in AF with rapid ventricular response. According to the electrophysiology role, the longer the cycle, the longer the refractory period and vice versa so after a long pause preceding a beat if there is a short cycle beat it shows RBBB pattern. This is because usually, the right bundle has a longer refractory period than the left bundle branch [3].

Case 24

Twenty years old man with dyspnea on exertion (Fc, II), fixed splitted second heart sound and II/VI ejection systolic murmur in left sternal border.

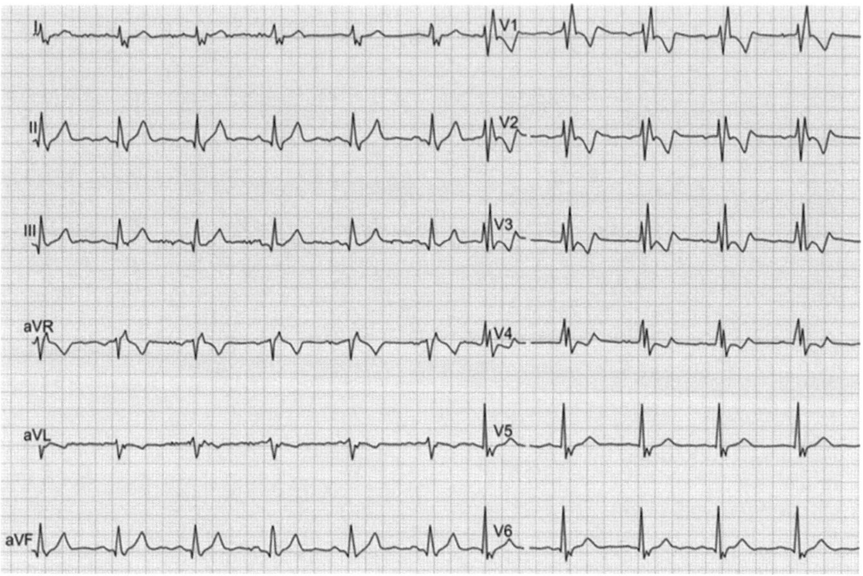

- ECG: NSR 100/min.
- Normal axis.
- Terminal r delay in D1.
- rSr' pattern in lead v1.
- s wave in lead I>/40 ms wide, and late intrinsicoid (prolonged time to peak r' wave in v1 is indicative of RBBB in v1).
- Diagnosis: Right bundle branch block most probably due to atrial septal defect secundum [1].

Case 25

Thirty-five years old lady with history of rheumatic fever and severe mitral stenosis since many years ago.

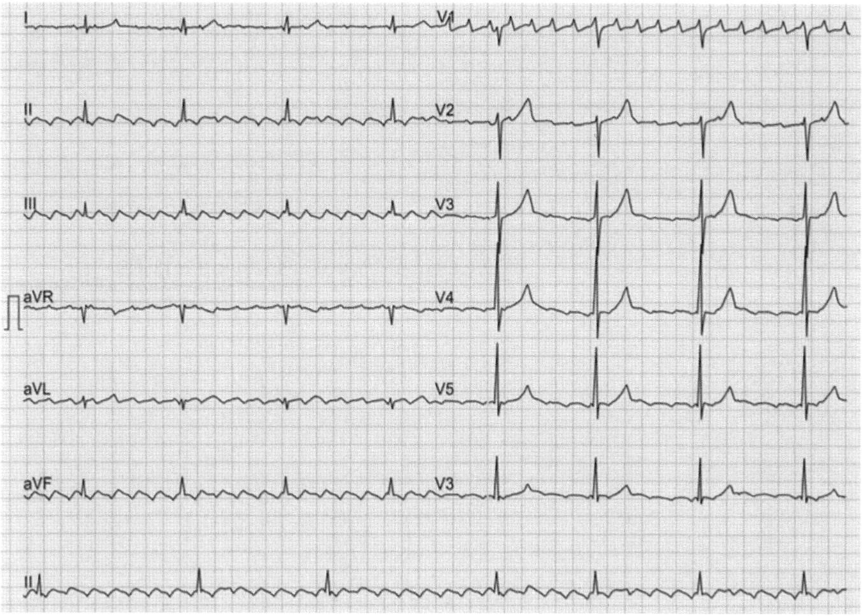

- ECG.
- HR: 55 min.
- Normal axin.
- Negative flutter wave in inferior lead and upright in v1.
- Counter clockwise atrial flutter with varied AV conduction.
- Dx: atrial flutter with slow ventricular response [4].

Case 26

Thirty years old pregnant woman who has been admitted due to severe dyspnea since one night before.

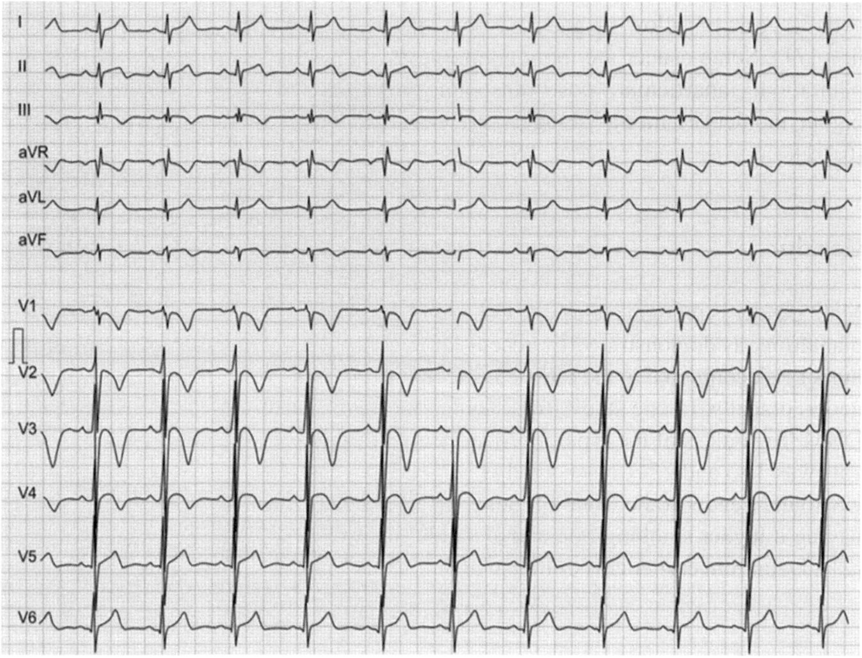

- ECG: NSR, 70/min.
- S1 Q3 T3 pattern, RAD.
- T wave inversion in v1-v4 suggesting RV overload, incomplete RBBB.
- Dx: ECG pattern compatible with submissive pulmonary embolism considering patient history [7].

Case 27

Forty years old asymptomatic man with history of longstanding hypertension.

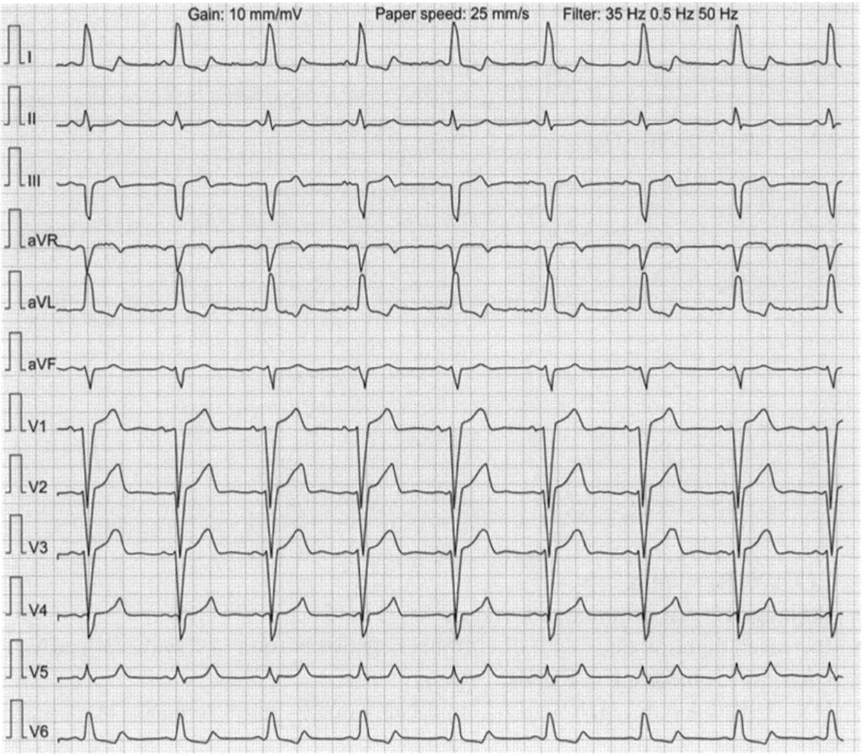

- ECG.
- NSR, 75/min.
- LAD.
- Broad R wave in leads I, AVL, V5, and V6.
- Absent initial r wave in v1.
- Absent septal q wave in lead I, V5, and V6.
- Dx: complete left bundle branch block (LBBB) [3].

Case 28

Thirty years old woman with history of Rheumatic fever (RF (who has been referred due to DOE (FC II) and palpitation since 1-year ago.

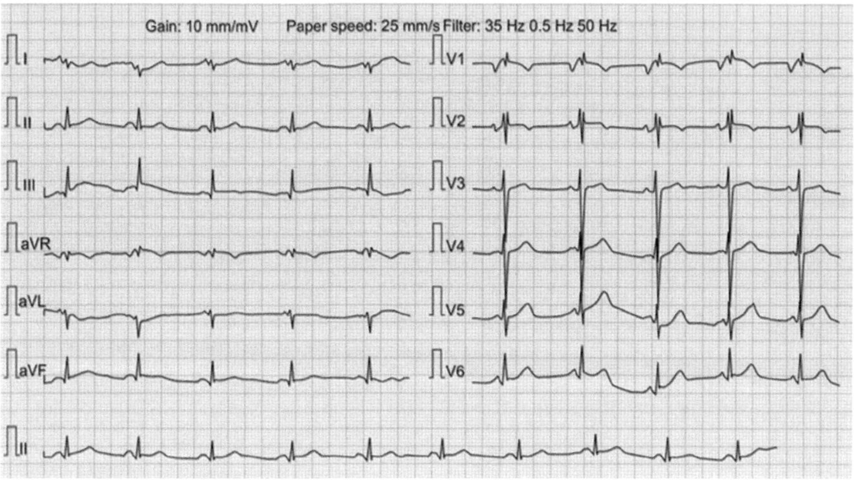

- ECG: NSR, 80/min.
- Prolonged P wave duration in lead II.
- Increased duration and depth of terminal negative portion of P wave in lead V1.
- LAA, RAD, incomplete RBBB.
- DX: NSR, LAA, RVH, RBBB most probably due to mitral stenosis [1].

Case 29

Twenty-five years old woman with history of RF in childhood. Physical exam showed diastolic rumble accentuated first heart sound (S1) and systolic murmur with inspiratory accentuation in the left sternal border.

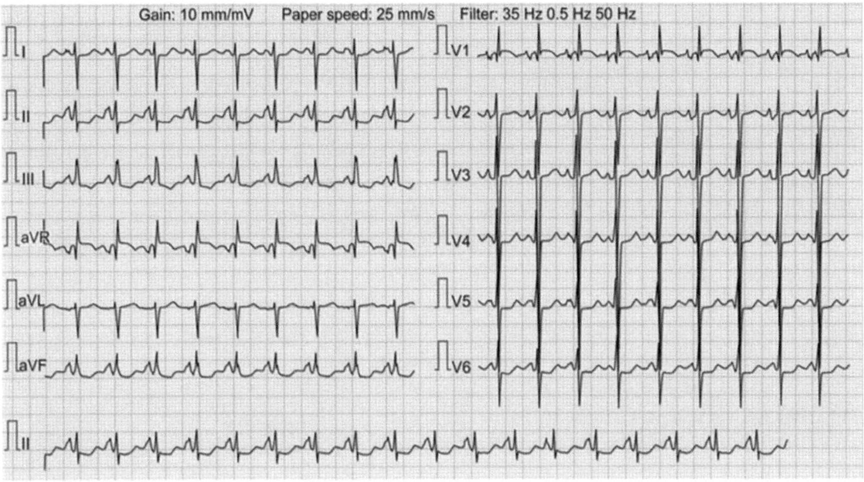

- ECG: Sinus Rhythm.
- HR, 140/min.
- RAD, tall P in lead II.
- Abnormal large terminal negative component of the P wave in V1 peaked P in II.
- DX: BAA, RAD, RVH probably due to mitral stenosis and tricuspid regurgitation [2].

Case 30

Thirty-five years old man with atypical chest pain with a diagnosis of extensive Ischemia and probable old myocardial infraction.

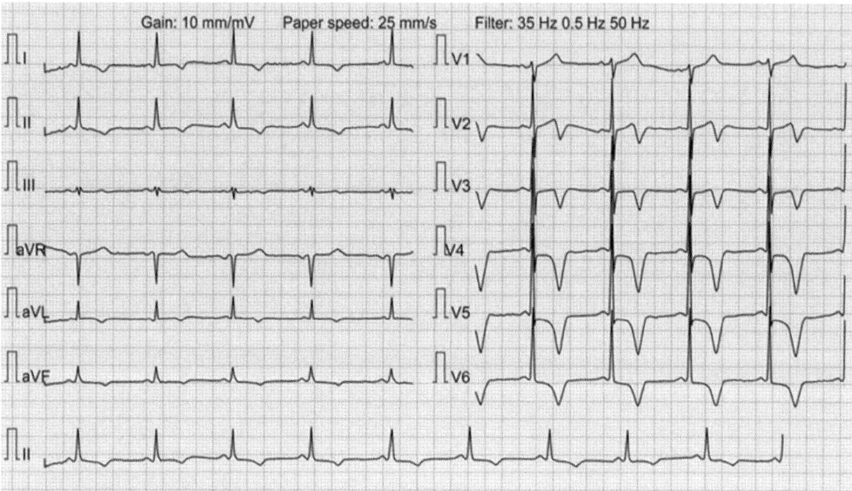

- ECG: NSR.
- Normal axis.
- HR: 90/min.
- Prominent downward ST-segment depression. Deep asymmetrical T wave inversion in precordial leads.
- DX: LVH most probably due to apical hypertrophic cardiomyopathy (HCM) (Yamaguchi Syndrome).
- Note: The echocardiogram confirmed the diagnosis and angiography showed normal coronary arteries [5].

Case 31

Twenty-five years old man with atypical chest pain.

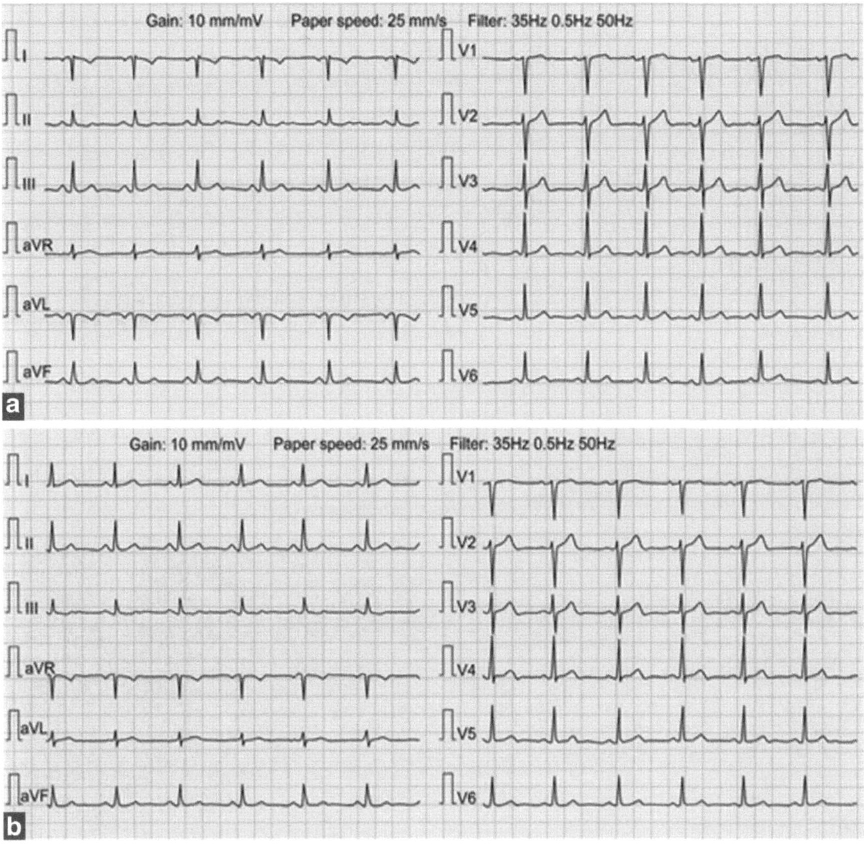

- ECG: Incorrect placement of limb leads (right and left arm reversal) in Figure A and the correct of the leads in a healthy individual in Figure B. Note to inversion in lead I, marked right axis deviation, reversal of leads II and III, reversal of leads aVR and aVL, and unchanged leads aVF and pericardial (A) as compared to normal ECG (B) [8].

Case 32

Forty years old obese woman who has been referred for a routine checkup.

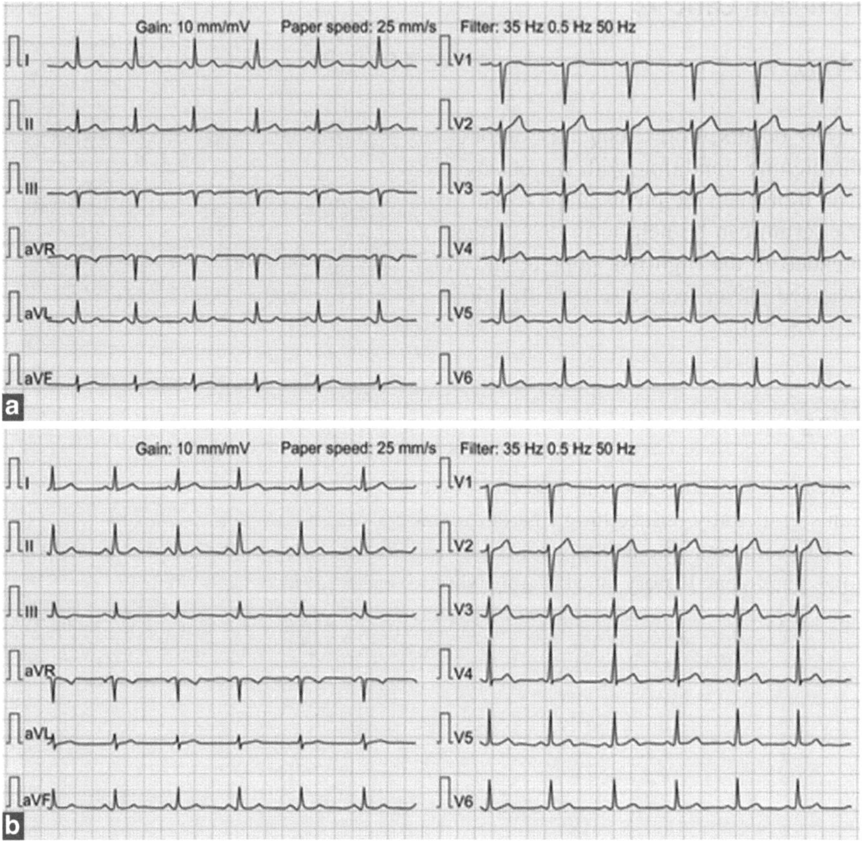

- ECG: Incorrect placement of limb leads (left arm and left leg reversal) in Figure A and the correct of the leads in a healthy individual in Figure B. Note to reversal of leads I and II, reversal of leads aVL and aVF, inversion of lead III, and unchanged leads aVR and pericordial (A) compared to normal ECG (B) [9]

Case 33

Eighteen years asymptomatic old boy who has been referred for evaluation of cardiovascular system due to ECG misdiagnosis.

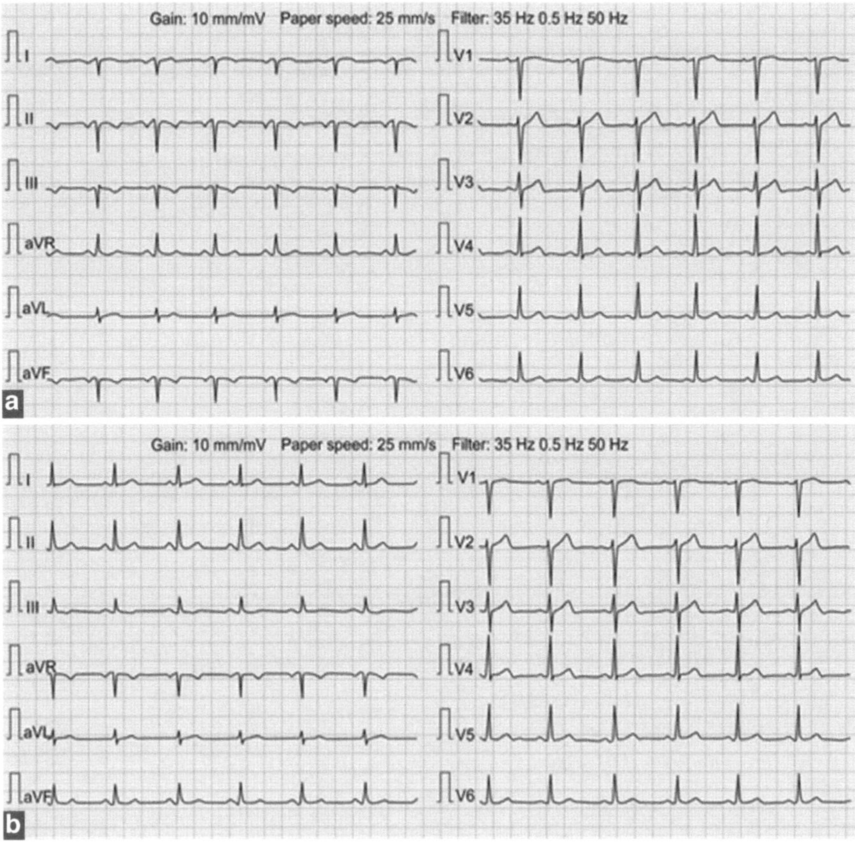

- ECG: Incorrect placement of limb leads (right arm and left leg reversal) in Figure A and the correct of the leads in a healthy individual in Figure B. Note to inversion of leads I, II, and III, reversal of leads I and III, reversal of leads aVR and aVF, and unchanged leads aVL and pericordial (A) compared to normal ECG (B) [8].

Case 34

Thirty-five years old man with atypical chest pain who has been diagnosis old lateral wall myocardial infarction by general practitioner.

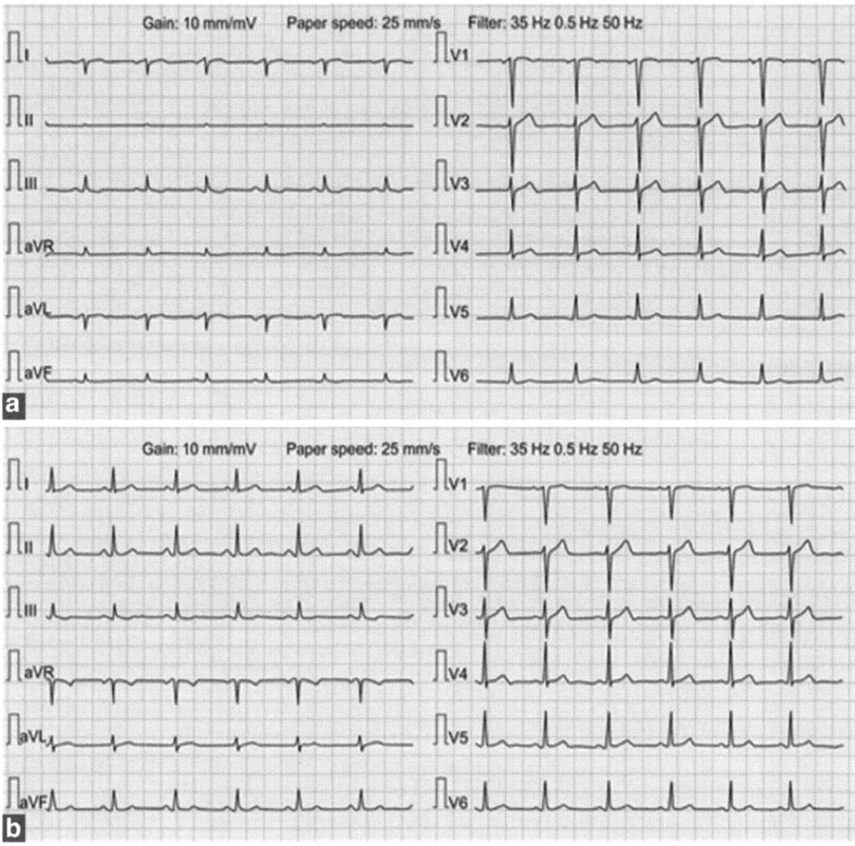

- ECG: Incorrect placement of limb leads (right arm and right leg reversal) in Figure A and the correct of the leads in a healthy individual in Figure B. Note to diminished signal (zero potential) in lead II, lead I that inverted lead III, leads aVR and aVF identical, lead aVL that approximates an inverted lead III, and unchanged precordial.
- leads (A) compared to normal ECG (B) [9].

Case 35

Thirty years old man with chest pain and misdiagnosis of inferior wall myocardial infarction by an intern in general hospital.

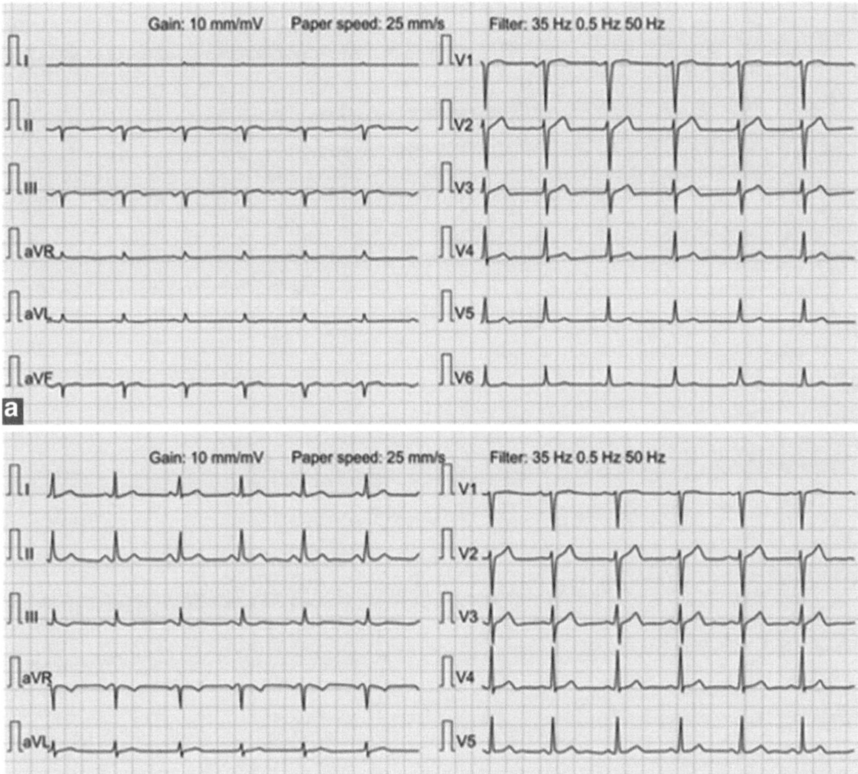

- ECG: Incorrect placement of limb leads (bilateral arm-leg reversal) in Figure A and the correct of the leads in a healthy individual in Figure B. Note to diminished signal (zero potential) in lead I, inversion of leads III, leads aVR and aVL that become identical, lead II and aVF that becomes approximately an inverted lead III, and unchanged precordial leads (A) compared to normal ECG (B) [9].

Case 36

Twenty years asymptomatic old boy with incidental finding in ECG.

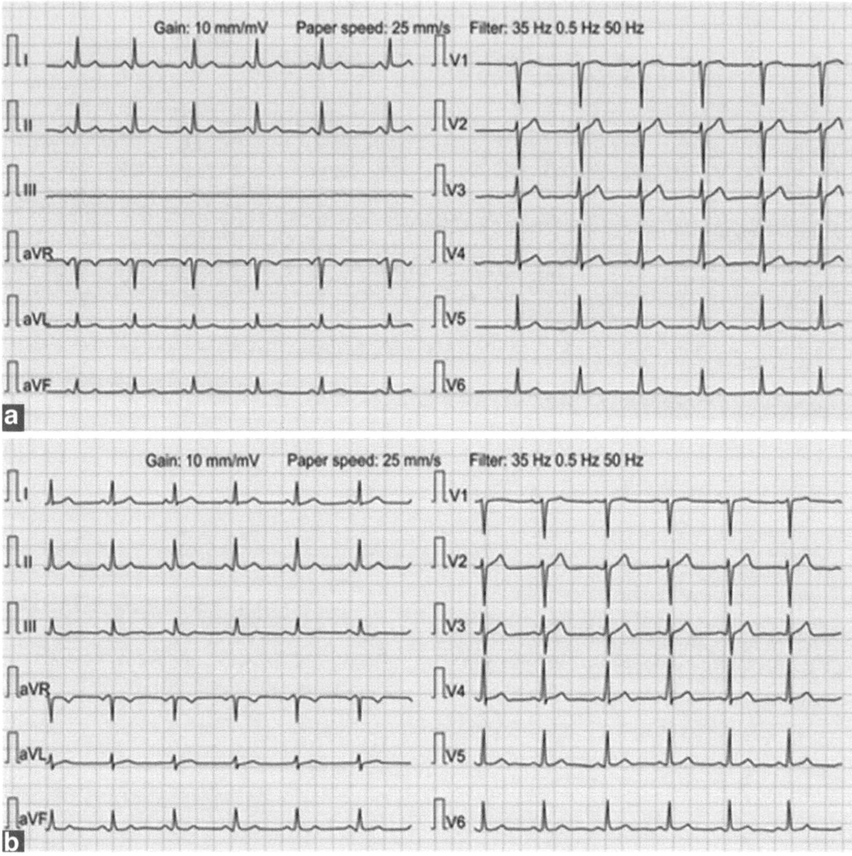

- ECG: Incorrect placement of limb leads (left arm and right leg reversal) in Figure A and the correct of the leads in a healthy individual in Figure B. Note to lead I that becomes identical to lead II, diminished signal (zero potential) in lead III, lead aVR that approximates to an inverted lead II, leads aVL and aVF that become identical, unchanged leads II and pericordial (A) compared to normal ECG (B) [8].

Case 37

Forty-five years old man with history of heavy smoking since 20 year ago. He has been referred due to Doe (Fc, II) with cough and sputum since 6 month ago.

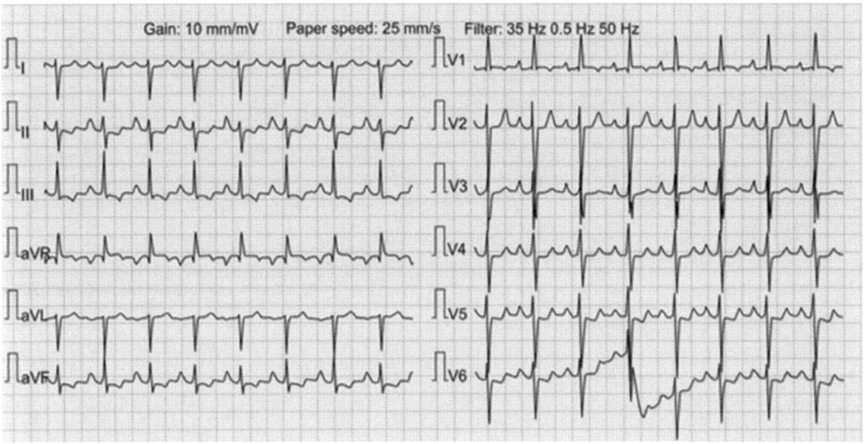

- ECG: NSR
- HR: 130/min
- Axis: RAD, large P wave in lead II and prominent initial positivity in V1 (p pulmonale) suggestive right atrial abnormality.
- Dominate R wave in V1 (7 mm tall and R/S in V1>1), dominant S more than r in V6. Reversal of normal R wore progression in precordial leads.
- Dx: RAA, RVH most probably due to cor pulmontal [10].

Case 38

Thirty-year-old woman with history of mitral stenosis and palpitation.

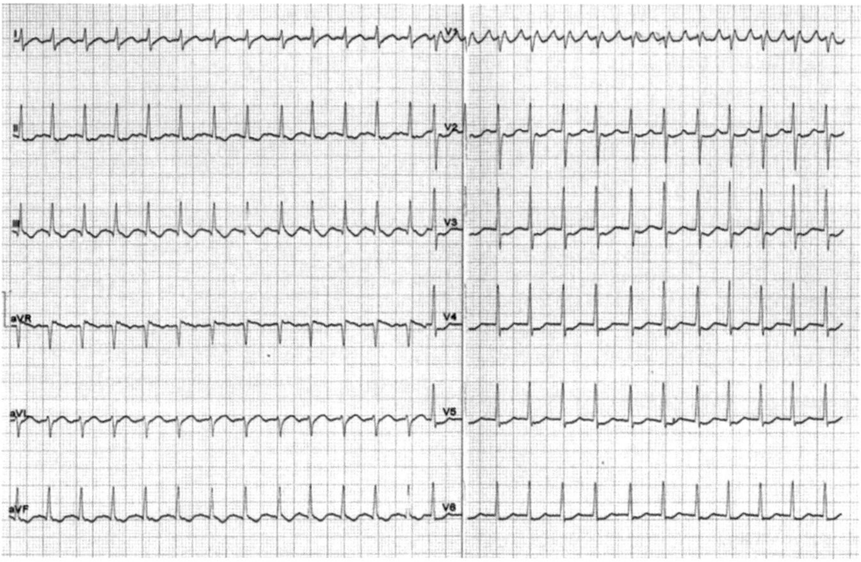

A counterclockwise atrial flutter. Note that the flutter waves are negative in inferior leads and upright in V1. The atrial rate is 300 beats/min and the ventricular rate is 150 beats/min (two-to-one AV conduction).

Case 39

Thirty-five years old man with history of rheumatic heart disease and frequent palpitation since a few months ago.

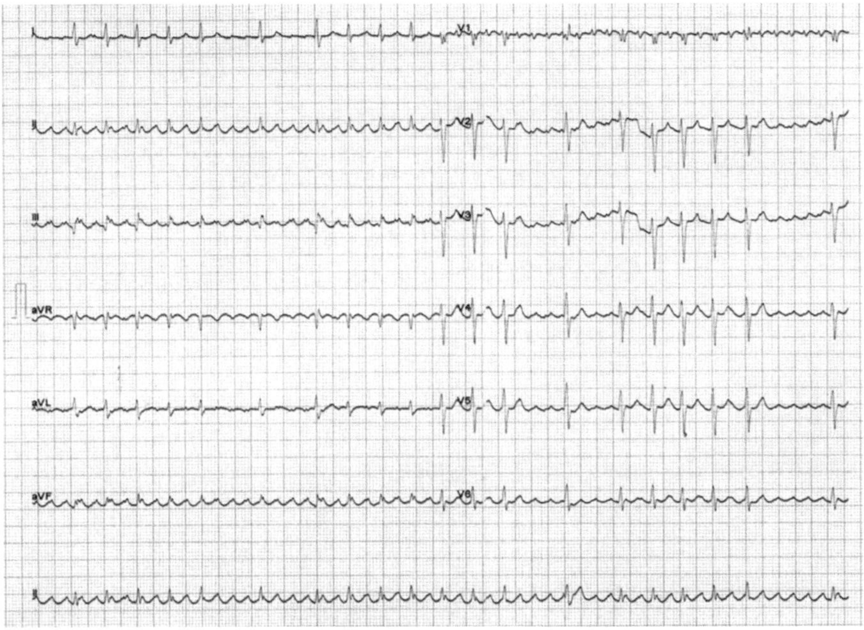

A clockwise atrial flutter with varied AV conduction. Note that the flutter waves are positive in inferior leads and negative in V1 [1].

Case 40

Forty years old lady with history of DOE (Fc: IIII) Since many years ago. She had recently atrioventricular septal defeat repair.

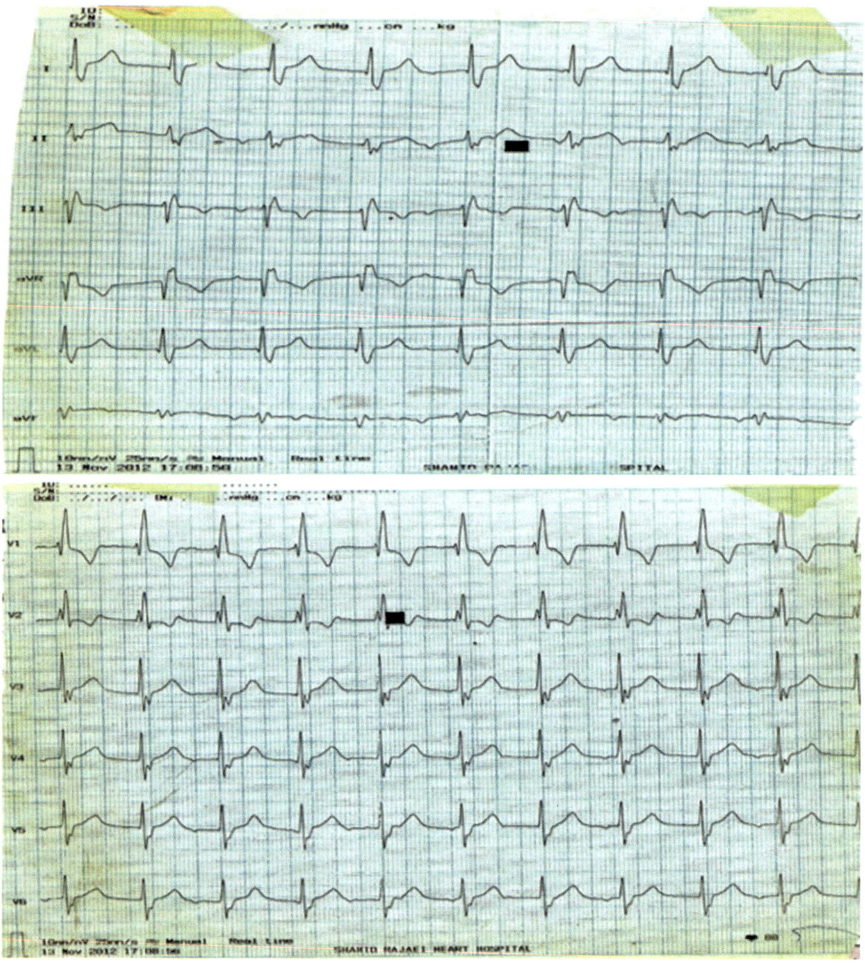

- ECG: wide QRS (RBBB pattern) with 85 bpm.
- Visible inverted P wave in leads II and III.
- Left axis deviation.
- Terminal S in DI rsr' in V1.
- Diagnosis: RBBB, LAHB, non-paroxysmal junctional tachycardia.
- Note: RBBB plus LAD in most often seen in endocardial cushion defect. NPJT in common after mitral valve repair or replacement, myocarditis, inferior MI.

Case 41

Eighteen years old girl with history of anorexia and vomiting.

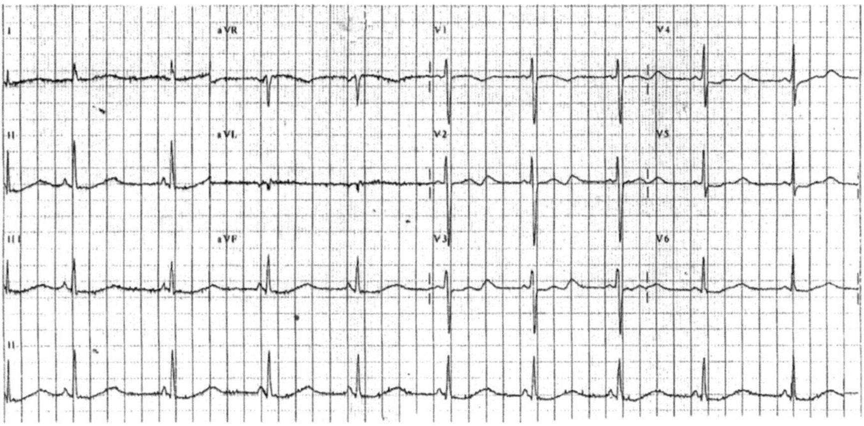

- ECG: Sinus bradycardia.
- 55 bpm.
- Normal axis.
- Small or T wave.
- Long QT.
- Note: Bulimia, vomiting, and hypokalemia in a young girl can cause Long QT interval and probably torsade de pointes [6].

Case 42

Fifty years old man with history of palpitation and DOE (Fc, II) Since 1 year ago. Echocardiogram in compatible with dilated cardiomyopathy.

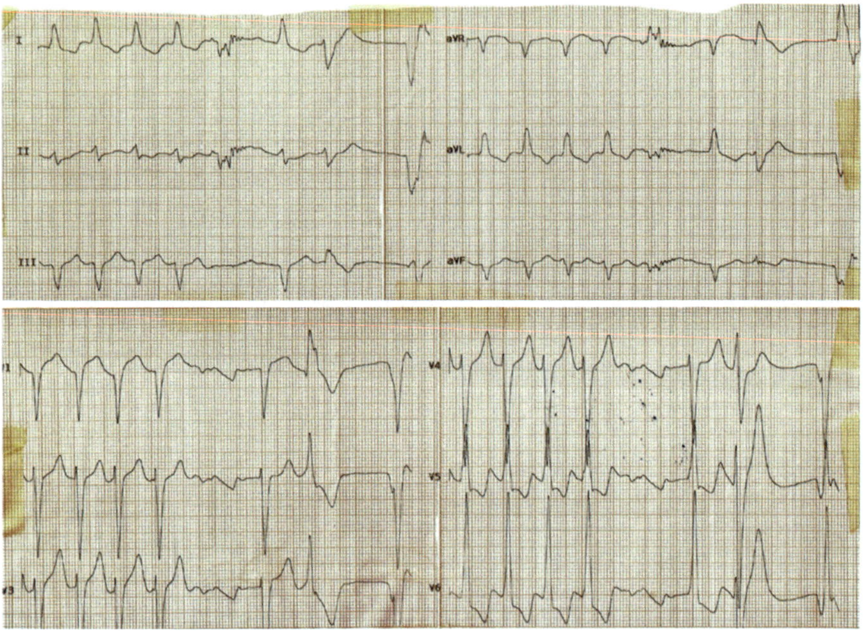

- ECG: AF with rapid ventricular response.
- Absence of Q wave in I, AVL, V4-v6.
- LBBB pattern.
- Occasional PVC.
- Note: Although there is long cycle, short cycle in V1 and wide QRS with RBBB pattern but in fact it is PVC because of already LBBB and wide QRS with compensatory pause. it is not Ashman phenomenon.

References

1. Maleki M, Alizadehasl A, Ansari MJA. Color Atlas of cardiology: Jaypee; 2017.
2. Mann DL, Zipes DP, Bonow RO. Braun Wald's HEART DISEASE: A TEXTBOOK OF CARDIOVASCULAR MEDICINE. Philadelphia: Elsevier Health Sciences; 2014.
3. Maleki M, Alizadehasl A, Haghjoo M, Ansari MJA. Practical cardiology: Elsevier; 2018.
4. Medi C, Kalman JM. Prediction of the atrial flutter circuit location from the surface electrocardiogram. Europace. 2008;10(7):786–96.
5. Jim MH, Chan AOO, Tang MO, Siu CW, Lee SWL, Lau CP. Angiographic and clinical implications of combined ST-segment elevation in anterior and inferior leads in acute myocardial infarction. Clin Cardiol. 2009;32(1):21–7.
6. Wellens HJ, Conover M. The ECG in emergency decision making. 2nd ed. Philadelphia: WB Saunders; 2006.
7. Goldberger AL. Deep T wave inversions: ischemia, cerebrovascular accident, or something else? ACC Curr J Rev. 1996;5:28.
8. Rowlands DJ. Inadvertent interchange of electrocardiogram limb lead connections. Analysis of predicted consequences. J Electrocardiol. 2008;41:84–90.
9. Garcia-Niebla J, Llontop-Garcia P, Valle-Racero JI, Serra-Autonell G, Batchvarov VN, De Luna AB. Technical mistakes during the acquisition of the electrocardiogram. Ann Noninvasive Electrocardiol. 2009;14:389–403.
10. Hancock EW, Deal BJ, Mirvis DM, Okin P, Kligfield P, Gettes LS. AHA/ACCF/HRS Recommendations for the Standardization and Interpretation of the Electrocardiogram: Part V: Electrocardiogram changes Associated with cardiac chamber Hypertrophy and Arrhythmias Committee, council on Clinical Cardiology. 2009
11. Goldberger AL, Goldberger ZD, Shvilkin A. Goldberger's clinical electrocardiography: a simplified approach. 8th ed. Philadelphia: Saunders; 2012.

Chapter 2
A Case of Mid-ventricular Obstructive Hypertrophic Cardiomyopathy

Azin Alizadehasl

Abstract Mid-ventricular hypertrophic obstructive cardiomyopathy is a rare type of hypertrophic cardiomyopathy that can be accompanied by an apical aneurysm.

Left heart catheterization and continuous-wave Doppler echocardiography revealed a pressure gradient between the apical and basal chambers of the left ventricle in concomitant with other important and prognostic echocardiographic findings.

Hypertrophic cardiomyopathy (HCM) is a genetic cardiac disorder characterized by marked variability in morphological appearance and natural history. The hypertrophic myocardium is frequently confined to the septum or lateral wall of the left ventricle (LV), however, it can also be encountered in the middle or apical regions of the LV myocardium [1–3].

Case Presentation

A 34-year-old woman presented with a history of chest pain and also shortness of breath producing important limitations on her daily activities. She had no history of hypertension, diabetes, and coronary artery disease. Her physical exam was unremarkable.

Transthoracic echocardiography (TTE) revealed normal systolic function and significant concentric LV hypertrophy that was greater in the mid-LV cavity region. There was high LV end-diastolic pressure; normal right ventricle function and normal pulmonary artery pressure (Fig. 2.1).

Our patient had persistent symptoms despite receiving optimized medical management, and a surgical approach was indicated for her. Coronary CT-angiography

A. Alizadehasl (✉)
Rajaie Cardiovascular Medical and Research Center, Cardio-Oncology Department and Research Center, Iran University of Medical Science, Tehran, Iran

M. Maleki, A. Alizadehasl (eds.), *Case-Based Clinical Cardiology*,
https://doi.org/10.1007/978-1-4471-7496-7_2

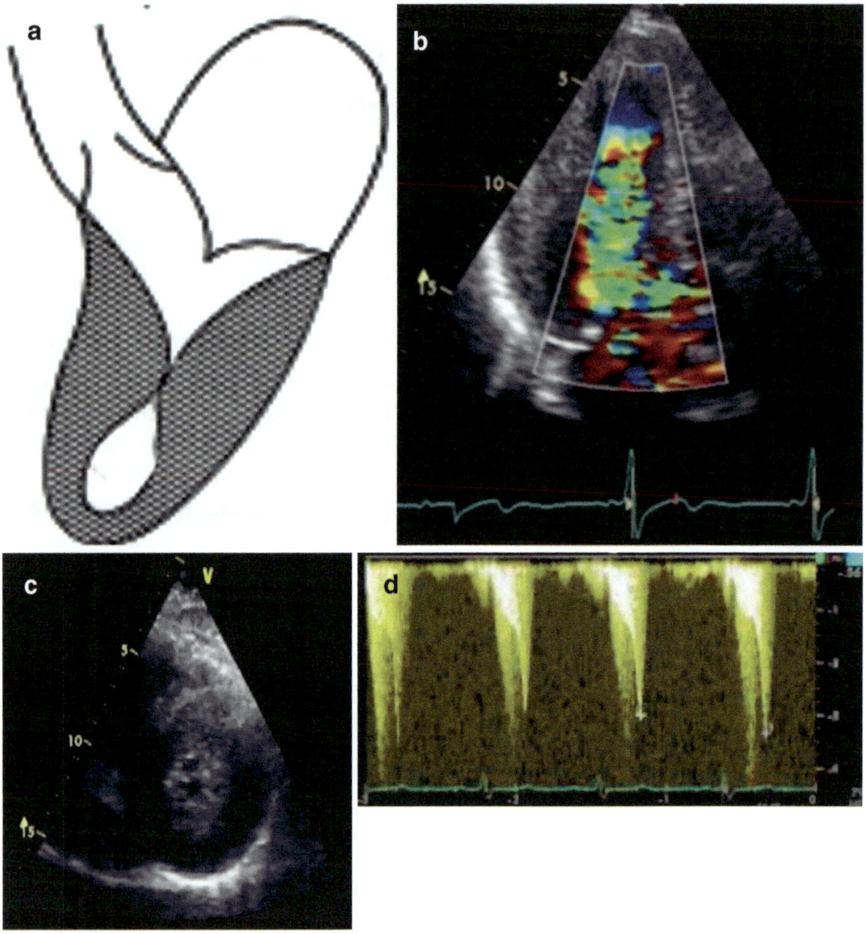

Fig. 2.1 (**a**) Mid-LV cavity hypertrophy, (**b**) Turbulent flow in mid-LV cavity in apical 3-chamber view, (**c**) LV short-axis view with significant hypertrophy, (**d**) High Doppler Flow gradient in mid-LV cavity

was normal; Precise myectomy surgery was done with preservation of papillary muscles and fortunately, no complications occurred after surgery, and her symptoms resolved completely.

In the follow-up beyond 1 month, the patient's NYHA class improved from III to I. Additionally, the medication being used was meaningfully reduced postoperatively. New TTE was performed after the surgery, and it confirmed the disappearance of the mid-ventricular pressure gradient.

Discussion

It might involve principally the proximal septum, or there can be diffuse LV hypertrophy. However, there are other forms, such as mid-ventricular and also apical hypertrophy. In the mid-LV cavity HCM pattern, there may be an intraventricular pressure gradient that creates an obstruction at the level of the papillary muscles, which may lead to apical myocardial infarction and an apical aneurysm. Mid-ventricular obstruction is defined as a ventricular gradient ≥30 mm Hg [1, 4] (Fig. 2.2).

Patients with mid-ventricular HCM are more symptomatic than HCM patients without obstruction or LV outflow tract obstruction. Moreover, the incidence of sudden death and arrhythmic events is relatively high in this pattern of HCM [3, 4]. Minami and colleagues, by using multivariate models, demonstrated that mid-ventricular obstruction is an independent determinant of HCM-related cardiac death [1, 5].

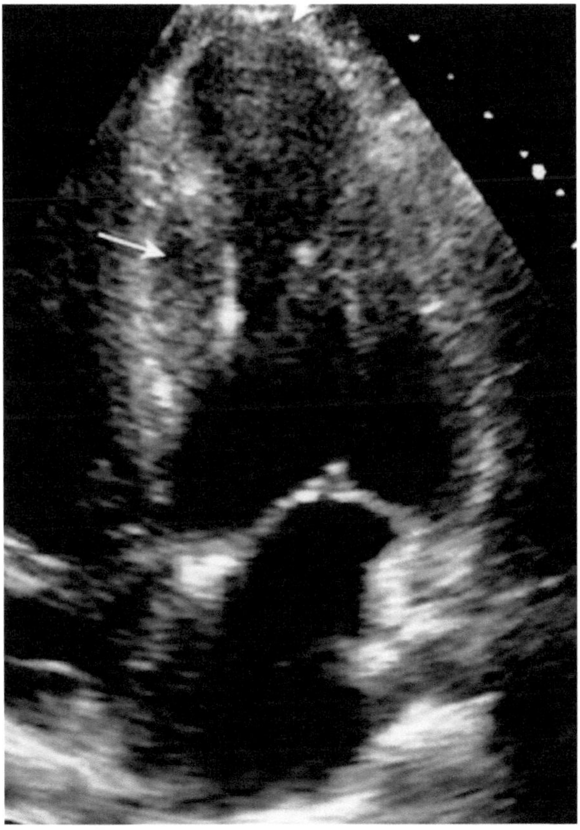

Fig. 2.2 Mid-LV cavity obstruction, apical four-chamber view, (white arrow)

The pharmacologic management of HCM, specially in obstructive variants, is based on β blockers, calcium-channel blockers, and disopyramide. This treatment is effective in many patients, however, those with mid-ventricular hypertrophy have worse results in terms of symptom relief. In these patients, the standard treatment is surgical resection of the hypertrophied portion of the ventricle or even cardiac transplantation [3–5].

Conclusion

Our patient had a mid-ventricular HCM with symptoms refractory to a optimize medical therapy. In addition, the patient's hypertrophy obstructed the cavity and created a significant intraventricular gradient. After consultation with the heart team, the surgical approach was chosen for her.

The procedure was performed without complications, and no damage in the mitral valve apparatus or disturbance in the left bundle branch was found too.

References

1. Minami Y, Kajimoto K, Terajima Y, Yashiro B, Okayama D, Haruki S, Nakajima T, Kawashiro N, Kawana M, Hagiwara N. Clinical implications of midventricular obstruction in patients with hypertrophic cardiomyopathy. J Am Coll Cardiol. 2011;57:2346–55. https://doi.org/10.1016/j.jacc.2011.02.033.
2. Kunkala MR, Schaff HV, Nishimura RA, Abel MD, Sorajja P, Dearani JA, Ommen SR. Transapical approach to myectomy for midventricular obstruction in hypertrophic cardiomyopathy. Ann Thorac Surg. 2013;96:564–70. https://doi.org/10.1016/j.athoracsur.2013.04.073.
3. Efthimiadis GK, Pagourelias ED, Parcharidou D, Gossios T, Kamperidis V, Theofilogiannakos EK, Pappa Z, Meditskou S, Hadjimiltiades S, Pliakos C, Karvounis H, Styliadis IH. Clinical characteristics and natural history of hypertrophic cardiomyopathy with midventricular obstruction. Circ J. 2013;77:2366–74. https://doi.org/10.1253/circj.CJ-12-1561.
4. Fifer MA, Vlahakes GJ. Management of symptoms in hypertrophic cardiomyopathy. Circulation. 2008;117:429–39. https://doi.org/10.1161/CIRCULATIONAHA.107.694158.
5. Maron BJ. Hypertrophic cardiomyopathy: a systematic review. JAMA. 2002;287:1308–20.

Chapter 3
Constrictive Pericarditis

Azin Alizadehasl

Abstract The diagnosis of constrictive pericarditis requires a high degree of clinical suspicion, for the signs and symptoms of this disease can be falsely attributed to other causes. Herein, we present A 67 year old woman, known case of breast cancer from 17 years ago, whose symptoms of right heart failure were initially attributed to cardio-toxicity due to chemotherapy.

Case Presentation

Herein, we present a 67-year-old woman, known case of breast cancer from 17 years ago, treated by surgery in 1381/8 and followed by 7 courses of chemotherapy and 27 courses of radiotherapy until 1382/2, after that she was followed by her oncologist.

She demonstrated dyspnea on exertion FCII from 2 years ago and orthopnea and abdominal distention from 4 months ago and was admitted to another center with impression of decompensating heart failure with a left ventricular ejection fraction of 30%.

She was discharged. One month later he presented with worsening breathlessness and ascites. Echocardiography, in our center revealed the diagnosis of constrictive pericarditis (CP) and CMR confirmed that. She underwent near-complete pericardiectomy and has made a good recovery. This case exemplifies the difficulty in diagnosing this condition, the investigation by echocardiography, and the benefit of surgery.

A. Alizadehasl (✉)
Rajaie Cardiovascular Medical and Research Center, Cardio-Oncology Department and Research Center, Iran University of Medical Science, Tehran, Iran

M. Maleki, A. Alizadehasl (eds.), *Case-Based Clinical Cardiology*,
https://doi.org/10.1007/978-1-4471-7496-7_3

Clinical and Echocardiographic Findings and Discussion

CP or Restrictive Cardiomyopathy (RCM) should be considered in any patient with the disproportional degree of right-sided HF with NL systolic and valve function. With a history of prior surgery, pericarditis, and radiation CP is more likely. Pericardial calcification seen on chest radiography is helpful but occurs in only 23% of patients and should raise the suspicion of TB pericarditis. Calcification per se is not diagnostic for CP.

The clinical and hemodynamic profiles of restriction (myocardial diastolic heart failure) and constriction (pericardial diastolic heart failure) are similar, although their pathophysiologic mechanisms are distinctly different.

Both are caused by limited or restricted diastolic filling, with relatively preserved global systolic function (Fig. 3.1).

Currently, the most common cause of constriction is previous cardiac surgery, followed by pericarditis, an episode of pericardial effusion, and radiotherapy. In the developed world the cause is most commonly idiopathic, postsurgical, or radiation injury.

In CP, diastolic dysfunction is related to a thickened or noncompliant pericardium, but Diastolic dysfunction in RCM or myocardial disease is the result of a stiff and noncompliant ventricular Myocardium, frequently RCM resulting from infiltrative cardiomyopathy is the easiest abnormality to diagnose typical 2D and biochemical features. A non-infiltrative type of RCM is more difficult to diagnose.

In CP Thickened, inflamed, adherent, or calcific pericardium forms a rigid shell that limits diastolic filling of the heart, in up to 20% of patients. The pericardial thickness is relatively normal but adherent to the epicardium pericardial thickness may be normal.

Atrial enlargement is less prominent in CP than in restrictive cardiomyopathy, but it can be as large.

To establish the diagnosis of CP, the following two hemodynamic characteristics need to be demonstrated either with 2D or Doppler echocardiography or with cardiac catheterization:

1. Disassociation between intrathoracic and intracardiac pressures and
2. Exaggerated ventricular interdependence

2D Echocardiographic Features of CP

- Thickened pericardium
- Abnormal ventricular septal motion

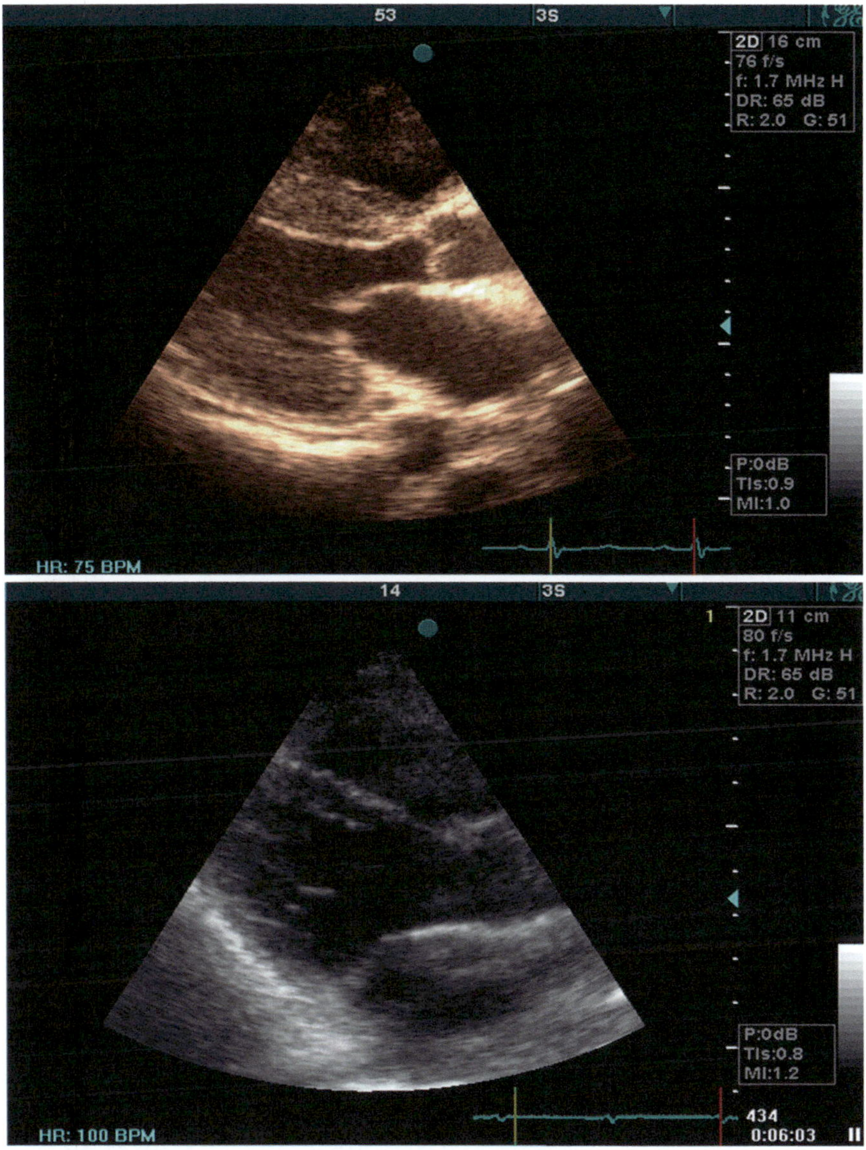

Fig. 3.1 Upper: Myocardial diastolic heart failure due to RCM. Lower: Pericardial diastolic heart failure due to CP and thickened pericardium

- Respiratory variation in ventricular size
- Dilated hepatic vein and inferior vena cava

But these findings are not sensitive or specific

M-Mode Echocardiographic Features of CP

- Flattening of the LV posterior wall during diastole and thickening (Fig. 3.2).
- Abrupt displacement of the IVS during early diastole (Septal bounce) Fig. 3.3, Upper.
- Septal motion reflects the competitive filling of the two ventricles Fig. 3.3, lower with constriction ventricles that may fill in an alternate fashion and produce a wavy pattern of diastolic septal motion.
- Premature pulmonic valve opening due to elevated RVEDP

Normally, with inspiration, intrathoracic pressure falls (normally 3–5 mm Hg) and the pressure in other intrathoracic structures (PVs, pulmonary capillaries) decreases to a similar degree. This inspiratory pressure change is not fully transmitted to the intrapericardial and intracardiac cavities.

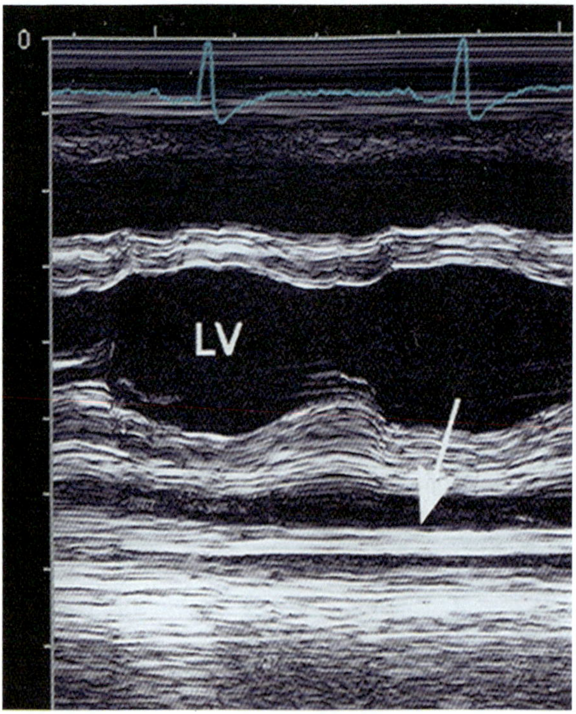

Fig. 3.2 Thickened pericardium in M-Mode Echocardiography (white arrow)

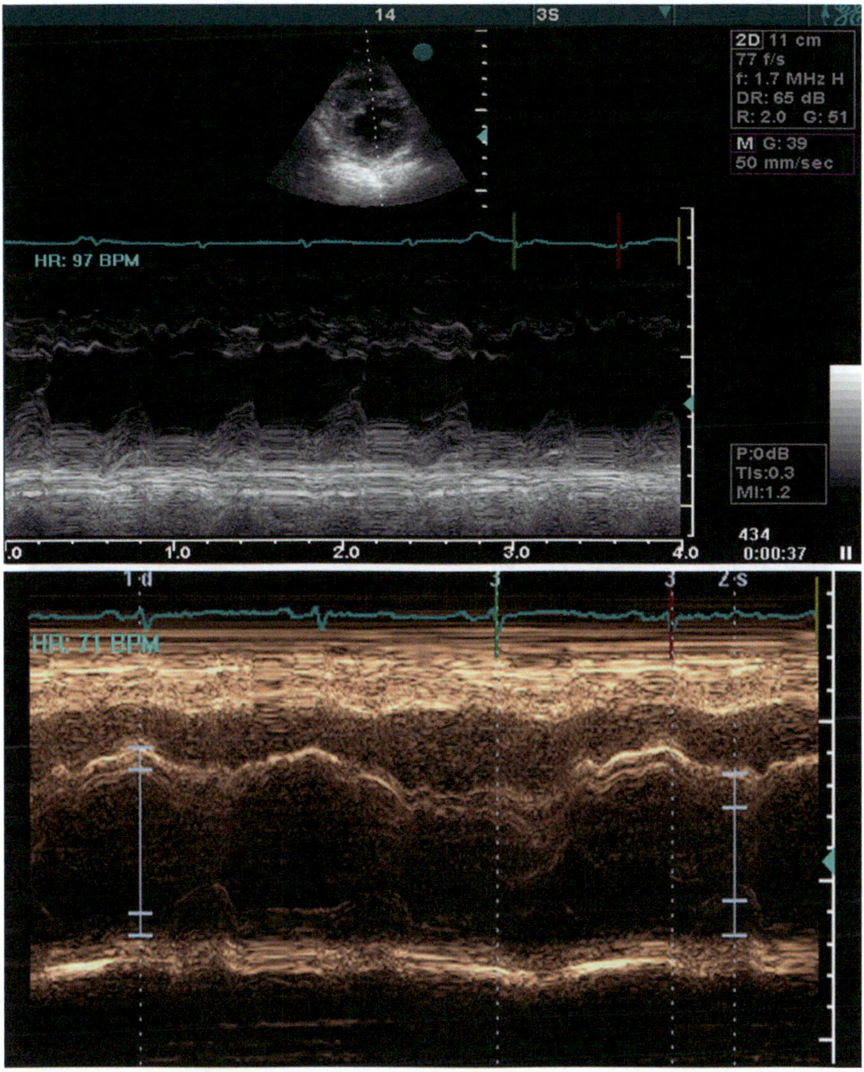

Fig. 3.3 Upper: Abrupt displacement of the IVS during early diastole (Septal bounce). Lower: Septal motion reflects a wavy pattern of diastolic septal motion

Consequently, the driving pressure gradient for LV filling decreases immediately after inspiration and increases with expiration.

In CP, a thickened or inflamed pericardium prevents full transmission of the intrathoracic pressure changes that occur with respiration to the pericardial and intracardiac cavities.

Diastolic filling (or distensibility) of the LV and RV relies on each other because the overall cardiac volume is relatively fixed within the thickened or noncompliant (adherent) pericardium, so there is exaggerated respiratory variation in heart chambers (Fig. 3.4).

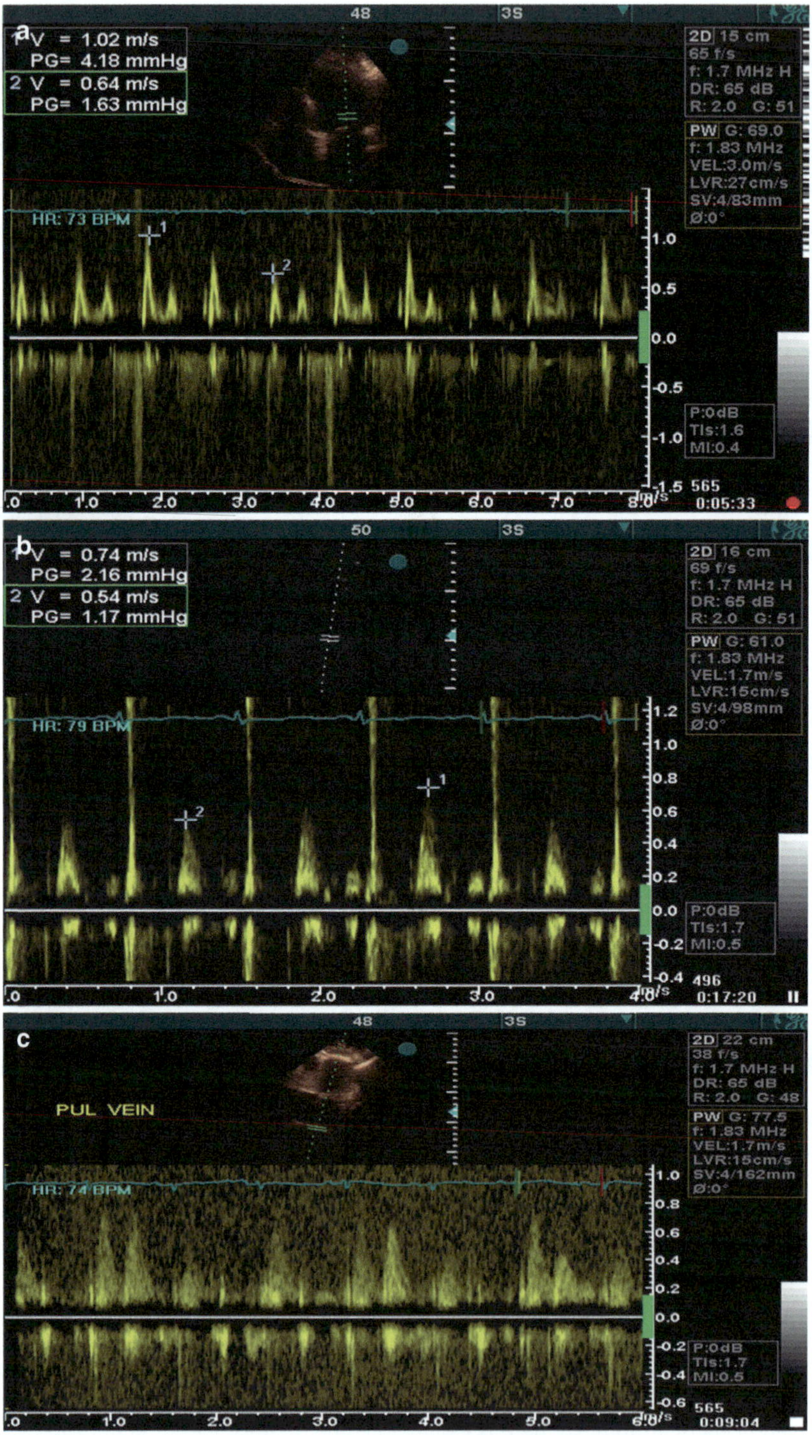

Fig. 3.4 Respiratory variation in (**a**) MV, (**b**) TV and in (**c**) pulmonary veins

Another important echocardiographic finding HV flow reversal after the onset of expiration, with decreased forward flow during diastole (D) (Fig. 3.5).

TDI is at least as sensitive as conventional echocardiography Doppler study. In myocardial disease, the mitral septal annulus velocity that reflects myocardial relaxation is decreased <7 cm/s because myocardial relaxation is abnormal; however, in constrictive pericarditis, the mitral annulus velocity, especially the septal annulus velocity, is relatively normal or even increased (Fig. 3.6).

Regional variations in deformation and strain include reduced LV circumferential strain, torsion, and early diastolic untwisting with preserved longitudinal strain and deformation.

In contrast, in restriction, circumferential strain and untwisting are preserved but these parameters are reduced in the longitudinal direction.

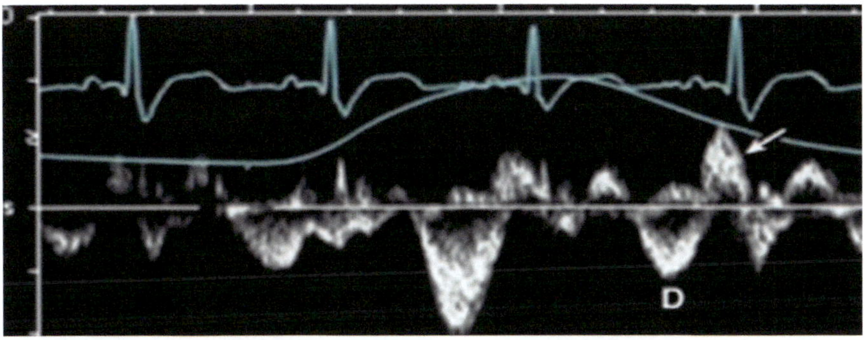

Fig. 3.5 Hepatic vein diastolic flow reversal after the onset of expiration

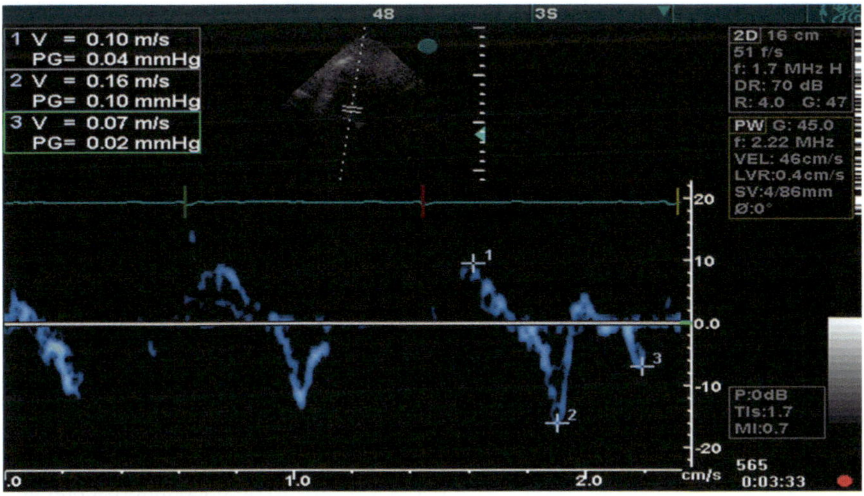

Fig. 3.6 Increase in MV septal annulus velocity in CP

When a comprehensive transthoracic echocardiographic study is diagnostic for constriction, no further diagnostic testing should be necessary. In equivocal cases, where noninvasive evaluation is inconclusive or discordant with clinical findings, hemodynamic assessment by cardiac catheterization should be performed [1–6].

Treatment

CP has a progressive but variable course. For most patients, surgical pericardiectomy is the definitive treatment.

Pericardiectomy for constriction has a relatively high perioperative mortality rate, ranging from 2% to nearly 20% in modern series.

Our case underwent near-complete pericardiectomy and has made a good recovery, and also echocardiography after surgery in the hospital and also 4 months later showed improvement in LV and RV function (Fig. 3.7) [4, 5].

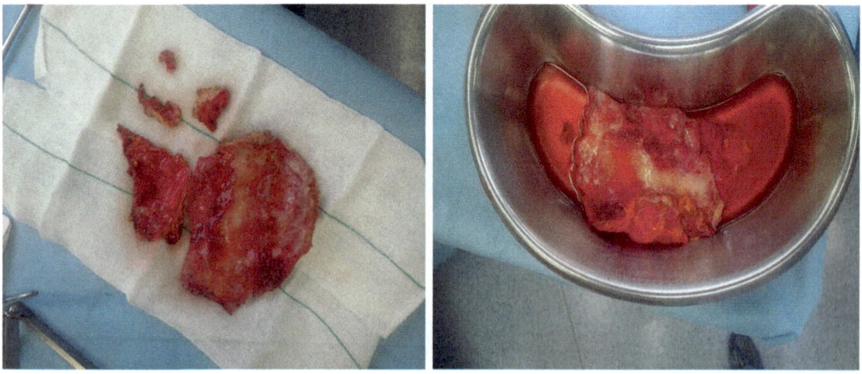

Fig. 3.7 Thickened pericardium after surgery

References

1. Garcia MJ. Constrictive pericarditis versus restrictive cardiomyopathy? J Am Coll Cardiol. 2016;67(17):2061–76.
2. Yared K, Baggish AL, Picard MH, Hoffmann U, Hung J. Multimodality imaging of pericardial diseases. JACC Cardiovasc Imaging. 2010;3(6):650–60.
3. Kaga S, Mikami T, Takamatsu Y, et al. Quantitative and pattern analyses of continuous-wave Doppler-derived pulmonary regurgitant flow velocity for the diagnosis of constrictive pericarditis. J Am Soc Echocardiogr. 2014;27:1223.
4. Choi JH, Choi JO, Ryu DR, et al. Mitral and tricuspid annular velocities in constrictive pericarditis and restrictive cardiomyopathy: correlation with pericardial thickness on computed tomography. JACC Cardiovasc Imaging. 2011;4:567.
5. Xu B, Kwon DH, Klein AL. Imaging of the pericardium: a multimodality cardiovascular imaging update. Cardiol Clin. 2017;35:491.
6. Maleki M, Alizadehasl A, Haghjoo M. Pericardial disease. In: Practical cardiology book. 1st ed. Elsevier; 2017.

Chapter 4
Ebstein Anomaly

Azin Alizadehasl

Abstract Ebstein's anomaly is an infrequent but fascinating congenital heart disorder accounting for <1% of all congenital heart disease. Since its depiction in 1866, dramatic developments in diagnosis and treatment have been made.

Ebstein's anomaly is a complex congenital disorder with a broad pathologic-anatomical and also clinical spectrum and no two patients are identical. So, precise knowledge of the different anatomic and hemodynamic variables, related malformations and management choices are essential. Managing Ebstein's anomaly patients is so complex. Thus, it is important that these patients are frequently seen by a cardiologist with expertise in congenital heart disease.

Here in we present a 24-year-old woman referred to our center due to frequent episodes of sudden-onset palpitation. He had a history of unknown congenital heart disease.

Keywords Ebstein's anomaly · Sail sound · Accessory conduction pathways · Complex congenital disorder · Right ventricular outflow tract obstruction

Clinical Presentation

A 24-year-old woman referred to our center due to frequent episodes of sudden-onset palpitation. She had a history of unknown congenital heart disease.

In physical exam, he was a well-developed young woman without distress, cyanosis, or clubbing. Blood pressure and pulses were normal. Jugular venous pressure was normal. PMI was in mid-clavicular line and, there was a widely split S1 with a loud tricuspid component (the "sail sound"), a widely split S2, a right-sided third heart sound, and a systolic murmur grade 2 in LSB (Fig. 4.1).

Diagnosis and differential diagnosis based on ECG:

A. Alizadehasl (✉)
Rajaie Cardiovascular Medical and Research Center, Cardio-Oncology Department and Research Center, Iran University of Medical Science, Tehran, Iran

M. Maleki, A. Alizadehasl (eds.), *Case-Based Clinical Cardiology*,
https://doi.org/10.1007/978-1-4471-7496-7_4

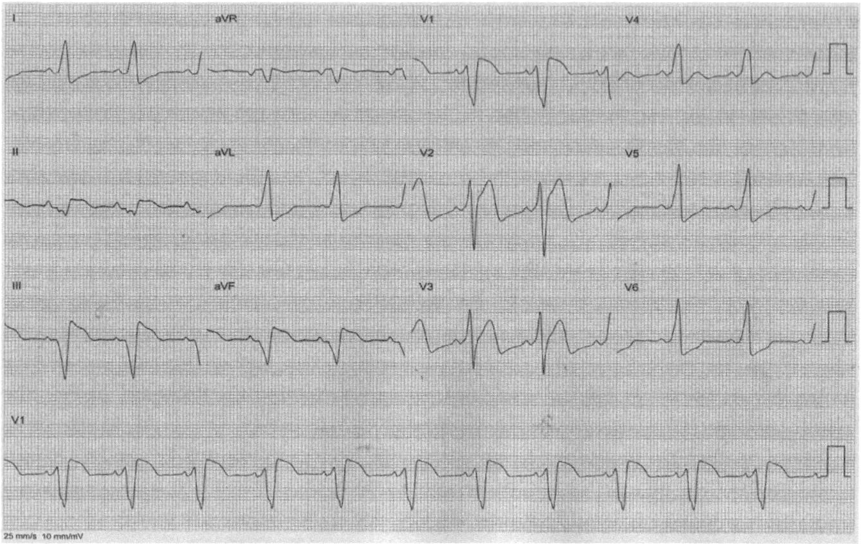

Fig. 4.1 ECG findings: Sinus rhythm; Rate = 80 bpm; Left axis deviation; No voltage criteria infavour of LA or RA abnormalities; Short PR interval; Wide QRS complex with atypical RBBB pattern; Negative QRS and delta wave in V1; Q wave in inferior leads (II, III, AVF); ST elevation with bi-phasic T wave (coved or brugada pattern) in leads V1–3 and inferior leads; ST depression in I, aVl, V4–6

- **DDX**: right posteroseptal accessory pathway: Ebstein anomaly or brugada syndrome type 1
- **Dx**: sinus rhythm, wide QRS complex, RBBB pattern, right posteroseptal accessory pathway: Ebstein anomaly (Fig. 4.2)

- **DDX:** "water bottle" or "box-shaped" heart
- R/O Ebstein anomaly; or Severe RA enlargement, or Severe TR, or Massive pericardial effusion
- **Dx**: Ebstein anomaly (Figs. 4.3 and 4.4)

Interestingly in this case the displacement of the posterior leaflet was more than the septal leaflet (5/2.2 cm) (Figs. 4.5, 4.6, 4.7 and 4.8).

Echocardiography allows accurate evaluation of the TV leaflets, the size of the right atrium, and size and function of both ventricles. The site and degree of TV regurgitation and the feasibility of valve repair are also assessed by echocardiography.

Associated anomalies with Ebstein's include PFO or ASD in approximately 50% of patients; accessory conduction pathways in 25% (usually right-sided); and, occasionally, varying degrees of right ventricular outflow tract obstruction, VSD, aortic coarctation, PDA, or mitral valve disease.

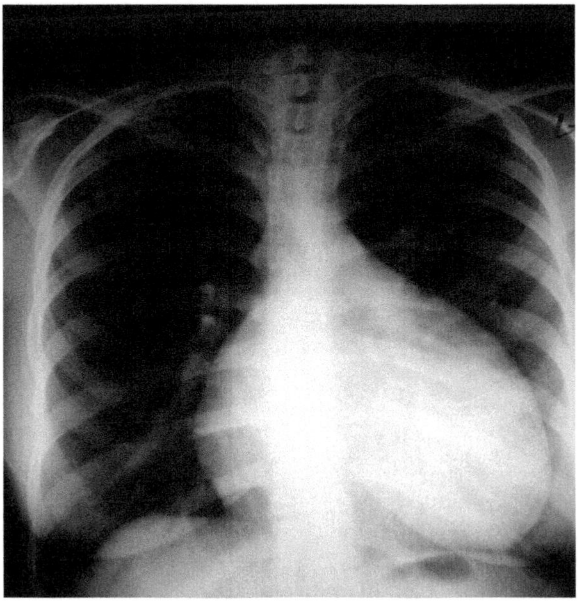

Fig. 4.2 PA x-ray in full inspiration and normal KV from a woman. Mild deviation to the left; Increased cardiothoracic (CT) ratio infavour of cardiomegaly indicative of enlargement of right-sided chambers; Normal position of gastric bubble and carinal angle; Normal pulmonary vasculature; No tracheal deviation

Current Indications for Intervention in Ebstein Anomaly

- Poor exercise capacity (NYHA class > II)
- Right heart failure
- Large heart size (cardiothoracic ratio > 64%)
- Important cyanosis (resting oxygen saturation < 90%)
- Severe symptomatic tricuspid regurgitation
- Transient ischemic attack, or stroke due to a paradoxic embolus, sustained atrial flutter, or fibrillation and atrial arrhythmias secondary to an accessory pathway.

Management

Medical

Patients with mild forms of Ebstein's anomaly may be followed medically for many years. Regular evaluation by a cardiologist with proficiency in congenital heart disease is suggested.

Endocarditis prophylaxis is commended in Ebstein's anomaly, although the risk of endocarditis is low.

In patients with Ebstein's anomaly and cardiac failure who are not candidates for surgery, we recommend standard heart failure treatment.

Heart transplantation is an alternative treatment option in select patients who are not candidates for standard surgical treatment.

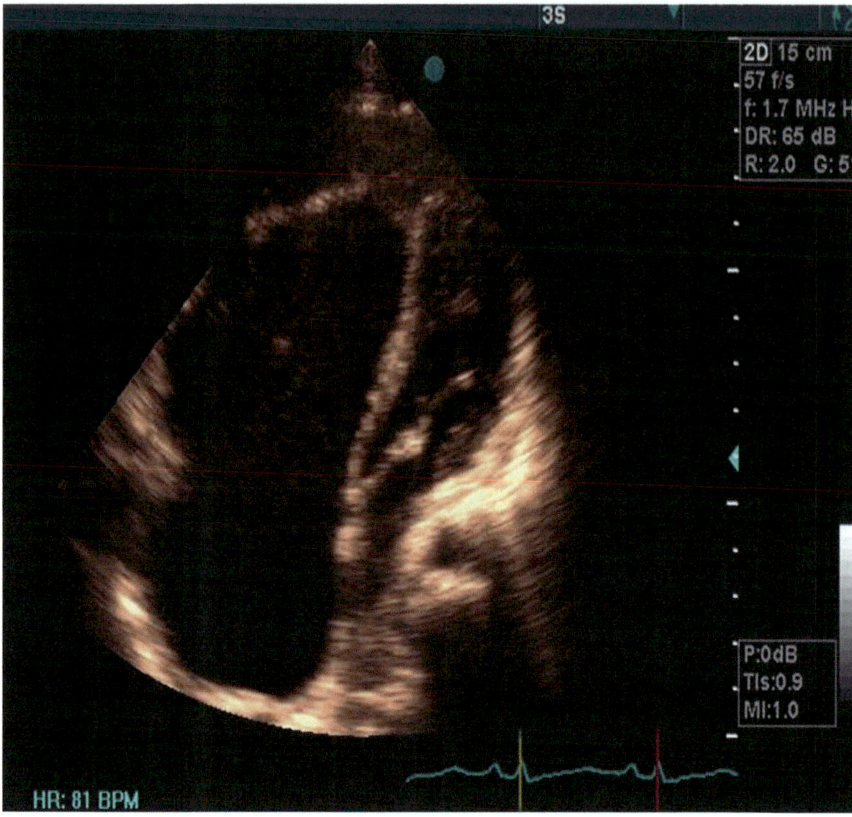

Fig. 4.3 Showing apical four-chamber view with significant apical displacement of septal tricuspid valve (TV) leaflet and tethered anterior TV leaflet

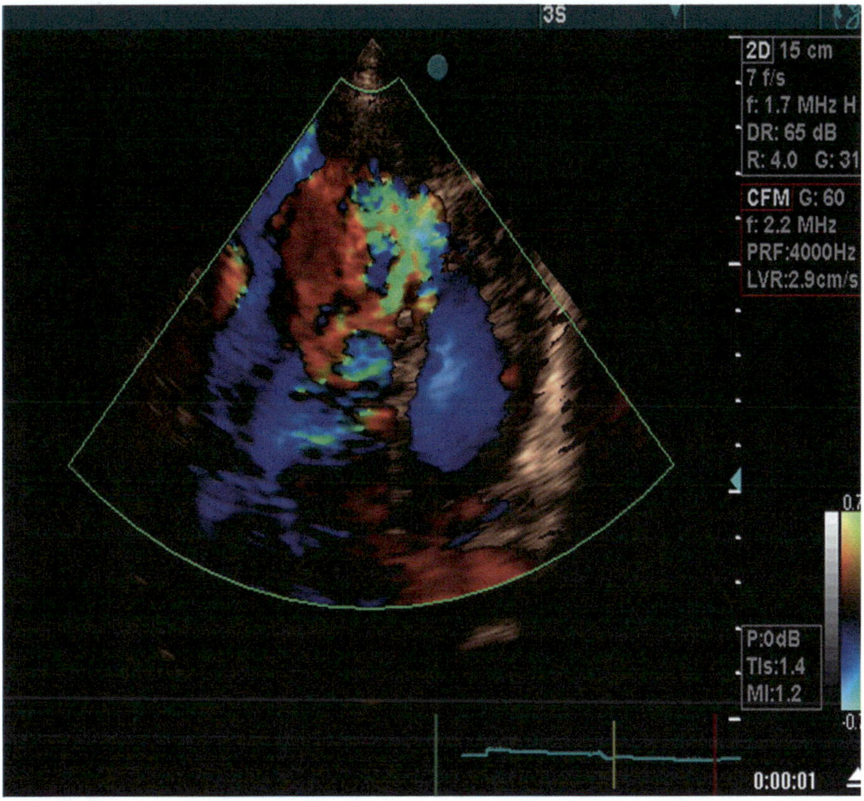

Fig. 4.4 Showing severe low-pressure TR

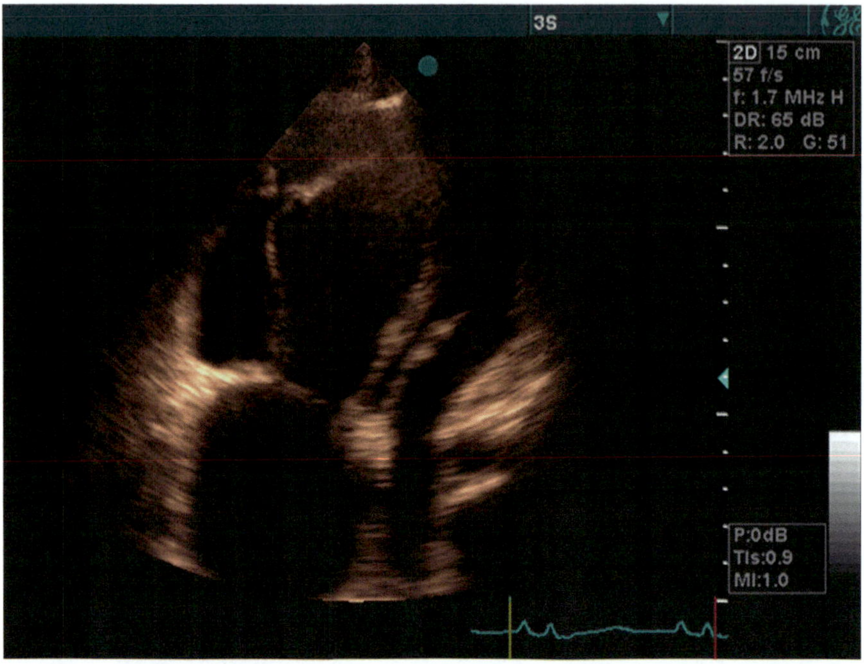

Fig. 4.5 Showing apical four-chamber view with tethered anterior TV leaflet

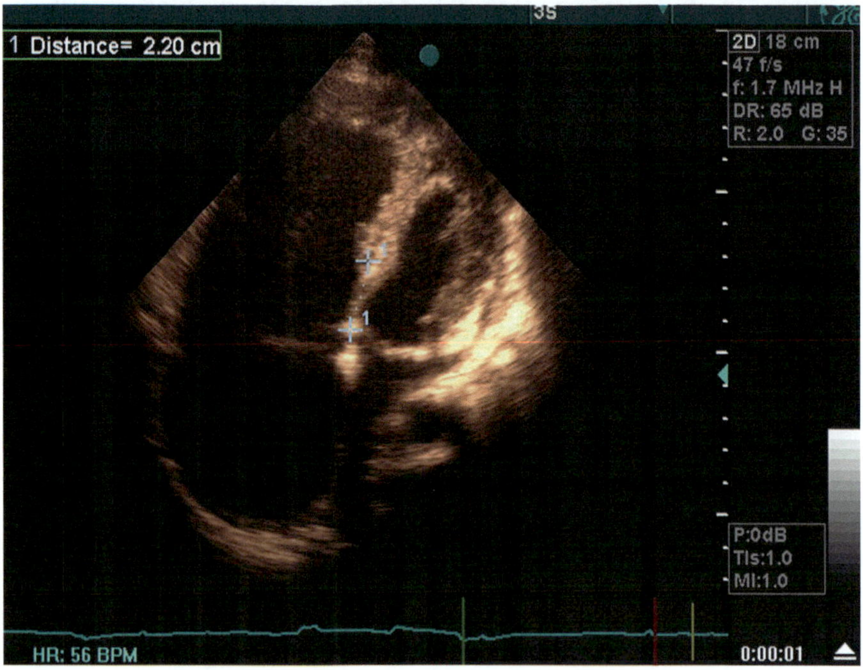

Fig. 4.6 Displacement distance of septal TV leaflet is 2.2 cm

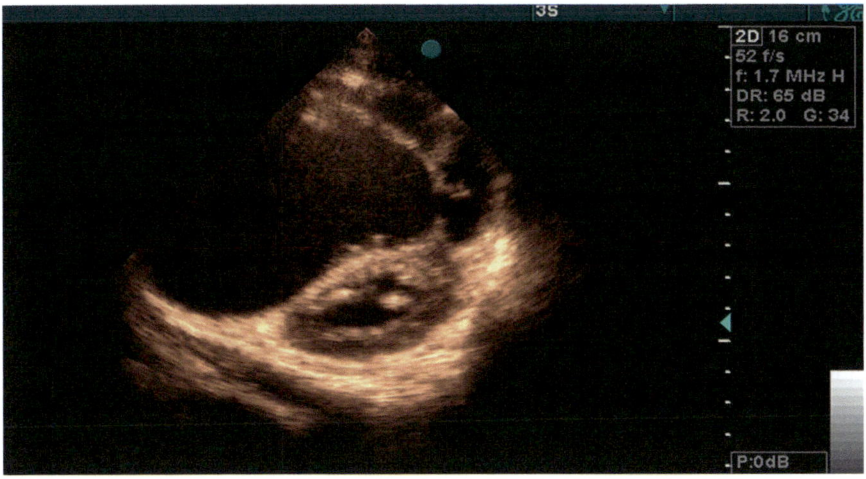

Fig. 4.7 Showing significant apical displacement of septal TV leaflet and tethered anterior TV leaflet

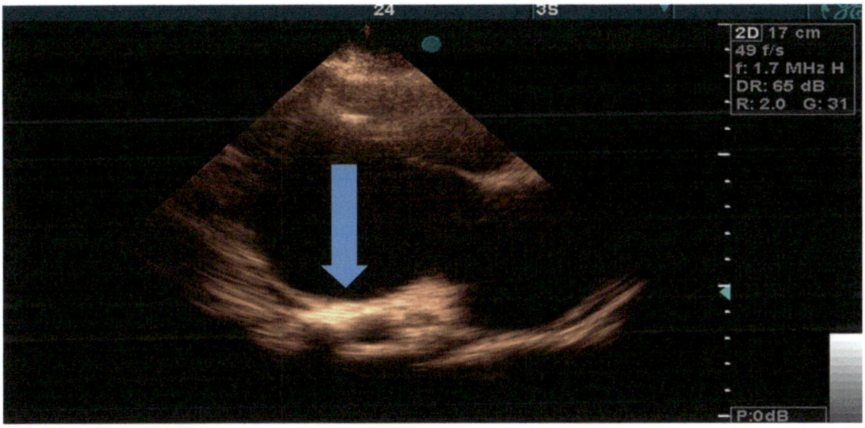

Fig. 4.8 Showing RV inflow view with significant apical displacement of posterior TV leaflet; Arrow: the insertion site of posterior TV leaflet

Catheter Interventions

Most patients with symptomatic WPW syndrome, with or without EA, must undergo electrophysiological assessment and maybe radiofrequency ablation of the accessory pathway(s); also, all types of supraventricular tachyarrhythmia associated with EA can be successfully ablated by the electrophysiologist.

Surgery

Several types of procedures can be used to surgically treat Ebstein anomaly and associated defects:

- Tricuspid valve repair.
- Tricuspid valve replacement. ...

The goal of this surgery is to fix the defective valve between the right atrium and the right ventricle so that the leaflets open and close correctly.

When there is enough tissue present, the valve can be repaired. This is the preferred treatment because it uses your own tissue. When the existing valve cannot be repaired, it is possible to replace it with a mechanical valve or one made of biologic tissue.

- Closure of the atrial septal defect.
- Maze procedure [1–6].

References

1. Paranon S, Acar P. Ebstein's anomaly of the tricuspid valve: from fetus to adult: congenital heart disease. Heart. 2008;94:237–43.
2. Ibrahim M, Tsang VT, Caruana M, et al. Cone reconstruction for Ebstein's anomaly: patient outcomes, biventricular function, and cardiopulmonary exercise capacity. J Thorac Cardiovasc Surg. 2015;149:1144–50.
3. Attenhofer Jost CH, Connolly HM, Dearani JA, Edwards WD, Danielson GK. Ebstein's anomaly. Circulation. 2007;115:277–85.
4. Yuan SM. Ebstein's anomaly: genetics, clinical manifestations, and management. Pediatr Neonatol. 2017;58:211–5.
5. Kron IL, Roeser ME. Management of Ebstein's anomaly. Ann Cardiothorac Surg. 2017;6:266–9.
6. Sadeghpour A, Alizadehasl A. The right ventricle: A comprehensive review from anatomy, physiology, and mechanics to hemodynamic, functional, and imaging evaluation. Review article. 2015;3(4):4–4. https://doi.org/10.5812/acvi.35717.

Chapter 5
Right Atrial Myxoma

Azin Alizadehasl

Abstract Right atrial myxoma accounts for 15–20% of cardiac myxomas and feet swelling is a rare manifestation. We present the case of an 59-year-old man with right atrial myxoma and progressive swelling of feet, and discuss the role of cardiac echocardiography in the diagnosis of myxomas.

Case Presentation

An 59-year-old man with a history of hypertension, hyperlipidemia, presented to the emergency department with progressive swelling of feet. Physical examination demonstrated normal and regular heart sounds, and normal respiratory rate and oxygen saturation. Echocardiogram described a well-circumscribed echo-dense pedunculated mass in the right atrial cavity, which was attached to the interatrial septum with short stalk and also with obstructing the tricuspid valve annulus, measuring 3.7 × 5.2 cm at its widest diameter (Figs. 5.1, 5.2, 5.3, 5.4, 5.5 and 5.6).

Discussion and Management

Myxomas are the most common type of adult primary heart tumor. Most myxomas arise sporadically (90%), and only about 10% are thought to arise due to inheritance.

About 10% of myxomas are inherited, as in Carney syndrome. Such tumors are called familial myxomas. They tend to occur in more than one part of the heart at a time and often cause symptoms at a younger age than other myxomas. Other abnormalities are observed in people with Carney syndrome include skin myxomas,

A. Alizadehasl (✉)
Rajaie Cardiovascular Medical and Research Center, Cardio-Oncology Department and Research Center, Iran University of Medical Science, Tehran, Iran

M. Maleki, A. Alizadehasl (eds.), *Case-Based Clinical Cardiology*,
https://doi.org/10.1007/978-1-4471-7496-7_5

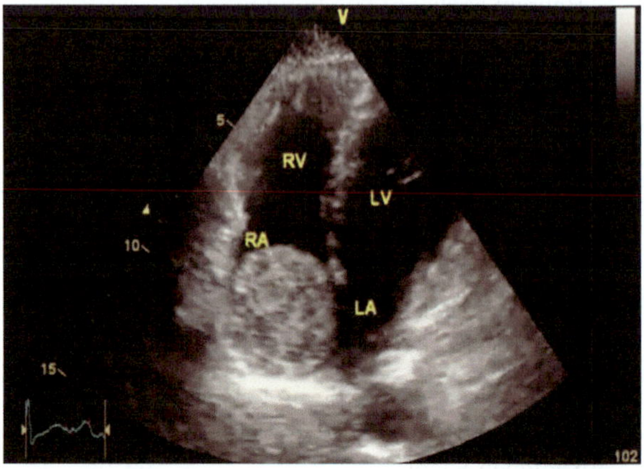

Fig. 5.1 Large well-circumscribed echo-dense mass in the right atrial cavity

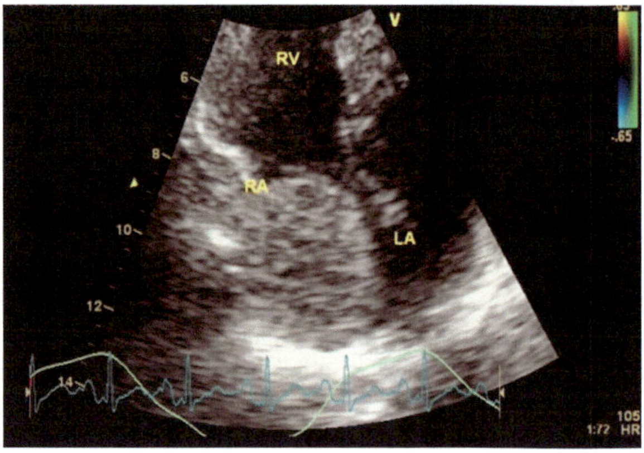

Fig. 5.2 Large well-circumscribed echo-dense mass that filled right atrial cavity

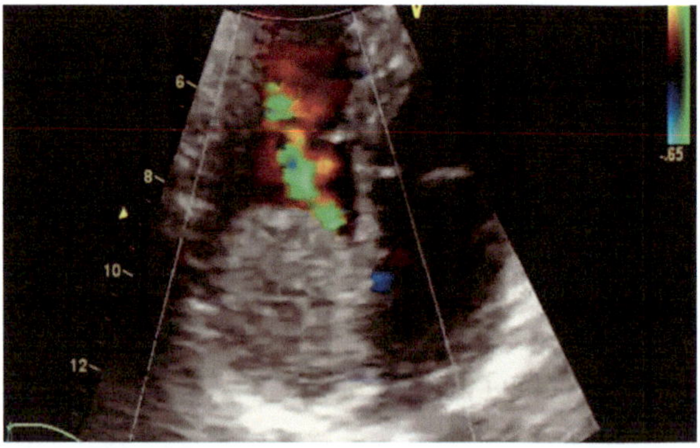

Fig. 5.3 Large well-circumscribed echo-dense mass that obstructing the tricuspid valve annulus

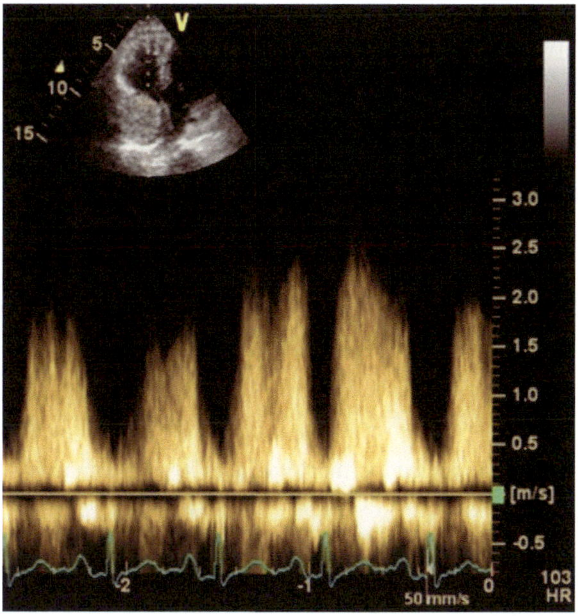

Fig. 5.4 Significant Doppler flow gradient due to large well-circumscribed echo-dense mass that obstructing the tricuspid valve annulus (Velocity: 2 m/s)

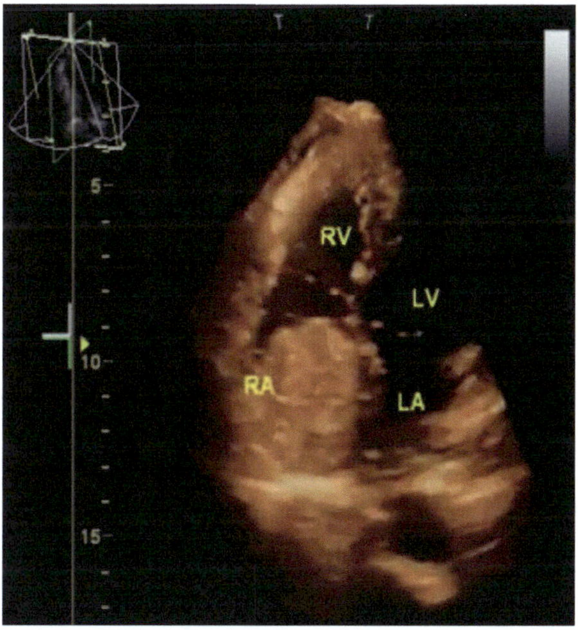

Fig. 5.5 3D view. Large well-circumscribed echo-dense mass in the right atrial cavity

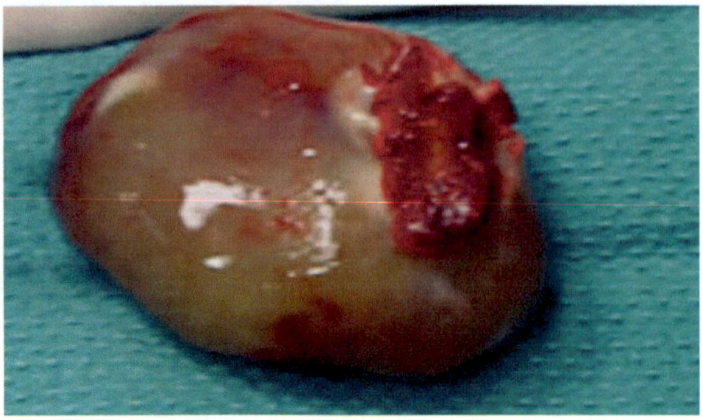

Fig. 5.6 Large extracted mass from RA in operating room

pigmentation, endocrine hyperactivity, schwannomas, and epithelioid blue nevi. Myxomas are more common in women than in men.

General symptoms of myxoma may also be present, such as:

- Cough
- Fever
- Cachexia—Involuntary weight loss
- General discomfort (malaise)
- Joint pain
- Blue discoloration of the skin, especially the fingers change color upon pressure, cold, or stress (Raynaud's phenomenon)
- Clubbing—Curvature of nails accompanied with soft tissue enlargement of the fingers
- Swelling—any part of the body

The symptoms and signs of left atrial myxomas probably mimic the mitral stenosis. Right atrial myxomas rarely produce symptoms until they have grown to be obstructive on TV.

The CMR of our patient confirmed the myxoma too and tumor surgically removed there is no need for TV repair. He discharged very well.

Some patients will also need their mitral or tricuspid valves to repair or replaced. This can be done during the same surgery, also myxomas may come back if the surgery did not remove all of the tumor cells [1–6].

References

1. Tzani A, Doulamis IP, Mylonas KS, Avgerinos DV, Nasioudis D. Cardiac tumors in pediatric patients: a systematic review. World J Pediatr Congenit Heart Surg. 2017;8:624–32. https://doi.org/10.1177/2150135117723904.
2. Akhundova A, Samedov F, Cincin A, et al. Giant left atrial myxoma with dual coronary supply presenting with recurrent stroke. http://link.springer.com/article/10.1007%2Fs00059-013-3999

3. Pinede L, Duhaut P, Loire P. Clinical presentation of left atrial cardiac myxoma. A series of 112 consecutive cases. Medicine (Baltimore) 2001;80:159–172. http://journals.lww.com/mdjournal/Fulltext/2001/05000/Infected_Cardiac_Myxoma__Case_Report_and.2.aspx.
4. Selkane C, Amahzoune B, Chavanis N, et al. Changing management of cardiac myxoma based on a series of 40 cases with long-term follow-up. Ann Thorac Surg. 2003;76:1935–38.
5. Hoffmeier A, Sindermann JR, Scheld HH, Martens S. Cardiac tumors. Deutsches Ärzteblatt Int. 2014;111(12):205–11.
6. Karabinis A, Samanidis G, Khoury M, Stavridis G, Perreas K. Clinical presentation and treatment of cardiac myxoma in 153 patients. Medicine. 2018;97(37):e12397.

Chapter 6
Pseudoaneurysm of the Mitral-Aortic Intervalvular Fibrosa (MAIVF)

Azin Alizadehasl

Abstract The region of the mitral-aortic continuity (MA inter-valvular fibroza; MAIVF) contains mostly fibrous and avascular tissue. MAIVF is the weakest segment of the aortic ring, prone to infection and trauma and creation of pseudoaneurysm.

TEE is the most sensitive technique.

Characteristic dynamic feature of pseudoaneurysm is its expansion during early systole and collapse in diastole. Confirmation of this diagnosis requires communication to the LVOT.

Keywords Pseudoaneurysm · Mitral-aortic intervalvular fibrosa (MAIVF) · Infective endocarditis · TEE · TTE · 3D echocardiography

Case Presentation

A 32-year-old woman with type 1 diabetes underwent TTE due to atypical chest pain.

She had had IE with *Streptococcus viridans* 3 years ago and fortunately improved just by medication and discharged with moderate aortic regurgitation.

In this visit TTE revealed an echolucent area adjacent to the aortic valve, raising suspicion of a Pseudoaneurysm of MAIVF (P-MAIVF).

TEE showed an echolucent area too measuring 23 mm in its widest dimension, which was freely communicating with the LVOT.

This cavity expanded during systole, bulging into the left atrium and collapsing during diastole. Doppler examination confirmed it. There was no fistulous communication to the left atrium or aorta.

She underwent surgical repair with the closure of the communication with the LVOT using a Dacron patch.

A. Alizadehasl (✉)
Rajaie Cardiovascular Medical and Research Center, Cardio-Oncology Department and Research Center, Iran University of Medical Science, Tehran, Iran

M. Maleki, A. Alizadehasl (eds.), *Case-Based Clinical Cardiology*,
https://doi.org/10.1007/978-1-4471-7496-7_6

Echocardiography Findings and Discussion (Figs. 6.1, 6.2, 6.3, 6.4 and 6.5)

Because TEE has come into routine use, there has been increasing recognition of this entity, although the number of patients in any series is quite small.

Pseudoaneurysm of the mitral-aortic intervalvular fibrosa (P-MAIVF) is a rare condition that has been reported as a sequela of endocarditis and surgical trauma.

It is defined as a pseudoaneurysm at the inter-annular zone between the mitral and aortic valves and its communication with the LVOT between the left coronary or non-coronary aortic cusp and the anterior leaflet of the mitral valve.

Our patient underwent surgical repair with the closure of the communication with the LVOT using a Dacron patch.

Endocarditis and aortic valve surgery were the two most frequently associated causative factors for PSA. In study, 46 patients (52%) had prosthetic aortic valves, either bioprosthetic (n = 6) or mechanical. Of the 43 patients (48%) with native valves, 14 (33%) had bicuspid valves, 1 had a unicuspid valve, and 27 had normal tricuspid aortic valves.

The shortest time reported after valve surgery to the development of a P-MAIVF was 9 days, but that patient had had a MAIVF abscess preoperatively. Pseudoaneurysms had developed within 1 month of valve surgery in two patients.

Aortic regurgitation has been suggested as a contributing factor for the development of P-MAIVF.

In other previous study Of the 87 patients, 42 were noted to have some degree of aortic regurgitation at the time of diagnosis. Diagnoses by TTE were made in 31 (54%), missed in 24 (42%). Diagnoses by TEE were made in all cases. 3D echocardiography was performed in five patients, with excellent visualization of the pseudoaneurysm. Computed tomography was performed in four patients CMR in six patients.

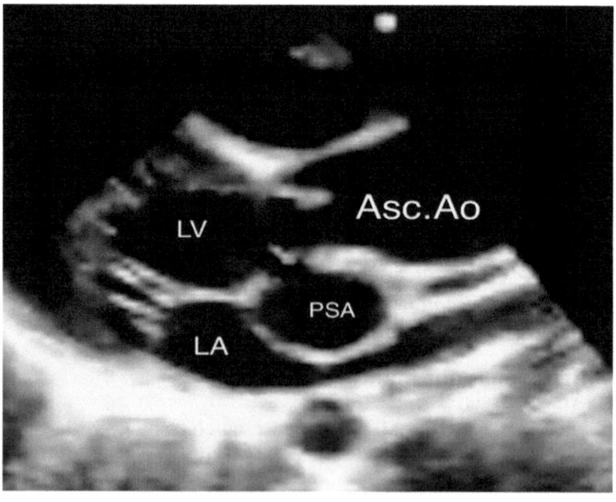

Fig. 6.1 TTE parasternal long-axis view showed an echolucent area adjacent to the aortic valve, a Pseudoaneurysm of MAIVF

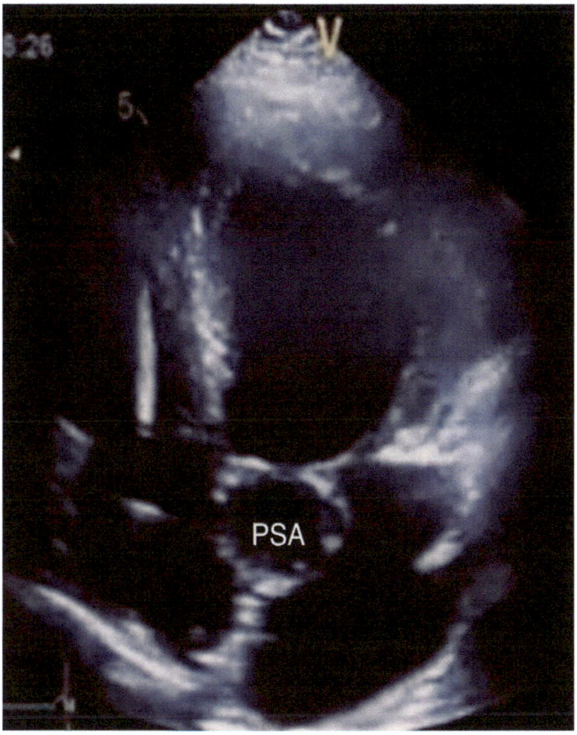

Fig. 6.2 TTE apical four-chamber view showed a Pseudoaneurysm of MAIVF

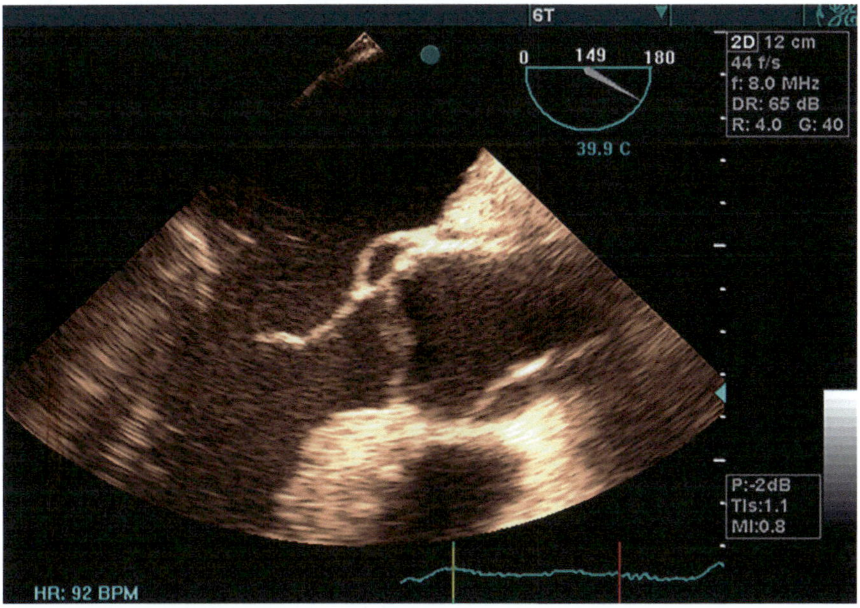

Fig. 6.3 TEE view showed an echolucent area (Pseudo-aneurysm of MAIVF)

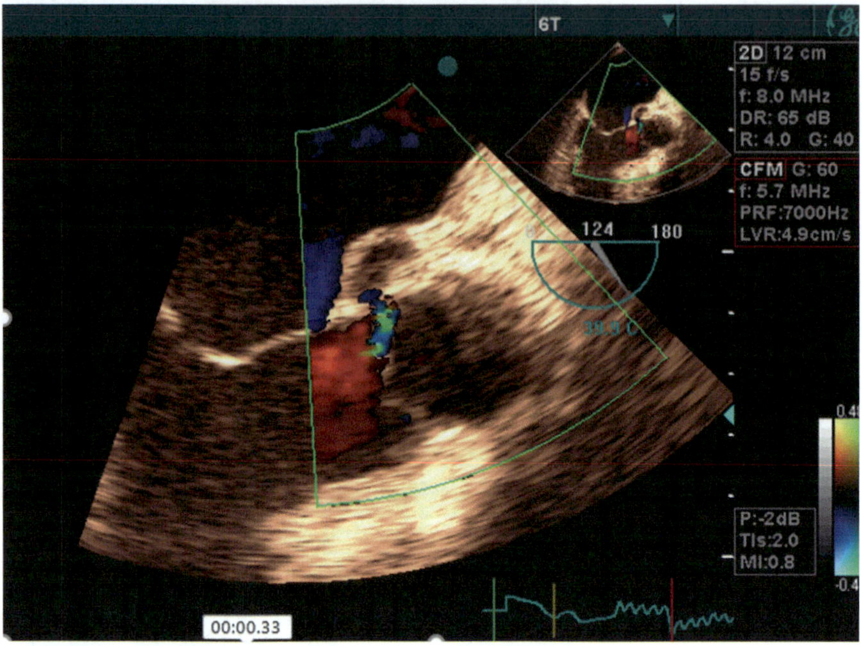

Fig. 6.4 Communication between LVOT and pseudoaneurysm

Fig. 6.5 3D TEE of P-AMIVF

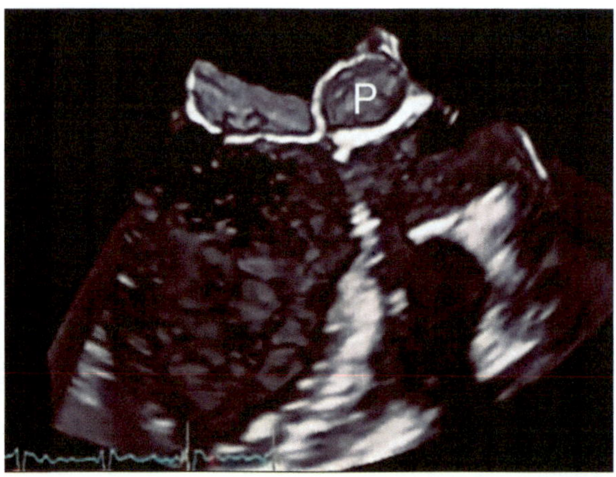

These modalities provided very good 3D information of the pseudoaneurysm size and its relationship to adjacent structures.

Surgery is currently the recommended treatment to prevent further enlargement and complications.

In this review the patient with 4-year follow-up, the P-MAIVF diameter increased from 1 to 1.7 cm and in two other patients, there were no changes in the pseudoaneurysm sizes at 10-month and 3-year follow-up; so the natural course of uncomplicated P-MAIVF is not clear, but, most patients undergo surgery as soon as the diagnosis is made. This study considered two groups of patients who might be at higher risk for developing P-MAIVF: one group includes patients with infective endocarditis complicated by ring abscess, particularly in the area of the MAIVF and the other group includes patients with prosthetic valves and histories of IE.

Surgery may still be the recommended course of action, but in patients who are at high risk for surgery and in asymptomatic patients who refuse surgery, watchful observation may be considered after careful evaluation of associated high-risk features [1–6].

References

1. Grimaldi A, Ho SY, Pozzoli A, Sora N, Taramasso M, Benussi S, La Canna G, Alfieri O. Pseudoaneurysm of mitral-aortic intervalvular fibrosa. Interact Cardiovasc Thorac Surg. 2011;13(2):142–7. https://doi.org/10.1510/icvts.2011.269258.
2. Sudhakar S, Sewani A, Agrawal M, Uretsky BF. Pseudoaneurysm of the mitral-aortic intervalvular fibrosa (MAIVF): a comprehensive review. J Am Soc Echocardiogr. 2010;23(10):1009–18. https://doi.org/10.1016/j.echo.2010.07.015. quiz 1112.
3. Hasin T, Reisner SA, Agmon Y. Large pseudoaneurysms of the mitral-aortic intervalvular fibrosa: long-term natural history without surgery in two patients. Eur J Echocardiogr. 2011;12(3):E24. https://doi.org/10.1093/ejechocard/jeq183.
4. Takawira FF, Joshi JA, Du Plessis DJ. Development of a subaortic aneurysm secondary to disseminated tuberculosis in a child. Ann Thorac Surg. 2010;90(2):644–7. https://doi.org/10.1016/j.athoracsur.2010.01.070.
5. Xie M, Li Y, Cheng TO, Wang X, Lu Q, He L, et al. Pseudoaneurysm of the mitral-aortic intervalvular fibrosa. Int J Cardiol. 2013;166:2–7.3.
6. Sahan E, Gül M, Sahan S, Sokmen E, Guray YA, Tufekçioglu O. Pseudoaneurysm of the mitral-aortic intervalvular brosa. A new comprehensive review. Herz. 2015;40(Suppl 2):182–9.

Chapter 7
Arrhythmogenic Right Ventricular Cardiomyopathy/Dysplasia

Azin Alizadehasl

Abstract Arrhythmogenic right ventricular cardiomyopathy/dysplasia (ARVC/D) is an infrequent disease categorized by progressive fibro-fatty replacement of the myocardium, primarily involving the right ventricle (RV). The structural changes in the ventricular myocardium form a substrate for ventricular arrhythmia ranging from premature ventricular complexes to ventricular tachycardia characteristically of RV origin and might result in RV failure and progress to congestive heart failure at a future stage. ARVC/D is a documented cause of sudden cardiac death in young people; however, it might occur at any age.

Keywords Arrhythmogenic right ventricular cardiomyopathy/dysplasia (ARVC/D) · Right ventricle (RV) · RV failure · Echocardiography · Prominent RV Moderator Band

Case Presentation

Here in we present a 19 years old female that presented with near syncope attacks due to recurrent self-limiting monomorphic VT originating from the RV in the electrophysiological study. She had no RV failure signs and symptoms. But her ECG and Echocardiogram was typical for this disease (Fig. 7.1).

Transthoracic Echocardiography

► A TTE study is a perfect screening tool to assess the RV size and function in cases with probable ARVD-C. TTE can be done easily at a low cost, and not only is it readily available but it is also portable. Additionally, this modality is mainly valuable in following affected patients over time because of its ability to present serial imaging in cases with ICDs.

A. Alizadehasl (✉)
Rajaie Cardiovascular Medical and Research Center, Cardio-Oncology Department and Research Center, Iran University of Medical Science, Tehran, Iran

M. Maleki, A. Alizadehasl (eds.), *Case-Based Clinical Cardiology*,
https://doi.org/10.1007/978-1-4471-7496-7_7

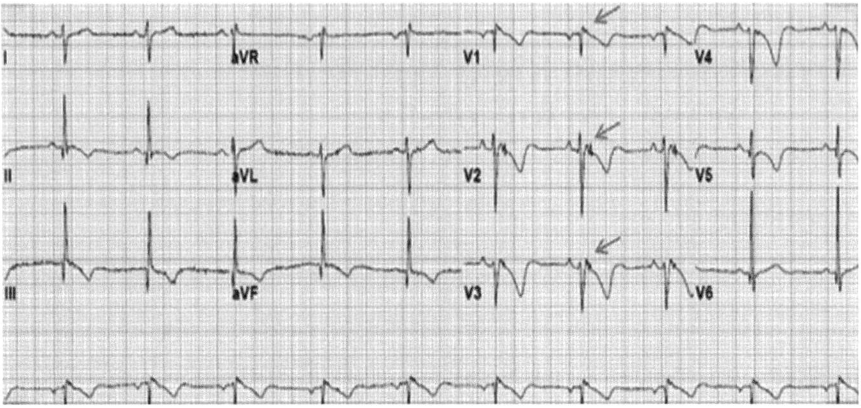

Fig. 7.1 ECG with classical Epsilon waves (Waves)

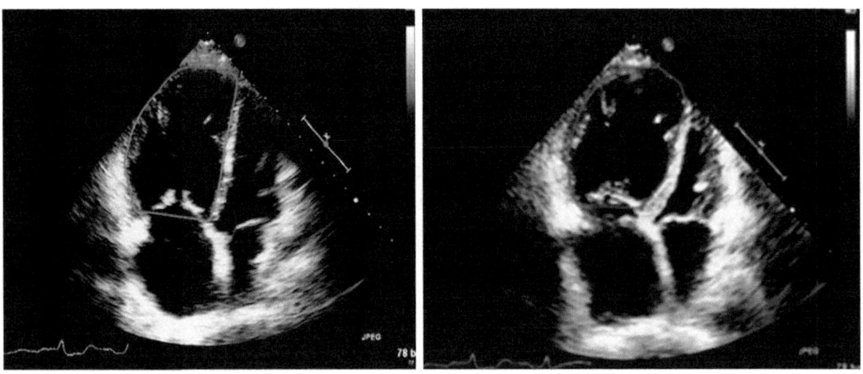

Fig. 7.2 RV enlargement in RV focus view

► TTE for ARVD-C study should be performed using the current American Society of Echocardiography's consensus and guidelines. Because the RV might be enlarged and, thus, not completely imaged on the standard imaging planes, additional off-axis views should be achieved to make sure that all parts of the RV free wall are well imaged and visualized. Given the patchy involvement, this is especially important to echocardiographers so that they do not miss small and localized aneurysms (Figs. 7.2, 7.3, 7.4, and 7.5).

Discussion

ARVC/D is a rare cardiac disease characterized by fibrofatty replacement of myocardial tissue. It affects the RV primarily, but an extension to the LV in more advanced stages of the disease may occur. At the molecular level, both ventricles are

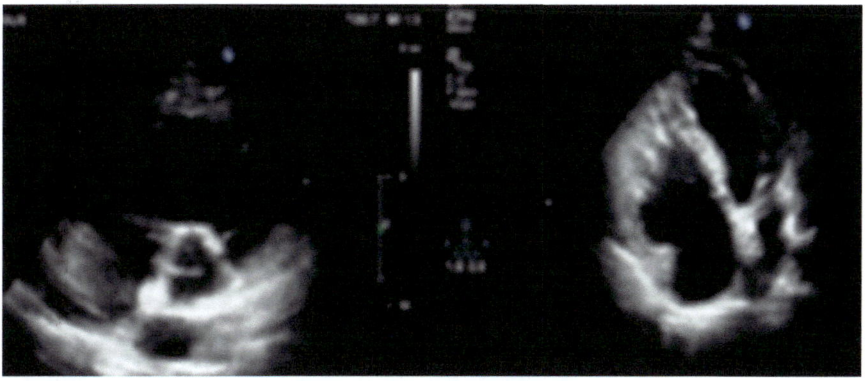

Fig. 7.3 RV dilation is often observed in cases with ARVD-C. Previous studies revealed that an enlarged right ventricular outflow tract (RVOT) was found in 100% of patients. A major criterion for ARVD-C is achieved when there is RVOT dilation on the parasternal long-axis view (≥32 mm) or in the short-axis view (≥36 mm), alongside localized akinesia, dyskinesia, or aneurysms in the RV free wall (the RVOT size of this case was 42 mm)

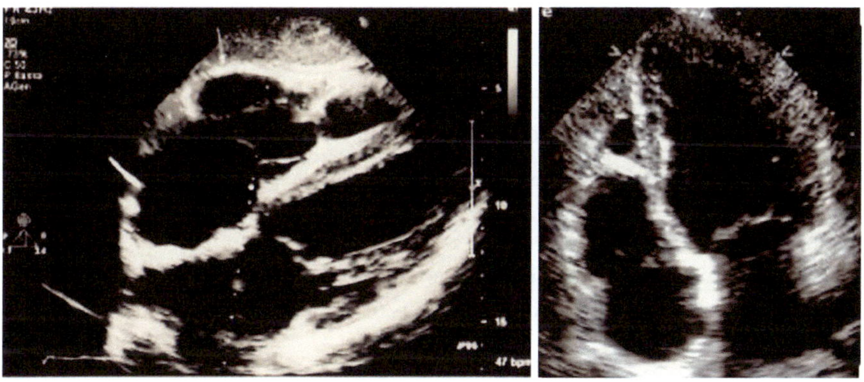

Fig. 7.4 Prominent RV Moderator Band in ARVD/C

affected, presumably in all stages of the disease. Its prevalence has been estimated to vary from 1:2000 to 1:5000. Patients typically present between the second and the fourth decade of life with VT episodes originating from the RV. It is also a major cause of SCD in young patients and athletes (Fig. 7.6).

Differential diagnosis of ARVC/D:

- RVOT tachycardia
- Sarcoidosis
- Idiopathic DCM
- Isolated myocarditis
- Adipositas cordis
- Uhi ANOMALY
- Congenital heart disease

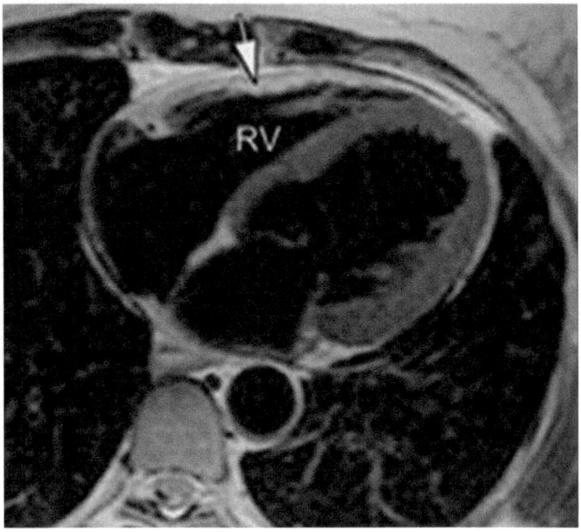

Fig. 7.5 Transmural fatty replacement in RV free wall at T1 weighted image of CMR

- RV infarction
- Carcinoid syndrome

Based on clinicopathologic and patients' follow-up studies, four different disease phases have been described for the classical form of ARVC/D:

- Concealed: No symptoms; Subtle structural changes
- Overt: Ventricular arrhythmias (PVCs/VT of LBBB morphology); RV structural abnormalities
- RV failure: Symptoms and signs of RV failure; Preserved LV function
- Biventricular failure: Symptoms and signs of LV failure; LV structural changes

LV involvement in ARVD has been increasingly described, with the prevalence reported as 16–76% [1–8].

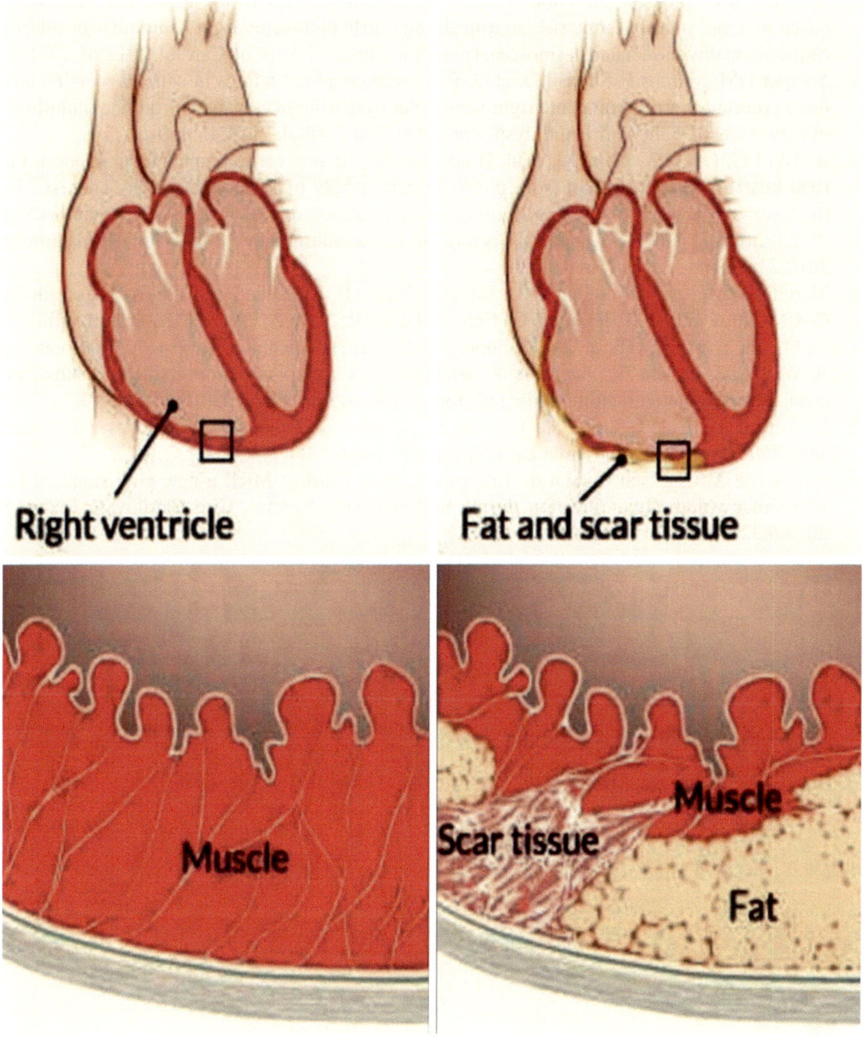

Fig. 7.6 Left: Normal; Right: ARVC/D. Fibrofatty change

References

1. Towbin JA, McKenna WJ, Abrams DJ, et al. 2019 HRS expert consensus statement on evaluation, risk stratification, and management of arrhythmogenic cardiomyopathy. Heart Rhythm. 2019;16:e301.
2. Marcus FI, McKenna WJ, Sherrill D, et al. Diagnosis of arrhythmogenic right ventricular cardiomyopathy/dysplasia: proposed modification of the task force criteria. Circulation. 2010;121:1533–41.

3. Te Riele AS, Bhonsale A, James CA, et al. Incremental value of cardiac magnetic resonance imaging in arrhythmic risk stratification of arrhythmogenic right ventricular dysplasia/cardiomyopathy-associated desmosomal mutation carriers. J Am Coll Cardiol. 2013;62:1761–9.
4. Yoerger DM, Marcus F, Sherrill D, et al. Echocardiographic findings in patients meeting task force criteria for arrhythmogenic right ventricular dysplasia: new insights from the multidisciplinary study of right ventricular dysplasia. J Am Coll Cardiol. 2005;45:860–5.
5. Rudski LG, Lai WW, Afilalo J, et al. Guidelines for the echocardiographic assessment of the right heart in adults: a report from the American Society of Echocardiography endorsed by the European Association of Echocardiography, a registered branch of the European Society of Cardiology, and the Canadian Society of Echocardiography. J Am Soc Echocardiogr. 2010;23:685–713, quiz 786–8.
6. Marcus FI, McKenna WJ, Sherrill D, Basso C, Bauce B, Bluemke DA, Calkins H, Corrado D, Cox MGPJ, Daubert JP, Fontaine G, Gear K, Hauer R, Nava A, Picard MH, Protonotarios N, Saffitz JE, Yoerger Sanborn DM, Steinberg JS, Tandri H, Thiene G, Towbin JA, Tsatsopoulou A, Wichter T, Zareba W. Diagnosis of arrhythmogenic right ventricular cardiomyopathy/dysplasia. Proposed modification of the task force Criteria. Eur Heart J. 2010;31:806–14.
7. Lindstrom L, Wilkenshoff UM, Larsson H, Wranne B. Echocardiographic assessment of arrhythmogenic right ventricular cardiomyopathy. Heart. 2001;86:31–8.
8. La Gerche A, Claessen G, Van de Bruaene A, et al. Cardiac MRI: a new gold standard for ventricular volume quantification during high-intensity exercise. Circ Cardiovasc Imaging. 2013;6:329–38.

Chapter 8
Cardiac Sarcoidosis

Azin Alizadehasl and Feridoun Noohi

Abstract Sarcoidosis is a systemic inflammatory disease of unknown etiology, characterized by non-caseating granulomas. It mainly affects people in the 3rd and 4th decades of life, but may also be found in children or elderly subjects.

Heart involvement has been reported in as many as 58% of patients and may be responsible for up to 85% of deaths due to sarcoidosis.

Various forms of echocardiography have been tried and features such as septal thinning, LV regional systolic dysfunction, pericardial effusion and commonly LV diastolic dysfunction determined, but these abnormalities only seem to be present in advanced heart involvement.

Keywords Sarcoidosis · Systemic inflammatory disease · LV regional systolic dysfunction · Non-caseating granulomas · Septal thinning · Pericardial effusion

Case Presentation

A 59-year-old woman with sarcoidosis was admitted to hospital for assessment of severe dyspnea, palpitation, and limb edema. Echocardiography showed severe LV and RV dysfunction and the following figures (Figs. 8.1, 8.2, 8.3, 8.4, 8.5, 8.6, 8.7, and 8.8):

A. Alizadehasl (✉)
Rajaie Cardiovascular Medical and Research Center, Cardio-Oncology Department and Research Center, Iran University of Medical Science, Tehran, Iran

F. Noohi
Interventional Cardiologist; Rajaie Cardiovascular Medical Center, Iran University of Medical Sciences, Tehran, Iran

M. Maleki, A. Alizadehasl (eds.), *Case-Based Clinical Cardiology*,
https://doi.org/10.1007/978-1-4471-7496-7_8

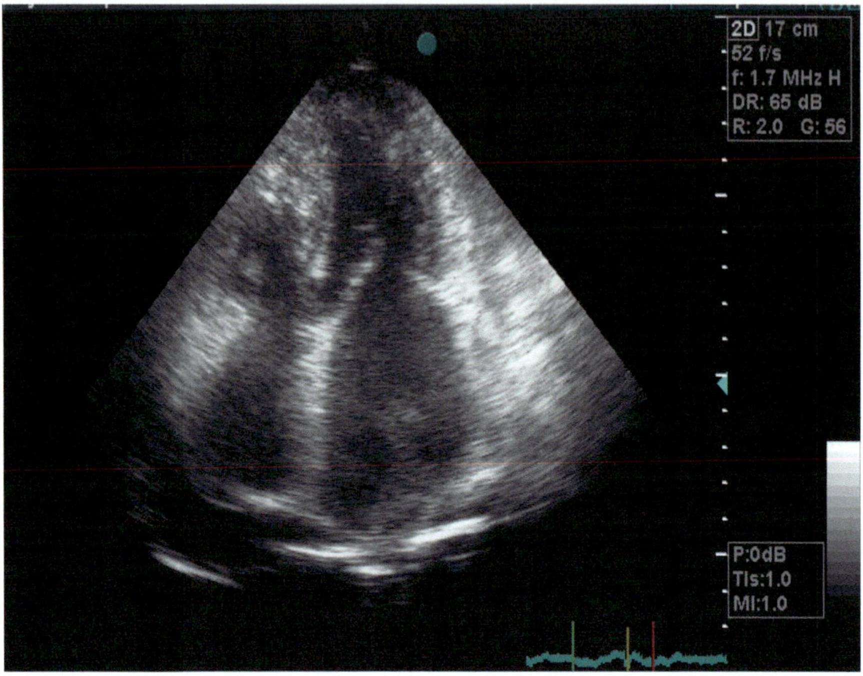

Fig. 8.1 Apical four-chamber view; Biatrial enlargement, LA thrombosis, Pericardial effusion

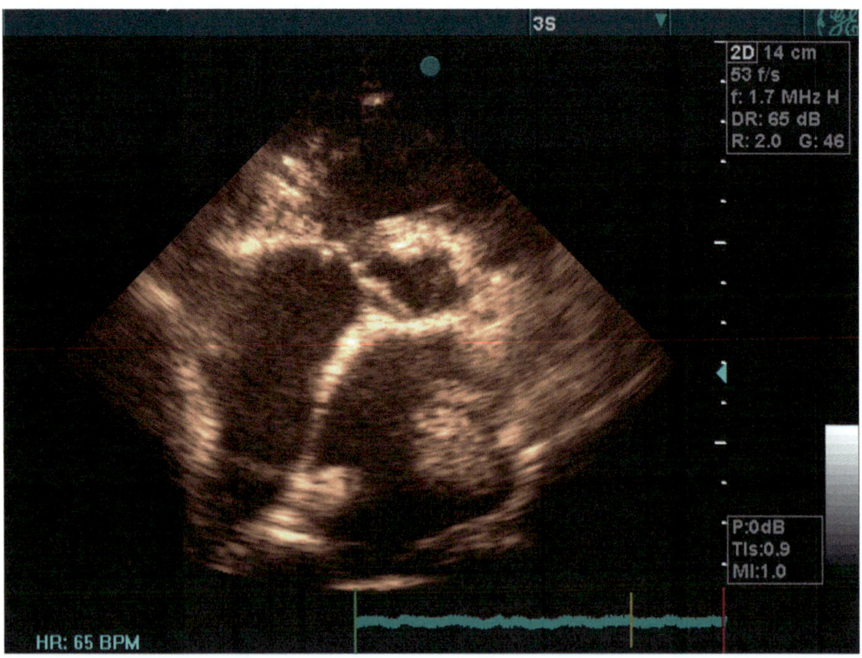

Fig. 8.2 Biatrial enlargement, LA thrombosis, Aortic, and tricuspid valve leaflets thickening

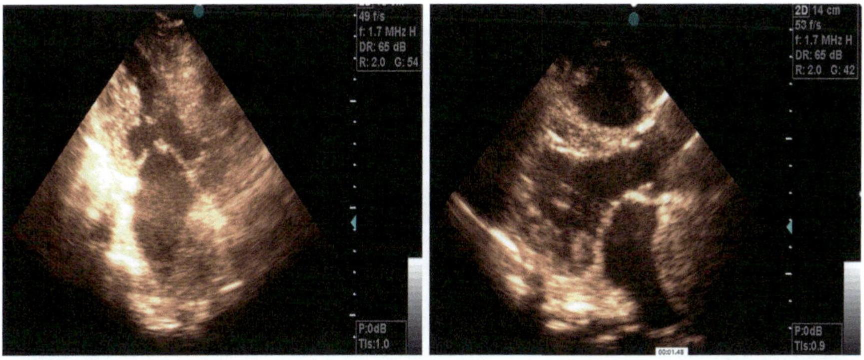

Fig. 8.3 LA thrombosis, Mitral valve leaflets thickening; Aneurysm formation at the base of inferior wall

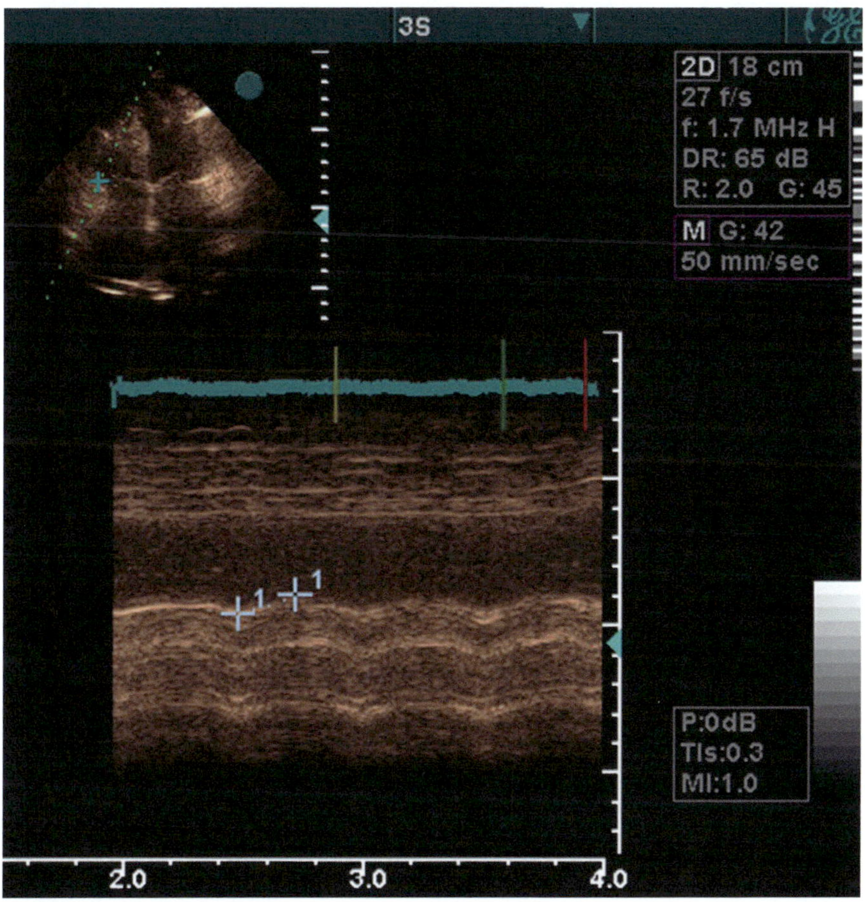

Fig. 8.4 Very reduced TAPSE = 0.6 cm (severe RV dysfunction)

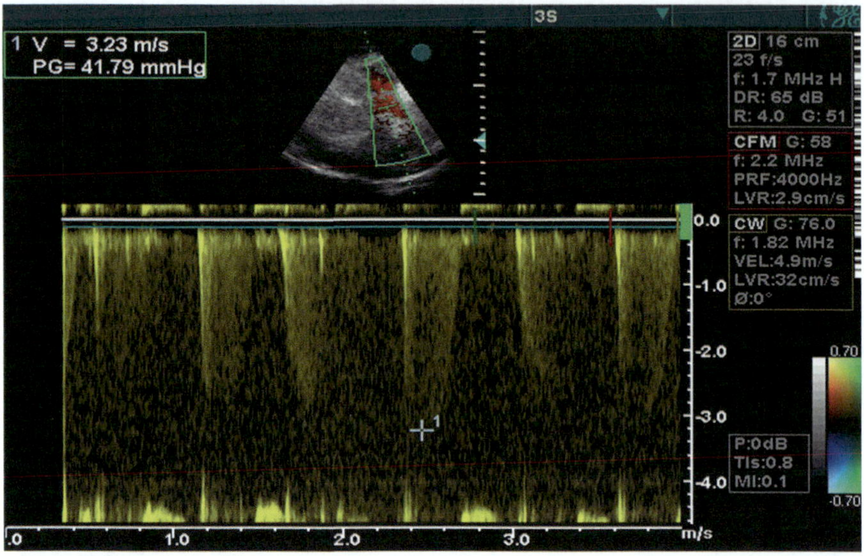

Fig. 8.5 TR gradient: 40 mmHg; Moderate to severe pulmonary hypertension

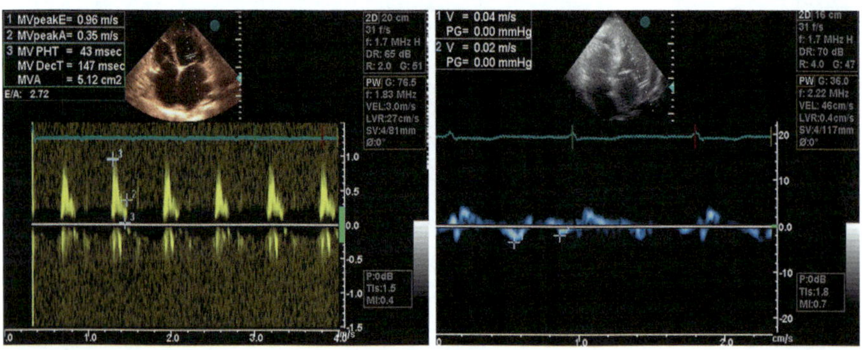

Fig. 8.6 Severe diastolic dysfunction; very reduced TDI velocities

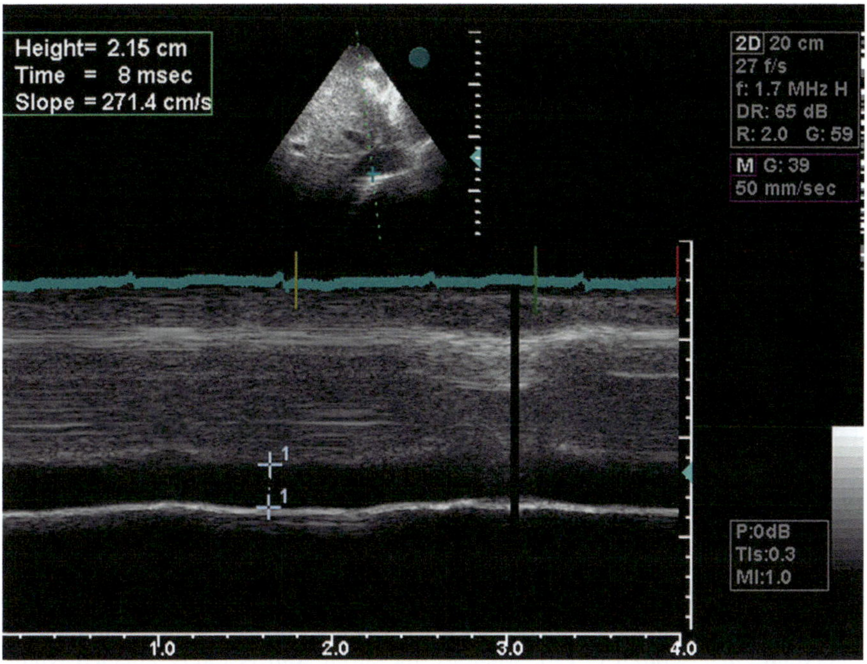

Fig. 8.7 Dilated IVC. High RA pressure

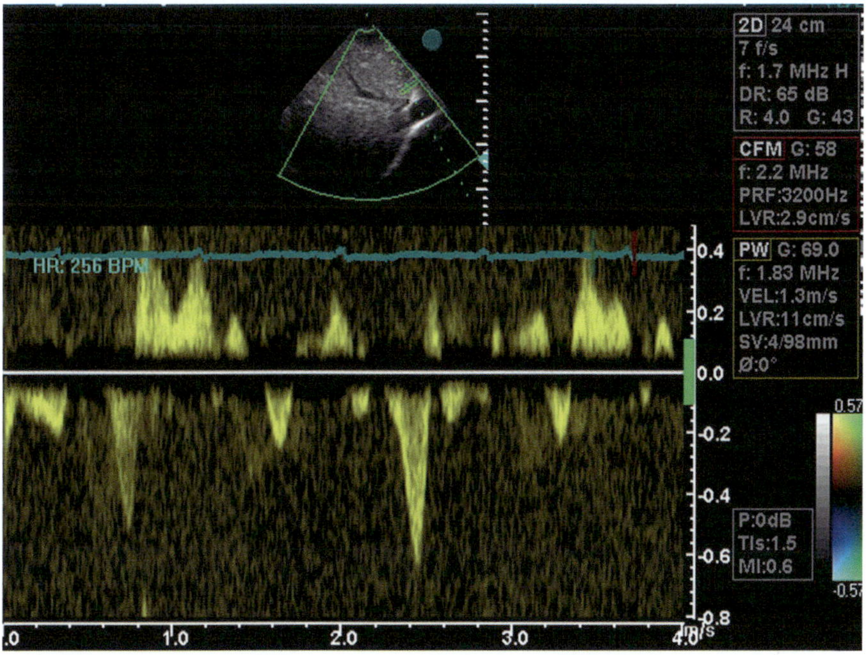

Fig. 8.8 Significant diastolic flow reversal of hepatic vein at inspiration

Discussion

The 2D echo features of myocardial involvement occur in less than 20% of sarcoid patients.

The heart is involved in as many as 50% of advanced cases including LV enlargement and regional wall motion abnormality (RWMA) in base and mid-levels.

In other study the echocardiographic findings are:

- RWMA
- Thining: at basal of posterior and lateral walls
- Posterobasal aneurysm
- Restrictive morphology
- Pulmonary hypertension and right-sided failure

Almost various forms of echocardiography have been tried and features such as septal thinning, LV regional systolic dysfunction, pericardial effusion, and commonly LV diastolic dysfunction determined, but these abnormalities only seem to be present in advanced heart involvement.

Pts with heart involvement may have had granulomas in the myocardial interstitium, which could stiffen the myocardium and damage ventricular Relaxation. Granulomas are most frequently located in the LV free wall (96%), followed by the interventricular septum (73%); whereas, the atrial wall is rarely affected (right, 11%; left, 7%).

Strain imaging demonstrated impaired longitudinal strain and strain rate of several lateral LV segments.

Finally, the frequency of is pulmonary hypertension ≈20% and the presence of Pulmonary hypertension contributed to poor outcomes in pts with sarcoidosis [1–5].

References

1. Kandolin R, Lehtonen J, Airaksinen J, et al. Cardiac sarcoidosis: epidemiology, characteristics, and outcome over 25 years in a nationwide study. Circulation. 2015;131:624–32.
2. Al-Kindi SG, Oliveira GH. Letter by Al-Kindi and Oliveira regarding article "Cardiac sarcoidosis: epidemiology, characteristics, and outcome over 25 years in a nationwide study". Circulation. 2015;132:e211.
3. Nery PB, Mc Ardle BA, Redpath CJ, et al. Prevalence of cardiac sarcoidosis in patients presenting with monomorphic ventricular tachycardia. Pacing Clin Electrophysiol. 2014;367:364–74.
4. Segura AM, Radovancevic R, Demirozu ZT, et al. Granulomatous myocarditis in severe heart failure patients undergoing implantation of a left ventricular assist device. Cardiovasc Pathol. 2014;23:17–20.
5. Schuller JL, Olson MD, Zipse MM, et al. Electrocardiographic characteristics in patients with pulmonary sarcoidosis indicating cardiac involvement. J Cardiovasc Electrophysiol. 2011;22:1243–8.

Chapter 9
Carcinoid Tumor and Echocardiography

Azin Alizadehasl

Abstract Carcinoid tumors are neuroendocrine tumors that have an estimated incidence of 1 to 8.4 cases per 100,000 people (2.5 to 5 cases per 100,000 population); these tumors release vasoactive compounds, including 5-hydroxytryptophan (serotonin) that fibroblast proliferative properties or transforming growth factor-b.

We are presenting a 75-year-old woman with neuroendocrine tumor with liver metastasis.

Keywords Carcinoid tumors · Neuroendocrine tumors · Liver metastasis · Intermittent flushing · Malignancy

A 75-year-old nice woman who presented to our clinic with complaint of dyspnea, fatigue, edema, and palpitation.

Medical history was remarkable for malignancy since 4 years ago. According to pathology sheet, it was neuroendocrine tumor with liver metastasis. She had received some medication from her oncologist.

Carcinoid tumors are neuroendocrine tumors that have an estimated incidence of 1–8.4 cases per 100,000 people; (2.5–5 cases per 100,000 population) these tumors release vasoactive compounds, including 5-hydroxytryptophan (serotonin) that fibroblast proliferative properties or transforming growth factor-b.

In 75% of patients, carcinoid tumors originate in the gastrointestinal tract, most often in the ileum or appendix, although they may also occur within the lungs, pancreas, and gonads.

Usually grow slowly, over years, commonly causing few or no symptoms until they are large or have metastasized to the liver and, less frequently, to other sites (e.g., the lungs or bone).

A. Alizadehasl (✉)
Rajaie Cardiovascular Medical and Research Center, Cardio-Oncology Department and Research Center, Iran University of Medical Science, Tehran, Iran

M. Maleki, A. Alizadehasl (eds.), *Case-Based Clinical Cardiology*,
https://doi.org/10.1007/978-1-4471-7496-7_9

Carcinoid Syndrome

In approximately 30% of patients with carcinoid tumors characterized by episodes of vasomotor changes:

- Intermittent flushing
- Hypotension
- Wheezing (due to bronchospasm)
- Diarrhea

Approximately two-thirds of patients with carcinoid syndrome develop carcinoid heart disease and up to 20% of patients with metastatic carcinoid tumors first present with carcinoid heart disease.

Carcinoid Heart Disease

Carcinoid heart disease is poorly understood, but it is believed to be due to the release of vasoactive substances from hepatic metastases into the systemic circulation.

Plasma serotonin and urine (5-hydroxyindoleacetic acid) (5-HIAA) levels are higher in patients with carcinoid syndrome with carcinoid heart disease.

Receptors for 5-HT play a pivotal role in the pathogenesis of carcinoid heart disease. These receptors are well represented in the heart, with the 5-HT2B receptor subtype being the most prevalent on cardiac valves. Mitogenic effects on fibroblasts and smooth muscle cells, triggering of inflammatory cytokines, and up-regulation of transforming growth factor-b1 are induced by 5-HT through activation of 5-HT receptors, especially subtype 2B.

The result is the deposition of plaque-like material on the endocardial surfaces of valve leaflets, subvalvular apparatus (chordae and papillary muscles), and cardiac chambers, and occasionally within the intima of the pulmonary arteries and aorta, as well as the venae cava.

Typical cardiac lesions are described as fibrous, plaque-like areas of endocardial thickening that lead to retraction of the valve leaflets, which causes a combination of stenosis and regurgitation (Table 9.1).

The Tricuspid Valve is the most commonly affected valve, followed by the pulmonic valve.

Table 9.1 Relative proportions of valvular pathologies in carcinoid heart disease

Heart valve	Most common	Less common
Tricuspid valve	Isolated regurgitation	Mixed stenosis and regurgitation
Pulmonary valve	Mixed regurgitation and stenosis	Isolated regurgitation or isolated stenosis
Left-sided valve	Isolated regurgitation	

The left side of the heart is affected less commonly and usually in the setting of:

- Right-to-left Shunts
- Large tumor burden
- Primary Bronchial Carcinoid Tumors (isolated left heart)

Because cardiac symptoms and signs are often subtle or absent early in the disease course, the diagnosis of carcinoid heart disease may be delayed if echocardiographic screening is not performed early in patients with carcinoid syndrome.

The imaging modality of choice for the diagnosis of carcinoid heart disease is transthoracic echocardiography (TTE) interpreted by a physician who is familiar with typical carcinoid heart disease valvular morphology.

Cardiac computed tomography (CT) and cardiac magnetic resonance (CMR) scanning may also be valuable adjuncts in the investigation of patients with the disease.

TTE remains the gold standard for the diagnosis and follow-up of carcinoid heart disease. It should be performed in all patients with carcinoid syndrome and high suspicion of carcinoid heart disease, such as those with clinical features or increased NT-pro BNP and/or 5-HIAA levels.

Pulmonary valve involvement is often underappreciated at the time of initial echocardiographic assessment. Special attention to the 2D/3D, color flow, and spectral Doppler features of the pulmonary valve is needed to provide a comprehensive assessment (Evidence Level 2, Grade B).

Advanced techniques, such as 3D TTE or 3D transesophageal echocardiogram, may be helpful in identifying and assessing valve pathology, as well as assessing right ventricular size and function (Evidence Level 2, Grade B).

- Thickened, Retracted and Malcoapted TV With Shortening Or Fusion Of The Chorda Resulted in Free Regurgitation and To Lesser Extent, Stenosis.
- The Leaflets May Be Affected Symmetric Or Asymmetric.
- Right, Atrial, And Ventricular Enlargement.
- A "Dagger-wave Form" With Early Peak Pressure & Rapid Decline In Doppler Study.
- Prolonged Pressure Half-time Consistent With TS (Figs. 9.1 and 9.2).

The involvement of the pulmonic valve is characterized by diffuse thickening of the arterial aspect of the valve leaflets, which results in reduced leaflet excursion and pulmonic stenosis, although pulmonic regurgitation (Fig. 9.3).

For established carcinoid heart disease, echocardiography should be performed if dictated by a change in clinical status; otherwise, it should be performed every 3–6 months, depending on the severity of established carcinoid heart disease and clinical status (Evidence Level 2, Grade B).

CMR imaging can be used to evaluate the pulmonary valve, identify cardiac metastases, and assess right ventricular size and function (Evidence Level 2, Grade B).

Cardiac CT imaging has a role for assessment of valvular pathology, especially of the pulmonary valve, right ventricular size, and function, and the pre-operative

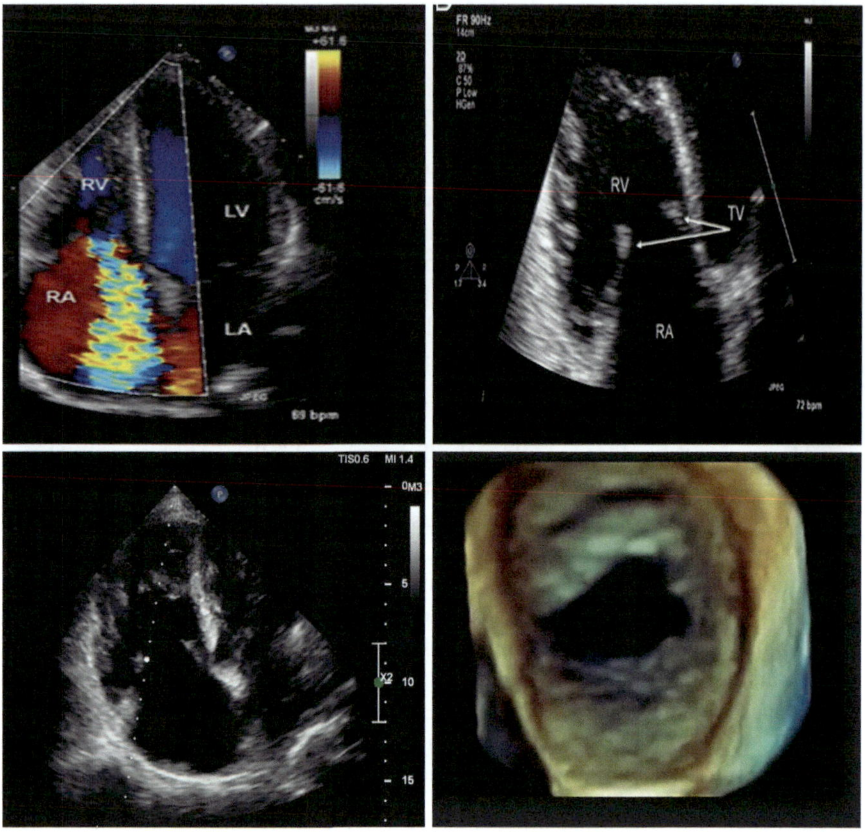

Fig. 9.1 Fibrotic and retracted tricuspid valve in 2D apical four-chamber view and also in 3D view, severe tricuspid regurgitation

assessment of coronary arteries, as well as relations of coronary arteries and cardiac metastasis (Evidence Level 3, Grade B).

Carcinoid heart disease is a marker for increased mortality in patients with carcinoid tumors who have a median survival of 14 months.

Treatment

The management of patients with carcinoid heart disease is complex because both systemic malignant disease and cardiac involvement have to be addressed at the same time. A multidisciplinary approach at an experienced center is recommended.

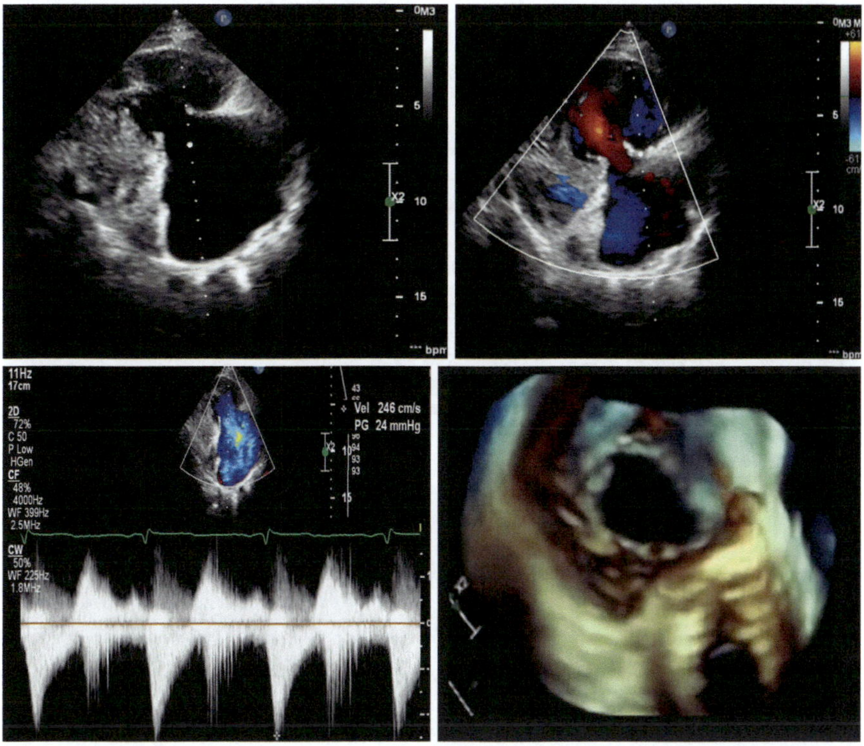

Fig. 9.2 Fibrotic and retracted tricuspid valve in 2D RV inflow view and also in 3D view, severe free tricuspid regurgitation

Therapeutic options include pharmacotherapy for heart failure, aggressive lowering of 5-HIAA levels (<300 mmol/24 h), and, in selected individuals, cardiac valve replacement.

Without treatment, the prognosis of carcinoid heart disease is poor, However, the prognosis of patients has improved over the past few decades, which may be due to advancements in cardiac imaging technologies, antitumor therapies, perioperative management, and cardiac surgery.

Symptomatic Tricuspid Regurgitation and Moderate To Severe RV Dilation & Failure associated with worse outcomes and are currently indications for TVR.

Recent data suggest that survival has improved over the past decades for patients with carcinoid heart disease who undergo earlier replacement surgery.

Generally, patients with carcinoid heart disease are referred for valve surgery when they develop symptoms or ventricular dysfunction and rarely in anticipation of hepatic surgery. By consensus, patients referred for cardiac surgery should have evidence of right heart failure, with at least 12 months of anticipated post-operative survival from their NET disease.

The choice of valve prosthesis is still a matter of debate. The decision on the type of prosthesis should be individualized.

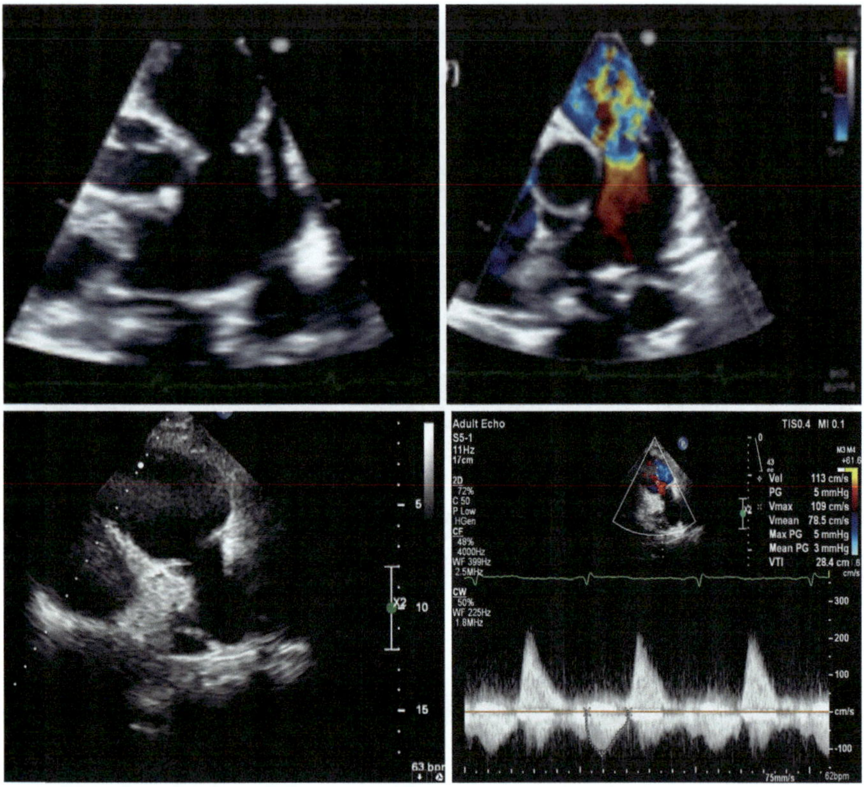

Fig. 9.3 Fibrotic and retracted pulmonary valve; severe free pulmonary regurgitation

Bioprosthetic valves are usually preferred (due to the inherently increased risk of bleeding in patients with advanced high-volume liver disease and hepatic dysfunction from carcinoid disease, the increased likelihood of invasive procedures requiring temporary discontinuation of anticoagulant agents, and to a lesser extent—the risk of right-sided mechanical valve thrombosis. Newer generation bioprosthetic valves may also be more durable.

The optimization of treatment of carcinoid syndrome after cardiac surgery may protect bioprosthetic valves from the adverse effects of vasoactive peptides by decreasing carcinoid activity, and patients with a biological prosthesis should receive anticoagulation therapy with warfarin for 3–6 months.

Also, balloon valvuloplasty for PS may be an option for patients with symptoms of pulmonic stenosis and elevated right-sided heart pressures to palliate symptoms and decrease the severity of tricuspid regurgitation [1–8].

References

1. Jensen RT, Norton JA, Oberg K. Neuroendocrine tumors. In: Feldman M, Friedman LS, Brandt LJ, editors. Sleisenger and Fordtran's gastrointestinal and liver diseases. 10th ed. Philadelphia: Elsevier Saunders; 2016. p. 501–41.
2. Kulke MH. Advances in the management of patients with carcinoid syndrome. Clin Adv Hematol Oncol. 2017;15:257–9.
3. Mansencal N, Mitry E, Bachet JB, Rougier P, Dubourg O. Echocardiographic follow-up of treated patients with carcinoid syndrome. Am J Cardiol. 2010;105:1588–91. https://doi.org/10.1016/j.amjcard.2010.01.017.
4. Robiolio PA, Rigolin VH, Wilson JS, Harrison JK, Sanders LL, Bashore TM, Feldman JM. Carcinoid heart disease: correlation of high serotonin levels with valvular abnormalities detected by cardiac catheterization and echocardiography. Circulation. 1995;92:790–5.
5. Lee KJ, Connolly HM, Pellikka PA. Carcinoid pulmonary valvulopathy evaluated by real-time 3-dimensional transthoracic echocardiography. J Am Soc Echocardiogr. 2008;21(4):407.e1–2.
6. Battacharyya S, Toumpanakis C, Burke M, Taylor AM, Caplin ME, Davar J. Features of carcinoid heart disease identified by 2- and 3-dimensional echocardiography and cardiac MRI. Circ Cardiovasc Imaging. 2010;3:103–11. https://doi.org/10.1161/CIRCIMAGING.109.886846.
7. Franzen D, Boldt A, Raute-Kreinsen U, et al. Magnetic resonance imaging of carcinoid heart disease. Clin Cardiol. 2009;32(6):E92–3. https://doi.org/10.1002/clc.20260.
8. Strosberg JR, Halfdanarson TR, Bellizzi AM, et al. The North American Neuroendocrine Tumor Society Consensus Guidelines for surveillance and medical management of midgut neuroendocrine tumors. Pancreas. 2017;46:707–14. Recent consensus paper from NANETs on management of midgut carcinoids.

Chapter 10
Aortic Coarctation and Complicated Infective Endocarditis

Azin Alizadehasl

Abstract Aortic coarctation is an example of congenital disorders with a high risk of development of endocarditis and endarteritis. In the presurgical era, infective endarteritis constituted a frequent complication of aortic coarctation and was responsible for 20% of death of these patients. Here in, we describe a case of coarctation endarteritis with pseudoaneurysm formation in an adult and review the echocardiographic findings of this condition.

Adult coarctation endarteritis is a rare entity but sometimes represents the initial presentation of coarctation. Diagnosis is critically important given the risk of rupture. Transesophageal echocardiography can be helpful in diagnosis and management.

Keywords Aortic coarctation · Infective endarteritis · Transesophageal echocardiography · Pseudoaneurysm · Aortic valve replacement

Case Presentation and Discussion

26-year-old young man with dyspnea and palpitation (FC II-III), Low aptitude, low-grade fever, and weight loss, Soft S1, SM II/VI in LSB, DM III/VI in LSB and specially in RUSB & low-Pitched apical diastolic murmur. Three sets of blood cultures grew viridans group streptococci. Here is the TTE and TEE findings (Figs. 10.1, 10.2, 10.3, 10.4, 10.5, 10.6, 10.7, 10.8, 10.9, 10.10, 10.11 and 10.12):

He underwent two-staged surgeries (at first repair for coarctation and then excision the pseudoaneurysm) and Aortic valve replacement 8 days later.

Macroscopic examination of the operative piece revealed a false aneurysm corresponding to the post stenotic dilatation communicating with the aortic lumen by a small hole.

A. Alizadehasl (✉)
Rajaie Cardiovascular Medical and Research Center, Cardio-Oncology Department and Research Center, Iran University of Medical Science, Tehran, Iran

M. Maleki, A. Alizadehasl (eds.), *Case-Based Clinical Cardiology*,
https://doi.org/10.1007/978-1-4471-7496-7_10

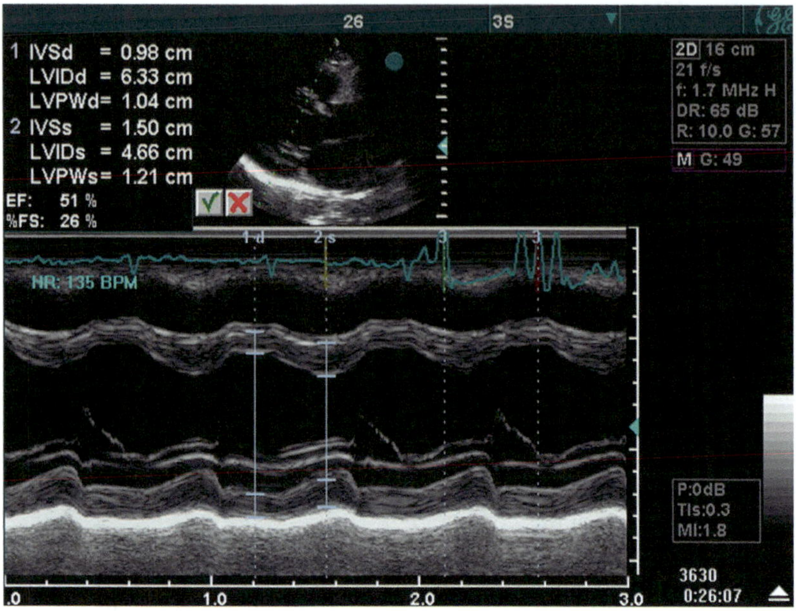

Fig. 10.1 M-mode tracing of LV, significant LV enlargement with LVEF = 50%

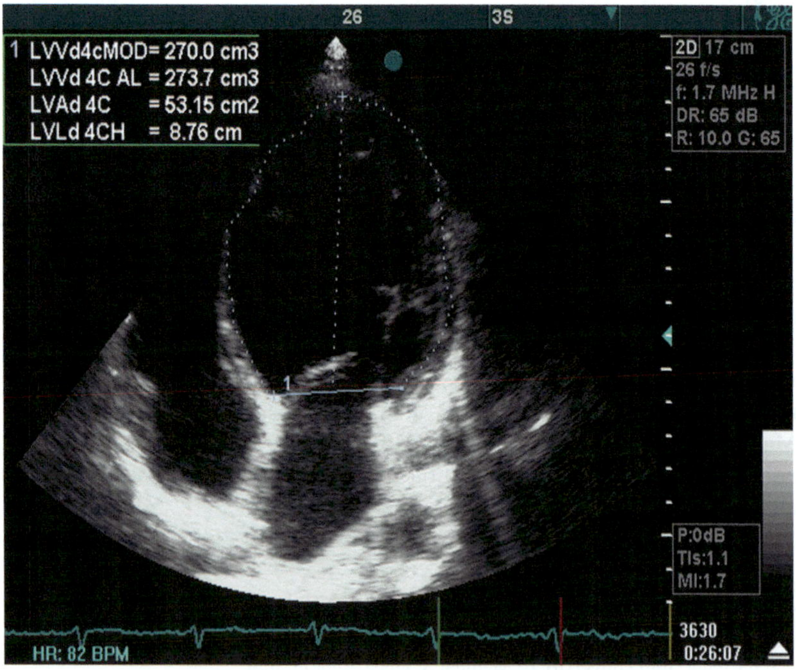

Fig. 10.2 Apical four-chamber view, severe LV enlargement with LVEF = 50%

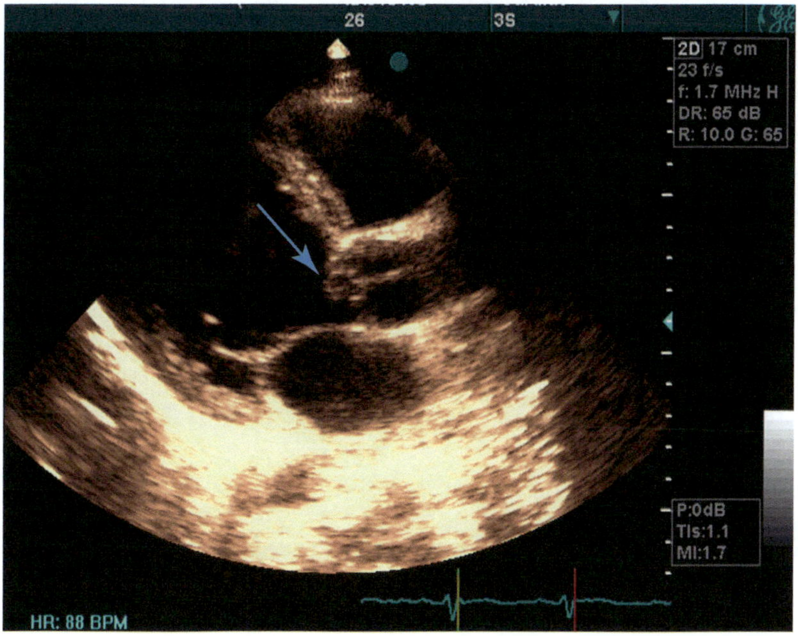

Fig. 10.3 Parasternal long-axis view, severe LV enlargement, bicuspid AV, vegetation on AV (arrow)

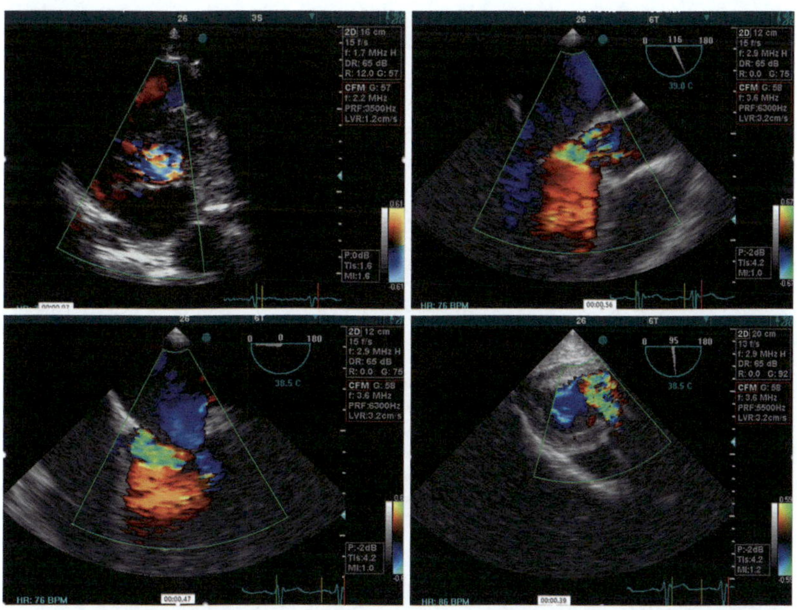

Fig. 10.4 Severe multi-jet AI due to destructed and perforated bicuspid aortic valve because of IE. Upper left: Parasternal short-axis view; Upper right: TEE, ME, 120′ view; Lower left: TEE, ME, 0′ view; Lower right: TEE, Trans-gastric, 90′ view

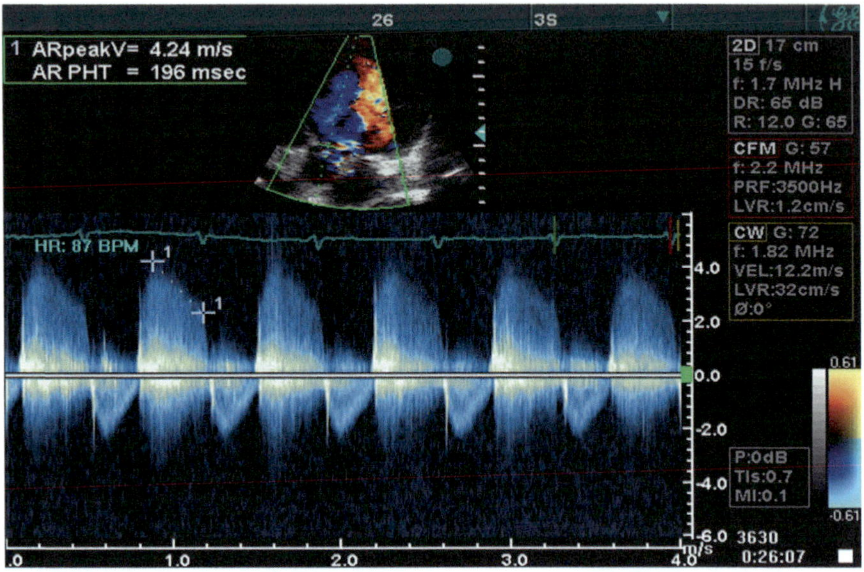

Fig. 10.5 Color-Doppler flow of Severe AI, AI flow PHT = 196 ms

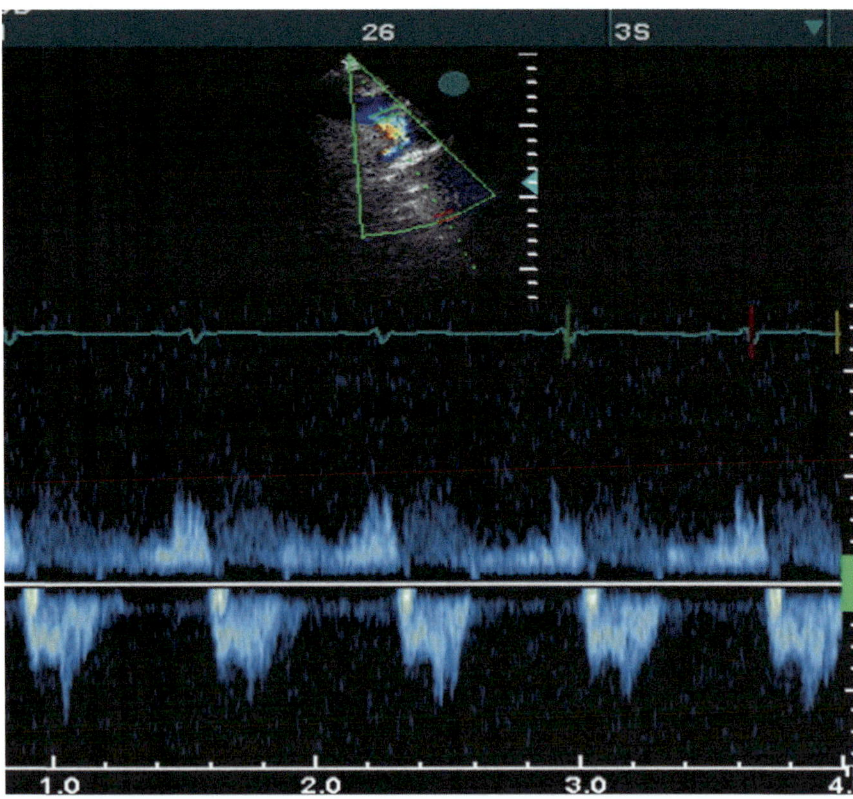

Fig. 10.6 Holo-diastolic flow reversal in the proximal part of descending aorta due to severe AI

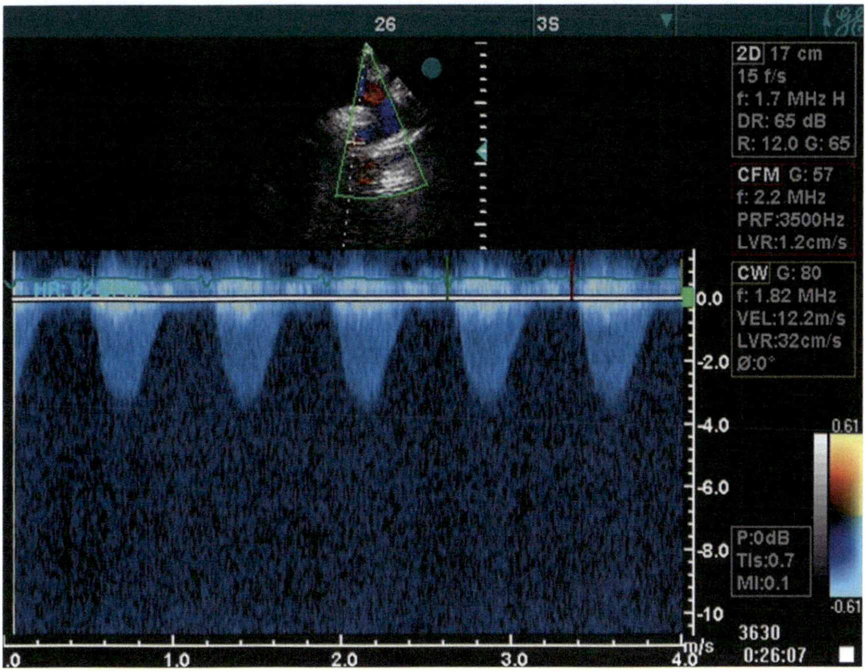

Fig. 10.7 Coarctation of aorta; flow velocity = 3.7 m/s

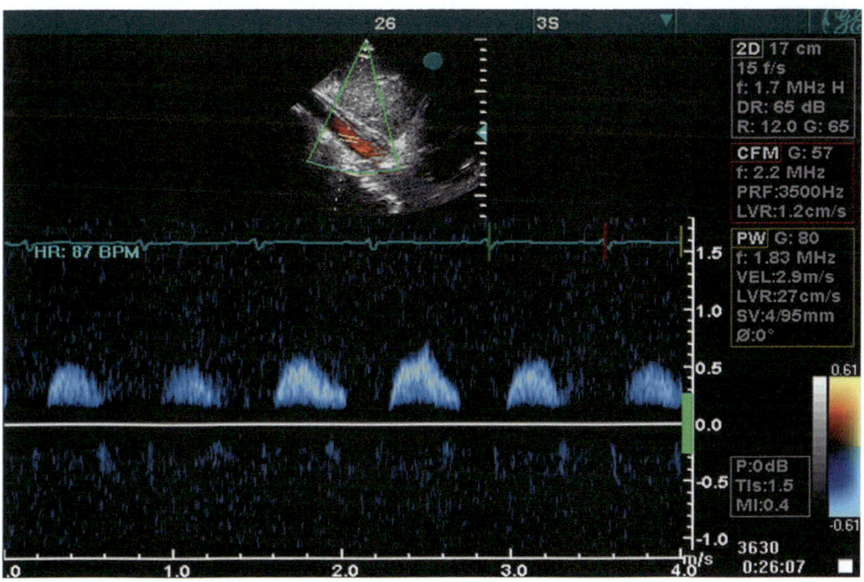

Fig. 10.8 Typical Doppler flow for aortic coarctation of abdominal aorta

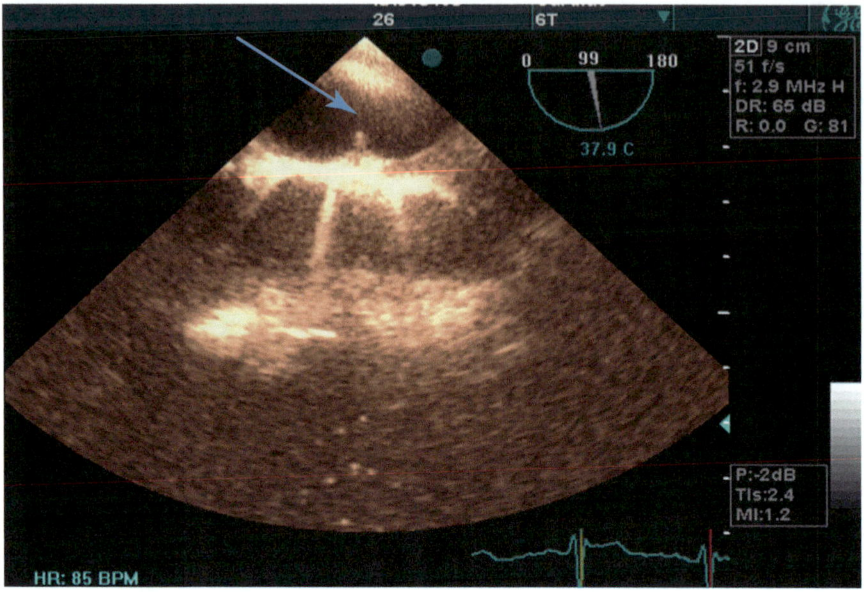

Fig. 10.9 TEE view. UE. 90′. Coarctation of aorta (arrow)

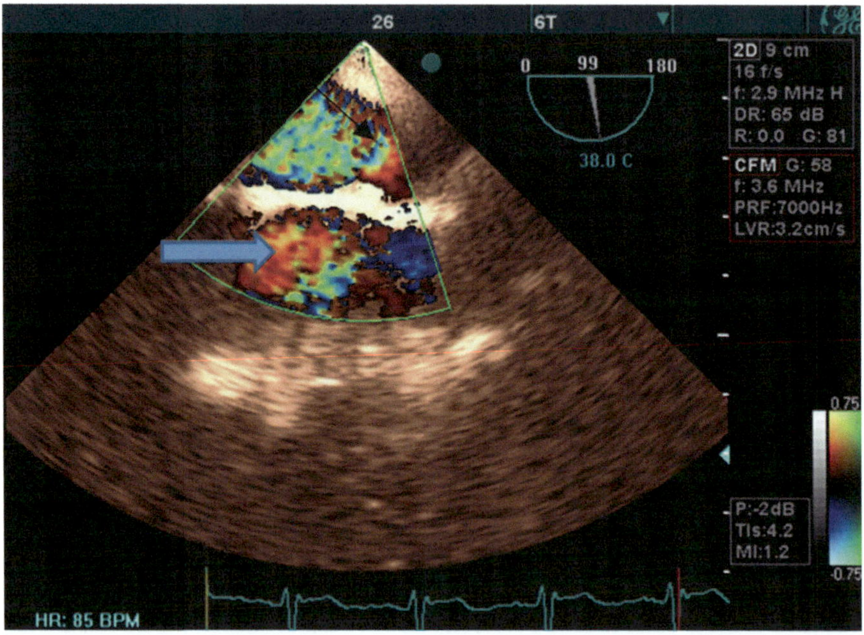

Fig. 10.10 Color flow of coarctation site (black arrow); Mirror artifact (wide arrow)

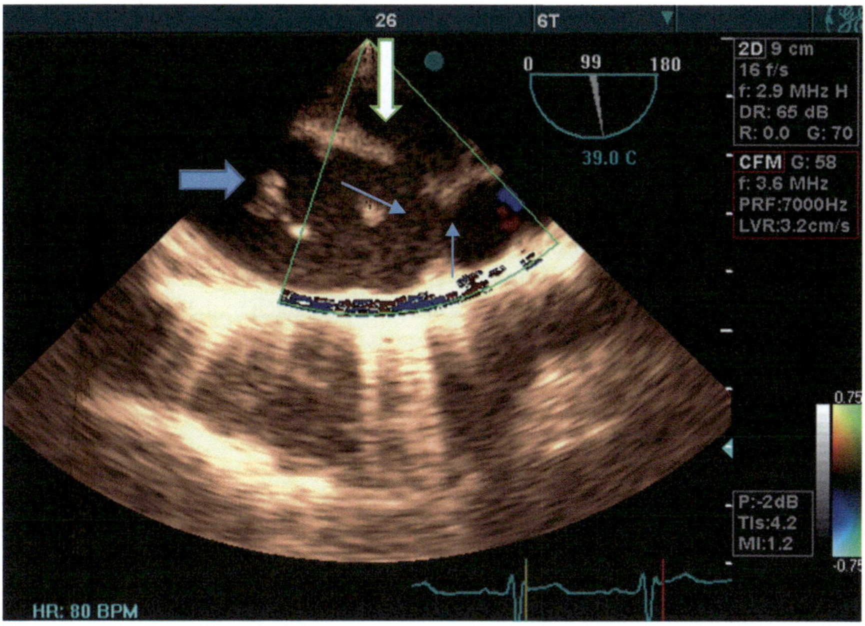

Fig. 10.11 Transesophageal echocardiography; descending aorta, Coarctation site (blue arrow); intraluminal vegetations (wide blue arrow); associated with a complex pseudoaneurysm (wide white arrow)

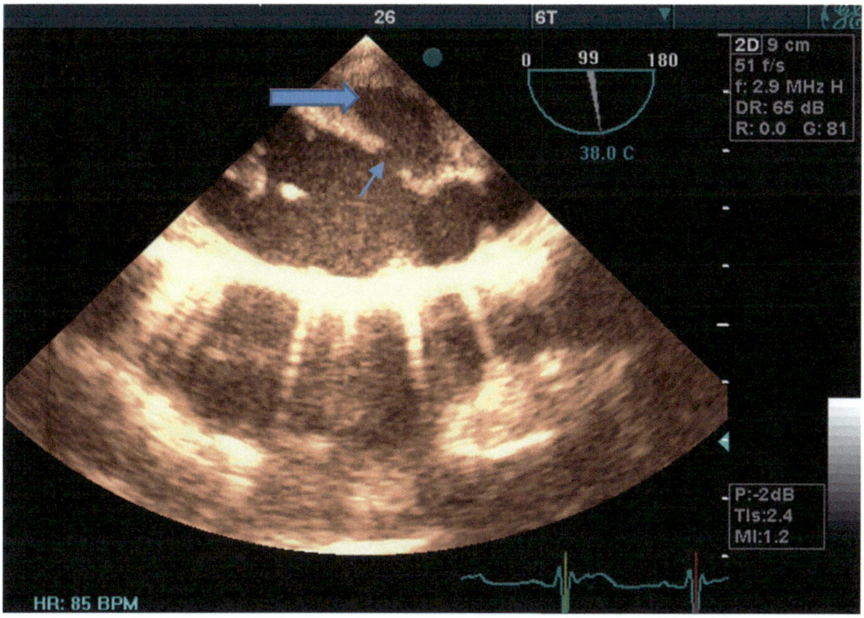

Fig. 10.12 Coarctation and vegetations and Pseudoaneurysm (wide blue arrow); also the neck of pseudoaneurysm is seen clearly (narrow arrow)

Postoperatively, the patient felt well with no complications. TEE study did not show any abnormality at the level of the dacron tube.

The last TTE before discharge includes: Severe LV enlargement and dysfunction (LVEF = 20–25%). Mild RV enlargement with moderate dysfunction. Acceptable AV prosthesis hemodynamic study with normal range of motion, no vegetation. Normal flow in Gore-tex and No PE.

So, aortic coarctation is an example of congenital malformation with a high risk of development of endocarditis-endarteritis. In aortic coarctation, blood flows through a narrowing in the aorta at high velocity, resulting in a lower-pressure "sink" in the area distal to the stenosis. Bacteria may attach to the aortic wall in this low-pressure region, especially when there is concurrent endothelial injury. In coarctation, endothelial injury is likely precipitated by shear stress forces [1–5].

References

1. Franco-Paredes C, Workowski K, Harris M. Infective endocarditis-endarteritis complicating coarctation of the aorta. Am J Med. 2002;112:590–2.
2. Jenkins NP, Ward C. Coarctation of the aorta: natural history and outcome after surgical treatment. QJM. 1999;92:365–71.
3. Anderson AM, Cabell CH, Sexton DJ. Aortic coarctation endarteritis in an adult: case report with cardiovascular magnetic resonance imaging findings and review of the literature. Clin Infect Dis. 2005;40:e28–31.
4. Ozkutlu S, Ozbarlas N, Bilgic A, Pasaoglu I. Mycotic aneurysm of the descending aorta diagnosed by echocardiography. Int J Cardiol. 1992;37:112–4.
5. Perez Day CM, Angela MP, Mangione SA, Furque JC. Coarctation of the aorta complicated by infectious endarteritis, mycotic aneurysm and rupture of the spleen. Rev Esp Cardiol. 1986;39:68–71.

Chapter 11
Symptomatic Mitral Prosthesis Paravalvular Leakage

Azin Alizadehasl

Abstract Prosthetic paravalvular leak is an uncommon but potentially serious complication following valve replacement surgery.

A 43-year-old man with history of prosthetic mitral valve replacement 8 years ago due to rheumatic valve disease. He presented with red urine and shortness of breath. A transoesophageal echocardiogram revealed a paravalvular leak at the prosthetic mitral valve, he underwent a repeat mitral valve replacement.

Keywords Prosthetic mitral valve · Paravalvular leakage · Rheumatic valve disease · Infective endocarditis · Mechanical hemolysis

Case Presentation and Discussion

A 43-year-old man with a history of prosthetic mitral valve replacement 8 years ago due to rheumatic heart disease. He presented with red urine and shortness of breath and sweating, he took warfarin as his only medication. He had a soft pansystolic murmur and an ejection systolic murmur. His chest was clear and also his abdomen was soft. A 12-lead ECG showed a sinus rhythm with no specific abnormalities. His echocardiographic findings are as follow (Figs. 11.1 and 11.2):

So, transesophageal echocardiography revealed an anterolateral mitral paravalvular leak (Figs. 11.3, 11.4 and 11.5). Left ventricular systolic function was near normal. As part of the standard pre-operative evaluation, the patient had an angiogram, which showed normal coronary arteries.

Active Infective endocarditis was ruled out. The patient should be screened for mechanical hemolysis because the paravalvular leak is a suspected cause of anemia and red urine. Normocytic anemia with raised lactate dehydrogenase, bilirubinaemia (with a raised unconjugated count) and reticulocyte count >2% can identified hemolysis.

A. Alizadehasl (✉)
Rajaie Cardiovascular Medical and Research Center, Cardio-Oncology Department and Research Center, Iran University of Medical Science, Tehran, Iran

M. Maleki, A. Alizadehasl (eds.), *Case-Based Clinical Cardiology*,
https://doi.org/10.1007/978-1-4471-7496-7_11

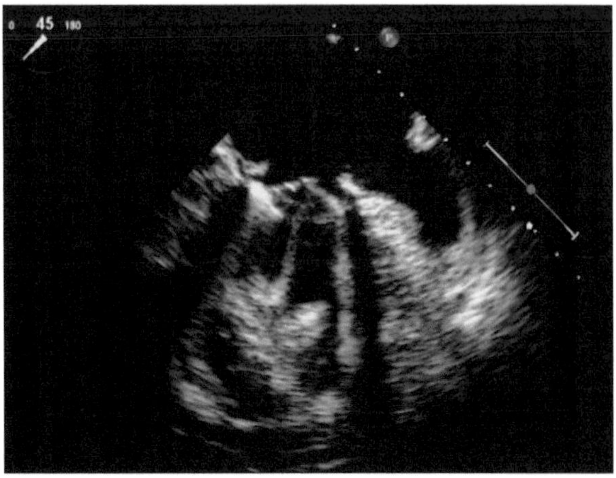

Fig. 11.1 TEE, Prosthetic MV

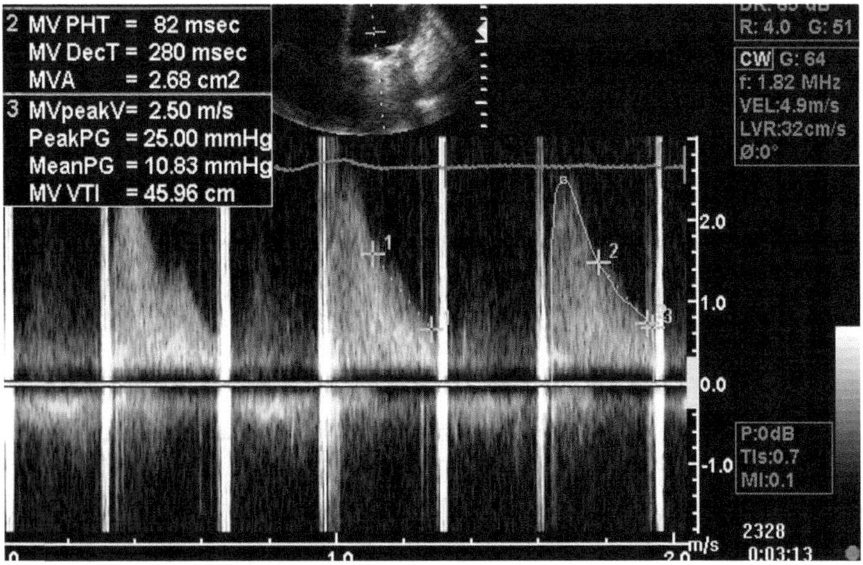

Fig. 11.2 Doppler flow showed high MV flow peak velocity and mean gradient and low-pressure half-time due to significant paravalvular leak

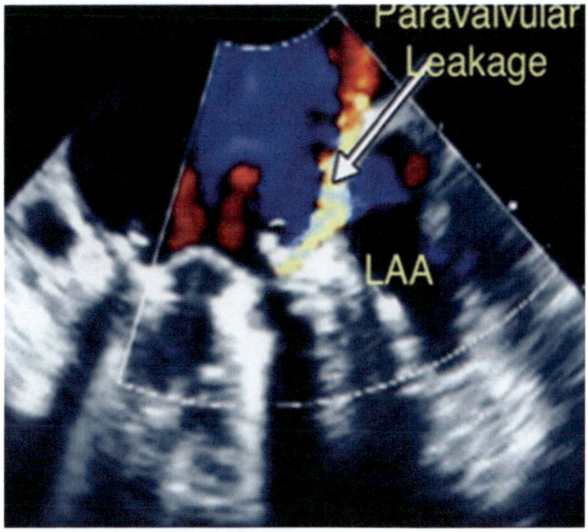

Fig. 11.3 TEE, 0′ view; Paravalvular leakage from the anterolateral side of prosthetic MV

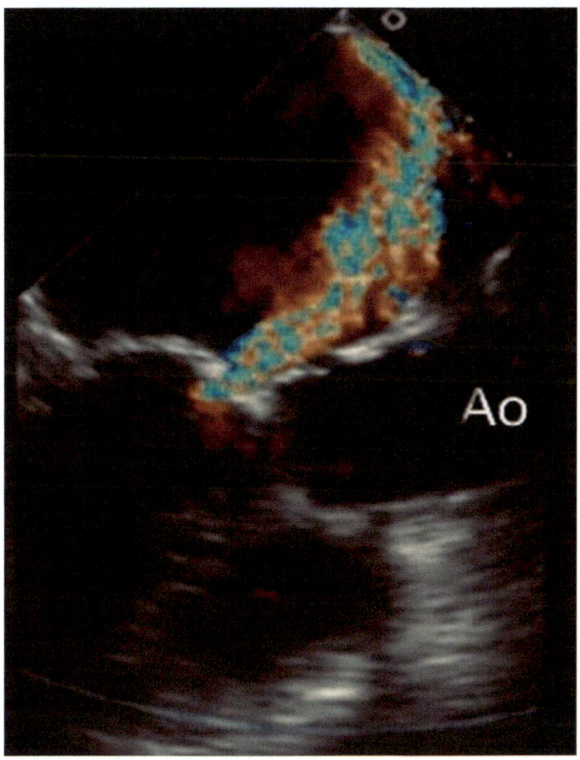

Fig. 11.4 TEE, 120′; significant paravalvular leakage more prominent at anterior side

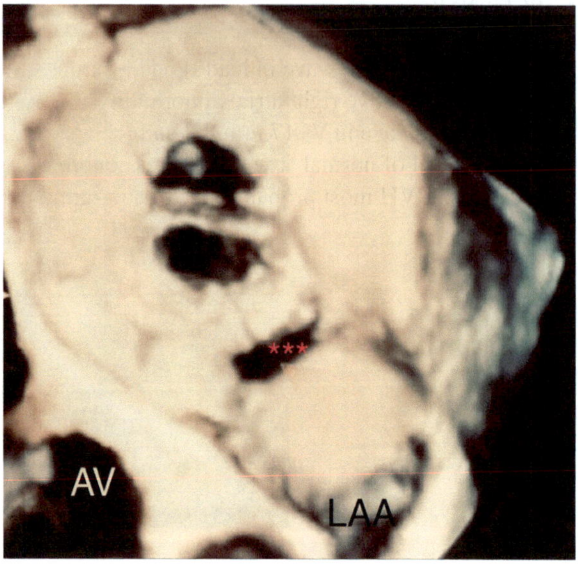

Fig. 11.5 3D TEE view with a paravalvular defect at the anterolateral side of the sewing ring (red stars). *LAA* left atrial auricule, *AV* aortic valve

Due to active hemolysis, the patient required blood transfusions. His warfarin was stopped and he was placed on an unfractionated heparin infusion awaiting surgery. With the possibility of percutaneous closure of the mitral paravalvular leak being negated because of his low risk for surgery and our case undergone surgical replacement of the mitral valve [1–5].

References

1. Kliger C, Eiros R, Isasti G, et al. Review of surgical prosthetic paravalvular leaks: diagnosis and catheter-based closure. Eur Heart J. 2013;34:638–49. https://doi.org/10.1093/eurheartj/ehs347.
2. Sorajja P, Cabalka AK, Hagler DJ, et al. Percutaneous repair of paravalvular prosthetic regurgitation: acute and 30-day outcomes in 115 patients. Circ Cardiovasc Interv. 2011;4:314–21.
3. Genoni M, Franzen D, Tavakoli R, et al. Does the morphology of mitral paravalvular leaks influence symptoms and hemolysis? J Heart Valve Dis. 2001;10:426–30.
4. Davila-Roman VG, Waggoner AD, Kennard ED, et al. Prevalence and severity of paravalvular regurgitation in the Artificial Valve Endocarditis Reduction Trial (AVERT) echocardiography study. J Am Coll Cardiol. 2004;44:1467–72. https://doi.org/10.1016/j.jacc.2003.12.060.
5. Maleki M, Alizadehasl A, Haghjoo M. Practical cardiology. Valvular Chapter.

Chapter 12
A 37-Year-Old Lady, Post-MVR, -AVR, -TVR and -AVNRT

Shabnam Madadi

Abstract In this chapter, some challenging and interesting Electrophysiology cases done in Rajaie Cardiovascular, Medical and Research Center were discussed. These cases include some interesting SVT and AFL, AF, PVC and accessory pathway cases. In each case, differentiating maneuvers were discussed. Some of them are simple arrhythmia cases but there was a challenge in ablation due to anatomical causes. The first case was a patient with prosthetic valves with SVT. The patient was a case of severe MS, severe AS, AI, and severe TR for whom AVR and MVR and TVR was done; 1 day after the operation she had revealed a regular narrow QRS tachycardia that was degenerated to AF; Amiodarone was administrated for her; about 3 h later, she had demonstrated torsade de point and with D/C shock had been converted to NSR and had revealed that QT was prolonged (about 500 ms) so sulfate magnesium was administrated and an epicardial pacemaker was programed in 70 VVI 85 bpm; then she had demonstrated three more episodes of narrow QRS tachycardia, mostly compatible with AVNRT (Fig. 12.1).

The patient was a case of rheumatic heart disease with severe MS, severe AS, AI, and severe TR for whom AVR and MVR and TVR was done; 1 day after the operation she had revealed a regular narrow QRS tachycardia degenerated to AF; Amiodarone was administrated for her; about 3 h later, she had demonstrated torsade de point and with D/C shock was converted to NSR and then revealed that QT was prolonged (about 500 ms) so sulfate magnesium was administrated and an epicardial pacemaker was programed in 70 VVI 85 bpm; then she had demonstrated three more episodes of narrow QRS tachycardia, mostly compatible with AVNRT (Fig. 12.1).

So we decided to ablate the arrhythmia, because we could not administer Beta-blocker or other antiarrhythmic drugs, due to long QT. EPS was done; we only used

S. Madadi (✉)
Rajaie Cardiovascular Medical and Research Center, Iran University of Medical Sciences, Tehran, Iran
e-mail: madadi@rhc.ac.ir

M. Maleki, A. Alizadehasl (eds.), *Case-Based Clinical Cardiology*,
https://doi.org/10.1007/978-1-4471-7496-7_12

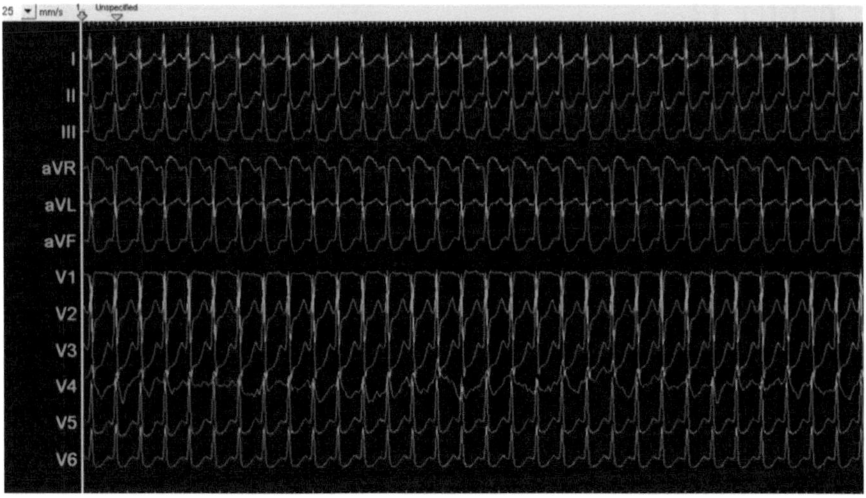

Fig. 12.1 Typical AVRT with pseudo S in inferior leads

a decapolar catheter in CS, epicardial temporary pacemaker was programmed to VVI 60 bpm. With CS pacing a narrow QRS tachycardia infavor of AVNRT was induced and RFA in the posterosetpal area, between CS ostium and prosthetic tricuspid valve resulted in junctional rhythm and RFA continued for 1 min. Then Isuprel was administrated and arrhythmia was not inducible after ablation (Fig. 12.2a, b).

Discussion

AVNRT is the most common type of supraventricular arrhythmia and usually presents with no visible P wave in narrow QRS tachycardia [1–3].

In typical AVNRT there is a long AH interval (>180 ms) during tachycardia, and the earliest retrograde atrial activity is at the fast (Beta) pathway; at the superior part of Koch's triangle, posterior to the Todaro tendon (Fig. 12.3) [4].

In most of the AVNRT patients, CS ostium is greater than normal subjects, and it may be a case of difference between slow and fast pathway conduction velocity and refractory periods and that could participate in the occurrence of AVNRT [5].

With HRA pacing prolongation of AH interval to more than 180 ms, is indicative of slow pathway conduction.

Some features of dual AV nodal physiology are as:

1. More than 50 ms increase in AH interval with 10 ms decrease in A1–A2 interval with atrial extrastimulation (Fig. 12.4).

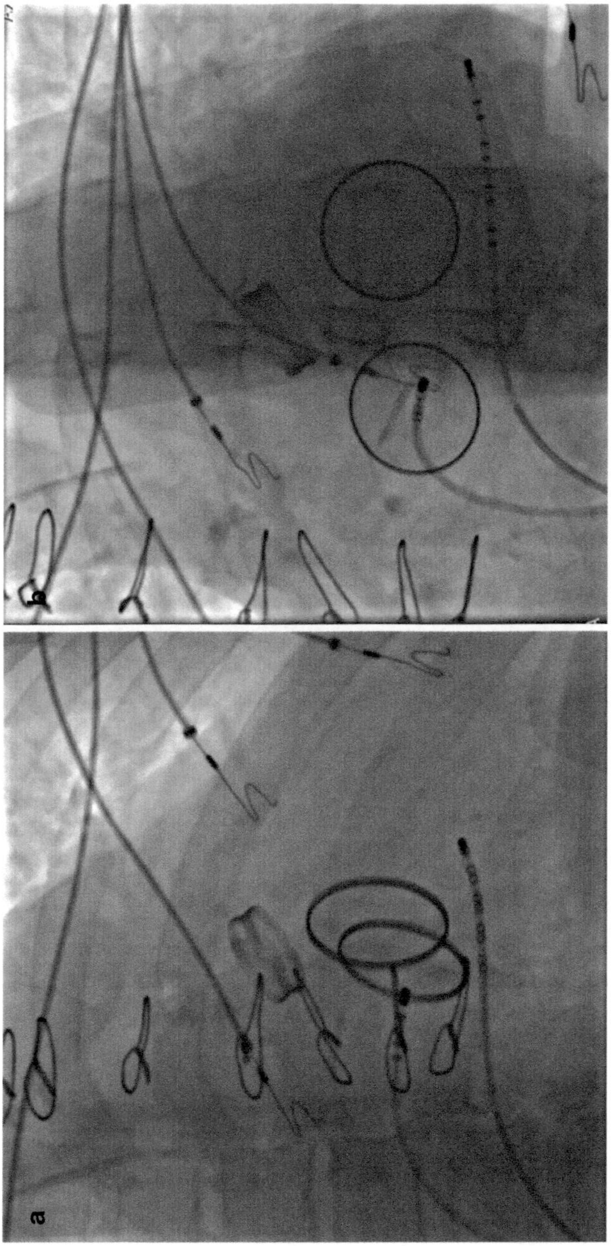

Fig. 12.2 (**a**, **b**) AP and LAO views of the position of ablation catheter in patient with prosthetic MV, AV, and TV valves

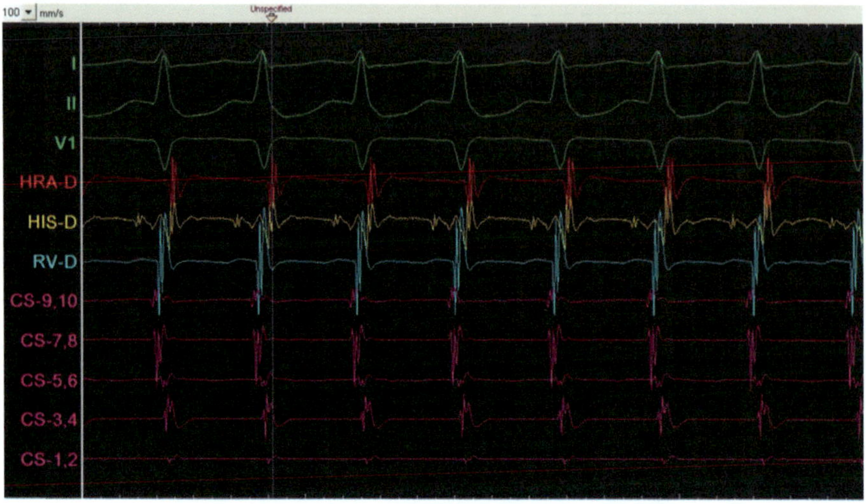

Fig. 12.3 Typical AVNRT, earliest site of retrograde atrial activation in His

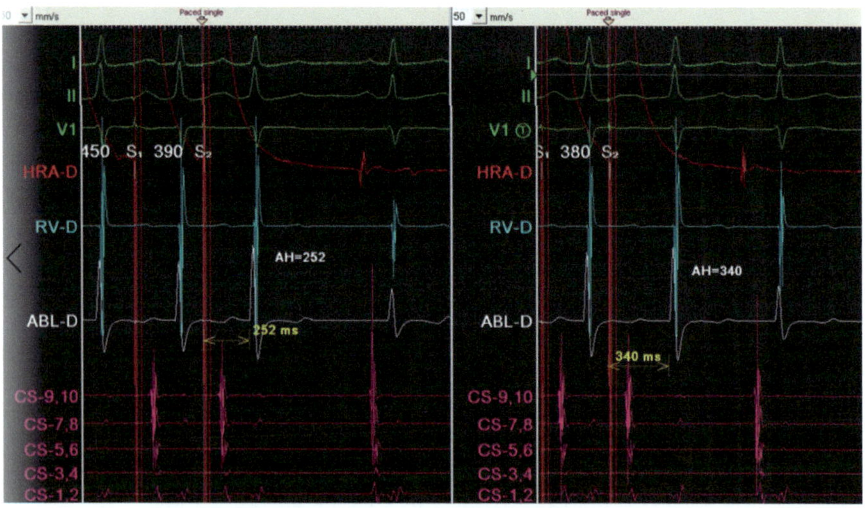

Fig. 12.4 AH jump, with 10 ms decrease in atrial extrastimulation, there is >50 ms in AH interval

In addition to the more common type of the AVNRT (slow–fast) type, there are two another less common types as: slow–slow and fast–slow types, which include about 3% and 2% of all AVNRT cases respectively [6–8].

2. Left-sided variant occur about 1.5% of all AVNRT cases who underwent ablation, and usually needs ablation from the left atrium (mostly via coronary sinuse). A short VA interval (<15 ms) and double response to atrial pacing are most frequent in this variant. The differential diagnosis of typical AVNRT is AT and

orthodromic AVRT via the anteroseptal accessory pathway. There are frequent maneuvers for differentiation of them, such as Morady maneuver (ventricular entrainment and VAV response with PPI–TCL (Post-pacing interval—Tachycardia cycle length) difference more than 110 ms and SA-VA difference more than 85 ms (Fig. 12.5) [9, 10].

Atrial pacing at TCL and AH interval difference between atrial pacing and during tachycardia more than 40 ms is infavor of AVNRT; between 20 and 40 ms is infavor of AVRT and less than 20 ms suggests AT.

At the beginning of all maneuvers, His pacing for evaluation about the nodal or extranodal response is more effective; and is sinus rhythm, para-Hision pacing could be done by low and higher amplitude for myocardial capture and his capture; if VA interval was the same during myocardial capture and His capture; there is evidence of extranodal response and in nodal conduction VA during His capture should be shorter than during myocardial capture (Fig. 12.6) [10].

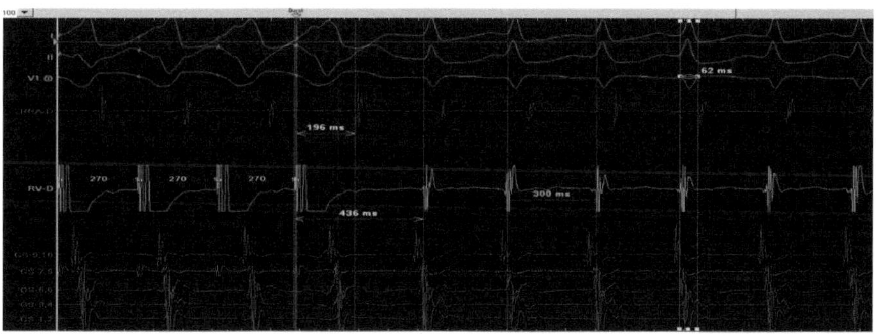

Fig. 12.5 Ventricular entrainment in AVNRT shows prolonged PPI–TCL difference

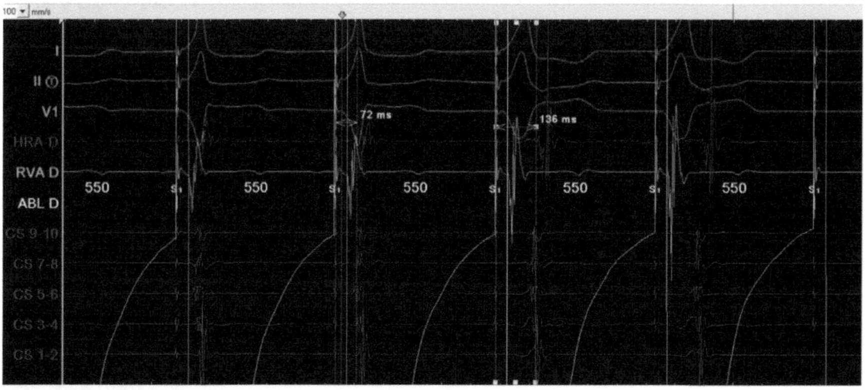

Fig. 12.6 His pasing shows nodal response in AVNRT

Junctional tachycardia (JT) is another arrhythmia that mostly occurs after ablation and should be differentiated from AVNRT for decision making about the termination of ablation. JT could be discriminated from AVNRT with early PAC that administered before His activation, and terminates the AVNRT, but could induce the JT [10].

Ablation of typical AVNRT is done by ablation of the slow pathway in CS ostium between CS and TV ring.

In this patient, we were very careful about prosthetic mechanical TV.

The atrial EGM in the ablation site should have multiple components and AV ratio should be about 1:3–1:10.

Ablation in the higher position and CS roof could result in AV block. The recommended power for initiation of ablation is 20–30 W with nonirrigated catheters, after 15 s the power could be gradually increased to 60 W with target temperature of 60 °C.

Junctional rhythm during ablation is a sensitive marker of success.

Cyoablation could be done with a lower risk of AV block but a higher rate of recurrence. No junctional rhythm is elucidated during cryoablation and it should be done during atrial pacing to demonstrate slow pathway conduction, and if eliminated, ablation should be continued 4 min at 60 °C.

It is recommended to give Isoproterenol after the ablation for all patients with AVNRT, regardless of the initial induction (with or without Isuprel).

References

1. Gonzalez M, Quiroga C, Fernandez P, Garro H, Chiale P. Different atrioventricular conduction times and cycle length alternans phenomenon of a typical AV nodal reentrant tachycardia. Arch Cardiol Mex. 2015;85:87–90.
2. Morady F. Catheter ablation of supraventricular arrhythmias: state of the art. Pacing Clin Electrophysiol. 2004;27:125–42.
3. Blomstrom-Lundqvist C, Scheinman MM, Aliot EM, et al. ACC/AHA/ESC guidelines for the management of patients with supraventricular arrhythmias–executive summary. A report of the American college of cardiology/American Heart Association task force on practice guidelines and the European society of cardiology committee for practice guidelines (writing committee to develop guidelines for the management of patients with supraventricular arrhythmias) developed in collaboration with NASPE-Heart Rhythm Society. J Am Coll Cardiol. 2003;42:1493–531.
4. Gonzalez MD, Contreras LJ, Cardona F, et al. Demonstration of a left atrial input to the atrioventricular node in humans. Circulation. 2002;106:2930–4.
5. Kiedrowicz RM, Kazmierczak J, Wielusinski M. The effect of atrial pacing site on electrophysiological properties of the atrioventricular junction and induction of atrioventricular nodal reentry in patients with typical atrioventricular nodal reentrant t achycardia. Kardiol Pol. 2017;75:221–30.
6. Yu WC, Chen SA, Chiang CE, et al. Effects of isoproterenol in facilitating induction of slow-fast atrioventricular nodal reentrant tachycardia. Am J Cardiol. 1996;78:1299–302.

7. Miller JM, Rosenthal ME, Gottlieb CD, Vassallo JA, Josephson ME. Usefulness of the delta HA interval to accurately distinguish atrioventricular nodal reentry from orthodromic septal bypass tract tachycardias. Am J. 1991;68:1037–44.
8. Knight BP, Zivin A, Souza J, et al. A technique for the rapid diagnosis of atrial tachycardia in the electrophysiology laboratory. J Am Coll Cardiol. 1999;33:775–81.
9. Knight BP, Ebinger M, Oral H, et al. Diagnostic value of tachycardia features and pacing maneuvers during paroxysmal supraventricular tachycardia. J Am Coll Cardiol. 2000;36:574–82.
10. Gonzalez-Torrecilla E, Arenal A, Atienza F, et al. First postpacing interval after tachycardia entrainment with correction for atrioventricular node delay: a simple maneuver for differential diagnosis of atrioventricular nodal reentrant tachycardias versus orthodromic reciprocating tachycardias. Rhythm. 2006;3:674–9.

Chapter 13
Slowly Conducting Posteroseptal Accessory Pathway

Shabnam Madadi

Abstract Long RP narrow QRS tachycardia with negative P waves in the inferior leads, in addition to CS ostium AT and atypical AVNRT be aware of PJRT.

PJRT

A 32-year-old lady, with frequent episodes of narrow QRS tachycardia and failed ablation elsewhere, presented to out clinic for more evaluation and redo ablation.

ECG revealed episodes of narrow QRS tachycardia, with rate about 110 bpm and long RP-short PR, negative P wave in the inferior leads. Patient had a history of frequent and long-standing episodes of palpitations. Echocardiography revealed mildly reduced LVEF.

EPS was done, using three quadripolar catheters, for recoding HRA, His and RV potentials, and a decapolar catheter for recording CS potentials. A long steerable sheet (Agillis) was used for the passage of the ablation catheter.

With AES a narrow QRS tachycardia was induced with a rate of about 110 pbm compatible with patient's clinical arrhythmia, with long RP-short RP; and 1:1 AV association. The earliest site of atrial activation was in CS 9–10; but VA signal was not so fused.

His refractory ventricular pacing was done during arrhythmia and resulted in the advancement and resetting of arrhythmia, consistent with the presence of a concealed AP's corporation in the arrhythmia (Fig. 13.1).

Another His refractory PVC resulted in the termination of the arrhythmia (Fig. 13.2).

HV interval was normal during sinus rhythm and with atrial overdrive pacing; suggesting that the accessory pathway had only retrograde conduction.

S. Madadi (✉)
Rajaie Cardiovascular Medical and Research Center, Iran University of Medical Sciences, Tehran, Iran
e-mail: madadi@rhc.ac.ir

M. Maleki, A. Alizadehasl (eds.), *Case-Based Clinical Cardiology*,
https://doi.org/10.1007/978-1-4471-7496-7_13

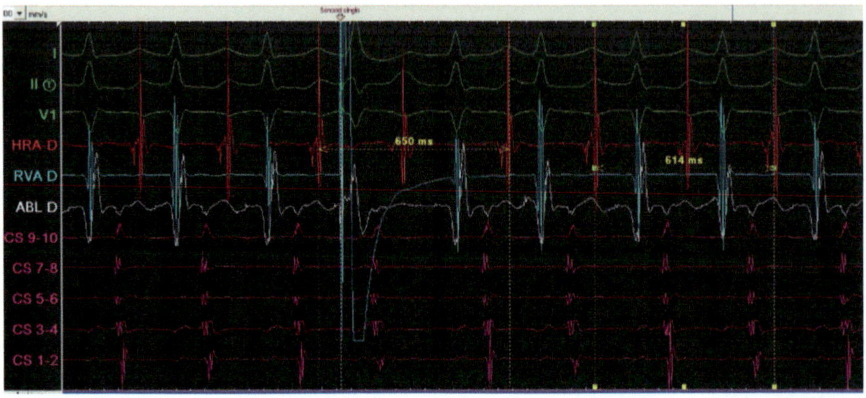

Fig. 13.1 His refractory pacing resulted in advancement and resetting of the arrhythmia infavor of the presence of an accessory pathway that is incorporating in the arryhthmia

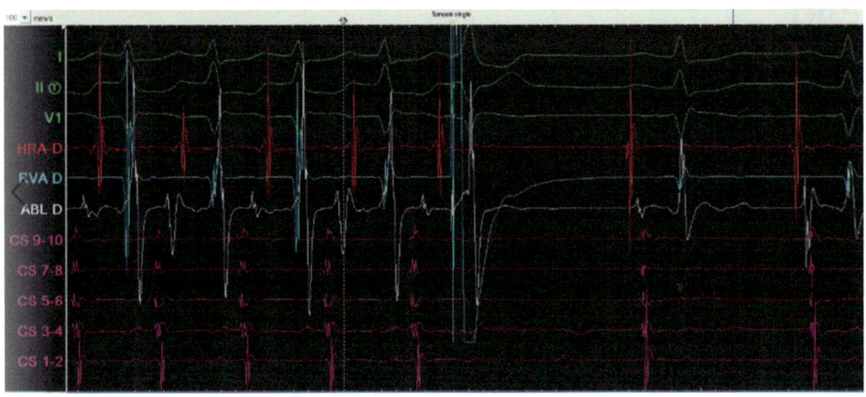

Fig. 13.2 Arrhythmia termination with His refractory PVC, that is strongly in favor of accessory pathway-mediated tachycardia that was PJRT in this case

Entrainment of the arrhythmia with ventricular overdrive pacing during arrhythmia was done and resulted in VAV response.

Also, His refractory ventricular pacing revealed the presence of an accessory pathway, but ventricular extra stimulation showed decremental conduction, so decremental, slowly conducting AP was considered as culprit pathway, resulting in PJRT.

In addition, AH interval during atrial pacing (after Isuprel infusion) at the tachycardia cycle length was within 20–40 ms of the tachycardia in PJRT, in contrast with atypical AVRNT, that is more than 40 ms (Fig. 13.3).

Results of differential septal sequential pacing were not conclusive.

Mapping of the right posteroseptal area for finding the earliest A was begun, after meticulous mapping, RF application in the site of atrial activation immediately

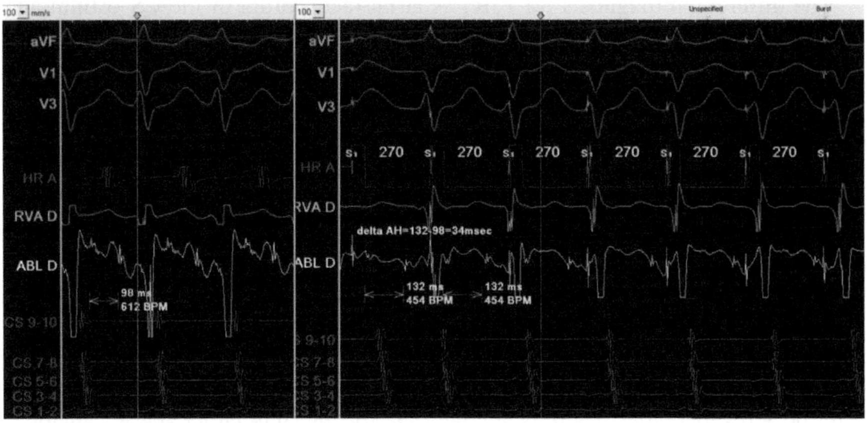

Fig. 13.3 AH interval during HRA pacing is within 20–40 ms of tachycardia AH interval (34 ms in this case)

resulted in the termination of the arrhythmia. Ventricular pacing showed VA dissociation immediately and after 30 min.

Half an hour after ablation VA was dissociated.

Discussion

Posteroseptal accessory pathways account for 25–30% of APs. Because of the complex anatomy of the posteroseptal area ablation of these types of APs is time consuming with greater fluoroscopic time [1].

The AP is located in the posteroseptal RA or CS proximal in 76% of cases, in 12% in mid septal location, and in the remainder is in right or left posterior or lateral [2, 3].

CS diverticula are present in about 9–10% of patients [3].

Patients often present with arrhythmia due to posteroseptal accessory pathways, but the presence of the CS diverticulum is not as reason for the presence of AP.

There are some electrocardiographic clues for discrimination of right from left septal accessory pathways in the WPW cases with antegrade conduction; such as negative or isoelectric delta wave in V1, with abrupt transition in V2 and deeply negative delta in III and aVF; but in left side delta is positive in V1 or $R > S$ in V1 is present, and aVF is less negative. These are not discriminating during orthodromic reciprocating tachycardia or in concealed accessory pathways [2, 3].

PJRT manifests as long RP tachycardia, for more than 12 h/day with typically inverted *P* waves in the inferior leads [4].

About 80% of the slowly conducting and decremental accessory pathways responsible for PJRT are located at the posteroseptal region [5, 6].

The differential diagnosis for PJRT is atrial tachycardia of the CS ostium and atypical from of AVNRT (fast–slow) type [7].

With ventricular overdrive pacing a VAAV post-pacing response indicates AT and could rule out PJRT.

With His refractory pacing, the atrial activation advancement or delay or termination of the arrhythmia without conduction to the atrium are in favor of PJRT, and could rule out atypical AVNRT and AT.

Differential septal sequential pacing as a variant of septal versus apical RV pacing has not been studied in patients with decremental APs [8].

In addition, AH interval during atrial pacing at the tachycardia cycle length is within 20–40 ms of the tachycardia in PJRT, in contrast with atypical AVRNT, that is more than 40 ms.

During ablation in long RP tachycardia, the target site for ablation is mostly the right posteroseptal area. There is another clue for the right target site for ablation, that is the presence of a sharp followed by blunt component of the earliest retrograde atrial electrogram, in contrast with blunt followed by sharp electrogram suggesting the left site of the septum as the target.

The shortest VA time and negative unipolar atrial electrogram are the best targets for ablation.

Despite the complex nature of the anatomy of the posteroseptal area, the success role for ablation is about 93%. Rarely heart block could be occurred due to damage to the AV nodal artery [9].

For ablation within the coronary sinus, the proximity to the right coronary artery may be problematic, and in such situations, coronary angiography is recommended. In sites with less than 2 mm distance of the coronary artery, cryoablation is the choice.

References

1. Anderson RH, Ho SY. Anatomy of the atrioventricular junctions with regard to ventricular preexcitation. Pacing Clin Electrophysiol. 1997;20:2072–6.
2. Calkins H, Kim YN, Schmaltz S, et al. Electrogram criteria for identification of appropriate target sites for radiofrequency catheter ablation of accessory atrioventricular connections. Circulation. 1992;85:565–73.
3. Amasyali B, Kose S, Aytemir K, Kilic A, Kursaklioglu H, Isik E. A permanent junctional reciprocating tachycardia with an atypically located accessory pathway successfully ablated from within the middle cardiac vein. Heart Vessel. 2006;21:188–91.
4. Gaita F, Haïssaguerre M, Giustetto C, et al. Catheter ablation of permanent junctional reciprocating tachycardia with radiofrequency current. J Am Coll Cardiol. 1995;25:648–54.
5. Rodriguez-Manero M, Fernandez-Lopez XA, Gonzalez-Melchor L, Garcia-Seara J, Martinez-Sande JL, Gonzalez-Juanatey JR. Permanent junctional reciprocating tachycardia in a patient with an atypically located accessory pathway in the left lateral mitral annulus. Rev Port Cardiol. 2016;35(59):e1–5.

6. Bennett MT, Leong-Sit P, Gula LJ, et al. Entrainment for distinguishing atypical atrioventricular node reentrant tachycardia from atrioventricular reentrant tachycardia over septal accessory pathways with long-RP [corrected] tachycardia. Circ Arrhythm Electrophysiol. 2011;4:506–9.
7. Haïssaguerre M, Montserrat P, Warin JF, Donzeau JP, Le Metayer P, Massiere JP. Catheter ablation of left posteroseptal accessory pathways and of "long RP" tachycardias with a right endocardial approach. Eur Heart J. 1991;12:845–59.
8. Sternick EB, Gerken LM, God EG. Concealed accessory pathway with long conduction times and incremental properties: a case report. J Cardiovasc Electrophysiol. 2001;12:103–7.
9. Ferro CR, de Assis CF, Mendonca MA, et al. Correlation of accessory pathway location with gender and their manifest or concealed presentation. Int J Cardiol. 2016;216:43–5.

Chapter 14
Anteroseptal Accessory Pathway

Shabnam Madadi

Abstract Antroseptal accessory pathways are sometimes challenging because of proximity to normal conduction system and risk of AV block. Sometimes they could be ablated via noncoronary cusp of aorta.

A 22-year-old lady; with frequent episodes of palpitations and near syncope; mildly reduced LVEF; manifest preexcited AF; with EPS elsewhere; considering antero-septal accessory pathway, without any attempt for ablation, referred for cryoablation, because of the risk of AV block.

EPS and Ablation

ECG revealed a narrow QRS tachycardia with rate about 200 bpm with 1:1 AV association and positive HV, earliest site of atrial activation in His (Fig. 14.1).

With ventricular pacing also earliest A was in His.

During sinus rhythm, HV was short about 10 ms.

With AES, AF rhythm was induced with SPERRI (shortest preexcited RR interval about 250 ms).

All of the above findings were infavour of need to ablation; because of the malignant type of the accessory pathway [1].

Cryoablation was inaccessible, so we tried for RF ablation.

During sinus rhythm the ventricular insertion site was targeted by searching the earliest site of ventricular activation time precedes the surface ECG delta wave by at least 15 ms, with a sharp QS deflection on the unipolar electrogram. We ablated on the atrial aspect of the annulus, with ratio of atrial to ventricular electrogram amplitude more than 0.4. We used a long steerable sheet to stabilize the position of the catheter tip.

S. Madadi (✉)
Rajaie Cardiovascular Medical and Research Center, Iran University of Medical Sciences, Tehran, Iran
e-mail: madadi@rhc.ac.ir

M. Maleki, A. Alizadehasl (eds.), *Case-Based Clinical Cardiology*,
https://doi.org/10.1007/978-1-4471-7496-7_14

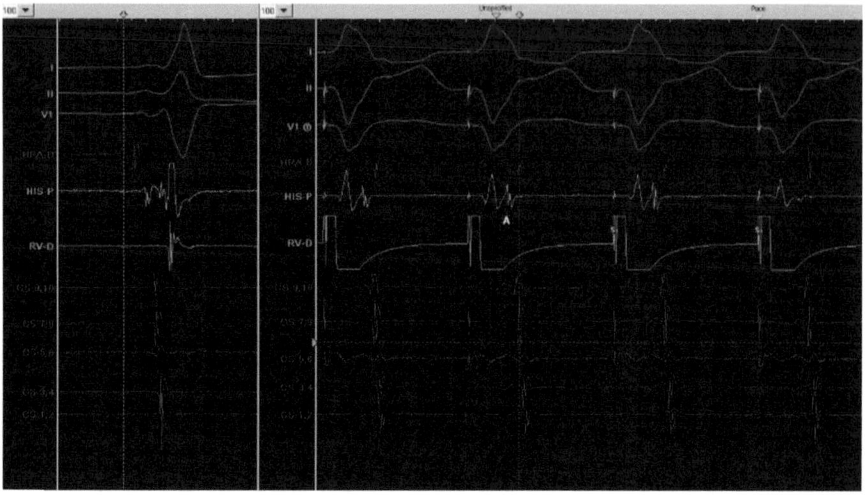

Fig. 14.1 Positive delta in I, II, short HV in sinus rhythm (left tracing), and earliest A in HIS during RV pacing (right tracing)

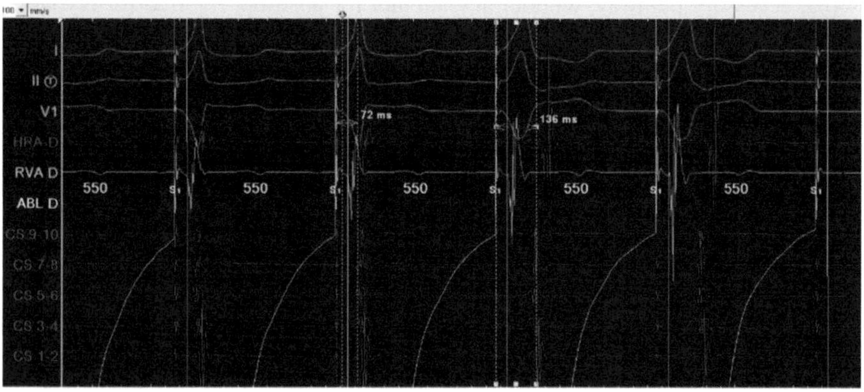

Fig. 14.2 Nodal response with HIS pacing after ablation

We started ablation with a relatively low power (10 W), and temperature 60 °C, and gradually increased the power to 30 W. In our lab, in any attempt, we do not continue for more than 5″ if the accessory pathway was present yet because of the possibility of edema formation and difficulty in the ablation.

In one attempt delta wave was disappeared abruptly so ablation was continued for 2 min.

His pacing after ablation showed nodal response (Fig. 14.2).

After 30 min waiting time, there was no evidence of AP conduction with Adenosine injection, so ablation was successfully terminated.

Discussion

Anteroseptal (superoparaseptal) accessory pathways comprise about 6–7% of all APs [2].

An antegrade conduction manifests as positive delta wave in the inferior leads, and negative delta in V1 with the early transition. In orthodromic SVT the P wave is positive in the inferior leads, also almost is buried in the ST segment [2].

The atrial activation sequence during SVT may similar to typical AVNRT; so in the case of concealed anteroseptal APs, there may be a challenge.

Introduction of ventricular premature His refractory extrastimulus could be diagnostic during tachycardia.

In case of non-sustained SVT, other maneuvers such as para-Hision pacing could be discriminating. Pacing from a location near His bundle could be done as follows: at low pacing outputs, ventricular capture occurs, whereas at higher outputs, His bundle capture occurs resulting in a narrower QRS. In the presence of a septal AP, the stimulus to atrial interval will be identical with and without His capture (extranodal responses) but in nodal response, the stimulus to atrial interval is longer with ventricular only capture than His capture [3–5].

With differential septal sequential pacing (DSSP), comparison of the stimulus to atrial intervals observed during apical versus basal RV pacing can demonstrate the presence of accessory pathway [3–5].

The apex is electrically closer to the atrium; although physically is distant; so RV apical pacing results in a shorter stimulus to atrial interval than RV basal pacing. However; in the presence of an accessory pathway, RV basal pacing results in a shorter stimulus to the atrial interval [4].

Comparison of the HA interval during tachycardia and RV pacing is also helpful for discrimination between AVNRT and ORT using an anteroseptal accessory pathway.

In ORT (orthodromic reciprocating tachycardia), HA interval during RV pacing is shorter than during arrhythmia, but in AVNRT, HA interval during RV pacing is longer than during arrhythmia. Because in QRT the sequence of Atrial, His, and Ventricular activation is in series and ventricular pacing results in a parallel activation of the Atrium and His, leading to a shorter HA interval, but in AVNRT, Ventricular, and Atrial activation is in parallel sequence and ventricular pacing results in series activation of the His and atrium, so HA should interval increases with ventricular pacing [4].

Ventricular Entrainment maneuvers also could help in differentiating between there; with ventricular overdrive pacing with cycle length about 20 ms less than arrhythmia CL, the difference between post-pacing interval (PPI) and tachycardia cycle length (TCL) in AVNRT is more than 110 ms and in AVRT is less than 110 ms.

Similarly, stimulus to atrial activation interval in ORT is less than 85 ms, but that is more than 85 ms in AVNRT.

In the presence of preexcitation, the ventricular insertion site can be targeted for ablation, in this situation pre-delta wave activation times are earlier in right-sided than in left-sided APs in general and that is true about anteroseptal (superoparaseptal) APs.

Ordinary, one should ablate on the ventricular aspect of the annulus, with lower risk of injury to the normal conduction system.

Cryomapping and ablation are introduced to avoid damage to the AV node, of note cryoablation does not result in accelerated junctional rhythm, however, this finding, should not be interpreted as lack of damage to normal conduction so ablation during HRA pacing with CL about tachycardia could help for monitoring of AV conduction during ablation [6].

There is about a 20% recurrence rate after cryoablation.

With Radiofrequency ablation, atrial aspect ablation with A/V EGM ratio of more than 0.4 may increase the risk of injury to the normal conduction system [7, 8].

There is one trick in the cases of a very close ablation site to His bundle, that the recording His catheter can be slightly advanced into the ventricle, leaving the insulated portion of the catheter as a potential physical barrier for His bundle.

Ablation during sinus rhythm allows monitoring of PR interval prolongation and accelerated junctional rhythm occurrence, indicating normal conduction injury.

In some cases, anteroseptal APs could be ablated in the left ventricular outflow tract and noncoronary sinus of valsalva [9].

Criteria for successful ablation are lack of preexcitation at rest (with adenosine injection), ventricular decremental pacing, and lack of retrograde conduction via accessory pathway.

Recurrence rate of AP conduction is about 15% for right-sided anteroseptal and mid septal APs.

References

1. Al-Khatib SM, Arshad A, Balk EM, et al. Risk stratification for arrhythmic events in patients with asymptomatic pre-excitation: a systematic review for the 2015 ACC/AHA/HRS guideline for the management of adult patients with supraventricular tachycardia: a report of the American College of Cardiology/American Heart Association task force on clinical practice guidelines and the Heart Rhythm Society. J Am Coll Cardiol. 2016;67:1624–38.
2. Gonzalez-Torrecilla E, Peinado R, Almendral J, et al. Reappraisal of classical electrocardiographic criteria in detecting accessory pathways with a strict para-Hisian location. Heart Rhythm. 2013;10(1):16–21.
3. Hirao K, Otomo K, Wang X, et al. Para-Hisian pacing. A new method for differentiating retrograde conduction over an accessory AV pathway from conduction over the AV node. Circulation. 1996;94(5):1027–35.
4. Miller JM, Rosenthal ME, Gottlieb CD, et al. Usefulness of the delta HA interval to accurately distinguish atrioventricular nodal reentry from orthodromic septal bypass tract tachycardias. Am J Cardiol. 1991;68(10):1037–44.
5. Michaud GF, Tada H, Chough S, et al. Differentiation of atypical atrioventricular node re-entrant tachycardia from orthodromic reciprocating tachycardia using a septal accessory pathway by the response to ventricular pacing. J Am Coll Cardiol. 2001;38(4):1163–7.
6. Wong T, Markides V, Peters NS, Davies DW. Clinical usefulness of cryomapping for ablation of tachycardias involving perinodal tissue. J Interv Card Electrophysiol. 2004;10(2):153–8.

7. Haïssaguerre M, Marcus F, Poquet F, Gencel L, Le Metayer P, Clementy J. Electrocardiographic characteristics and catheter ablation of parahissian accessory pathways. Circulation. 1994;90(3):1124–8.
8. Miyauchi Y, Kobayashi Y, Morita N, et al. Successful radiofrequency catheter ablation of an anteroseptal (superoparaseptal) atrioventricular accessory pathway from the left ventricular outflow tract. Pacing Clin Electrophysiol. 2004;27(5):668–70.
9. Brugada J, Puigfel M, Mont L, et al. Radiofrequency ablation of anteroseptal, para-Hisian, and mid-septal accessory pathways using a simplified femoral approach. Pacing Clin Electrophysiol. 1998;21(4 Pt 1):735–41.

Chapter 15
Mahaim Accessory Pathway

Shabnam Madadi

Abstract In any young patient with wide QRS tachycardia with LBBB pattern without structural heart disease, when SVT is considered be aware of Mahaim.

A 27-year-old man presented with frequent episodes of palpitation, without syncope. Some episodes of palpitations were during exercise and another episodes were occurred during rest without any known precipitating factor. Electrocardiography during palpitation revealed a wide QRS tachycardia with LBBB morphology and superior axis. Arrhythmia was adenosine sensitive and several episodes of arrhythmia were terminated with adenosine injection at the emergency ward. Patient was referred for ablation and electrophysiology study was revealed that arrhythmia is contributed to the atriofascicular accessory pathway (Mahaim) and successful ablation of the accessory pathway was done.

ECG demonstrated a wide QRS tachycardia with LBBB morphology with rate of about 170 bpm and left axis deviation. There is no evidence of AV dissociation. Morphology criteria were infavor of SVT. There was not any evidence of broad R wave in V1 or R/S nadir more than 70 ms in V1–V2 and QR or QS in V6.

EPS

Atrial overdrive pacing resulted in AH prolongation HV interval shortening and LBBB appearance of QRS (Fig. 15.1).

AES (Atrial extra stimulation) demonstrated LBBB morphology and AH prolongation with HV interval shortening all consistent with decremental conducting atriofascicular accessory pathway (Fig. 15.2).

S. Madadi (✉)
Rajaie Cardiovascular Medical and Research Center, Iran University of Medical Sciences, Tehran, Iran
e-mail: madadi@rhc.ac.ir

M. Maleki, A. Alizadehasl (eds.), *Case-Based Clinical Cardiology*,
https://doi.org/10.1007/978-1-4471-7496-7_15

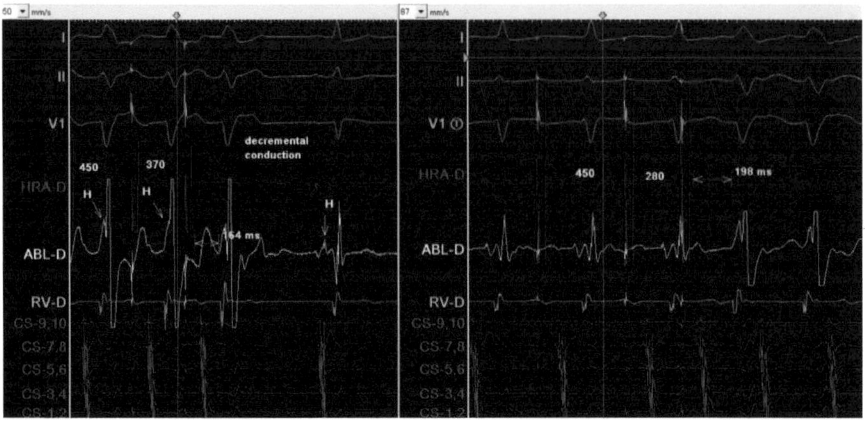

Fig. 15.1 With HRA pacing AH prolongation, HV shortening and LBBB pattern is seen

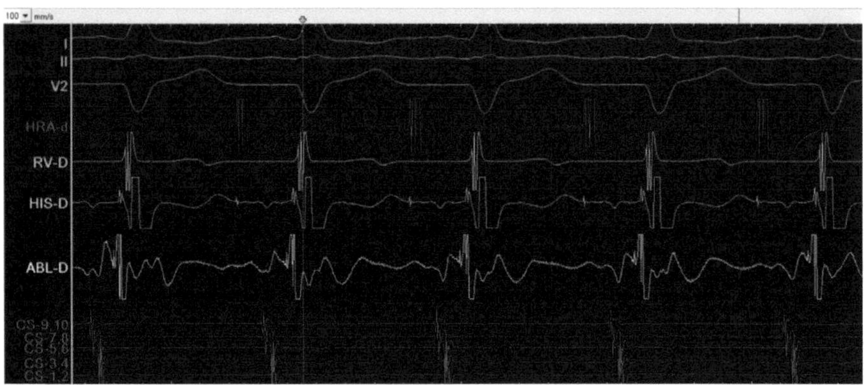

Fig. 15.2 LBBB pattern and HV shortening in Mahaim

With ventricular stimulation, a wide QRS tachycardia with LBBB morphology, similar to the patient's documented arrhythmia was initiated with negative HV interval (about 12 ms) and 1:1 AV association and earliest site of atrial activation in His consistent with antidromic AVRT due to right atriofascicular accessory pathway (Mahiam accessory pathway) (Figs. 15.3 and 15.4).

Patient's basic ECG evaluation demonstrated no evidence of preexcitation during sinus rhythm in favor of decremental conduction property of the accessory pathway.

Catheter ablation with radiofrequency was done during atrial stimulation with targeting the M potential in the lateral site of the tricuspid ring. During ablation ventricular automaticity was appeared, similar to the junctional rhythm during AVNRT ablation (Fig. 15.5).

After ablation no arrhythmia was inducible with AES or VES. Accessory pathway was not appeared as at the lateral side of the TV ring with atrial stimulation (Fig. 15.6).

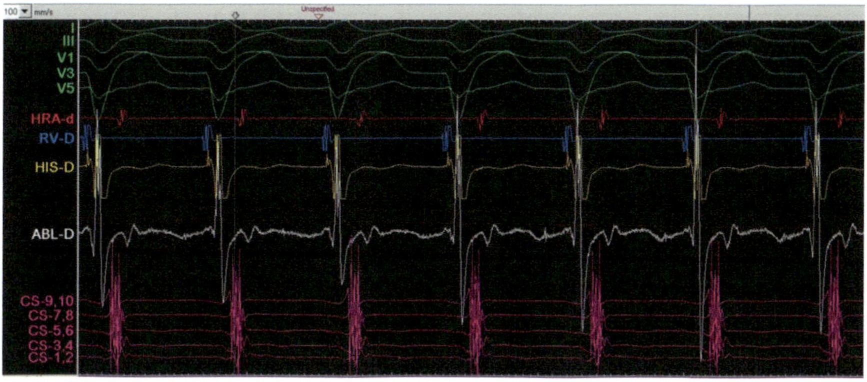

Fig. 15.3 Antidromic AVRT in Mahaim

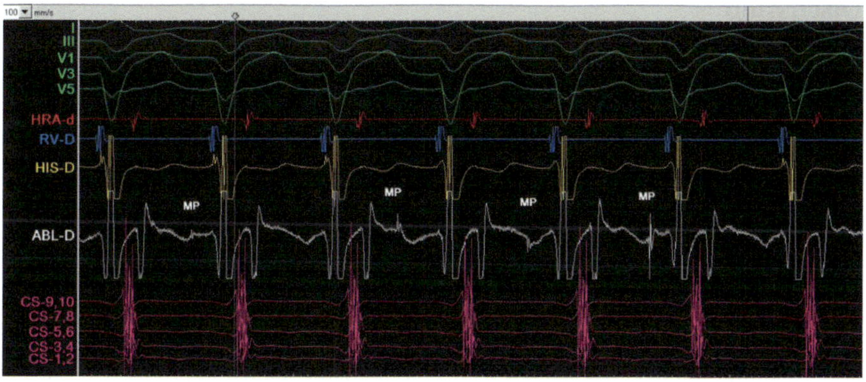

Fig. 15.4 Mahaim potential on the catheter ablation that is positioned in the lateral side if TV ring

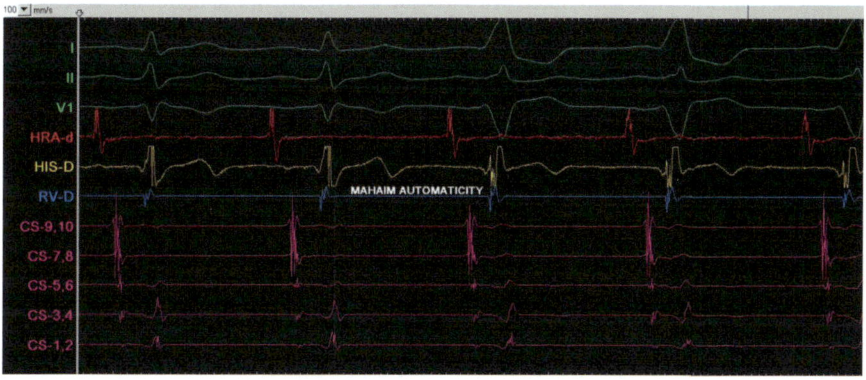

Fig. 15.5 Mahaim automaticity similar to AV automaticity during RFA

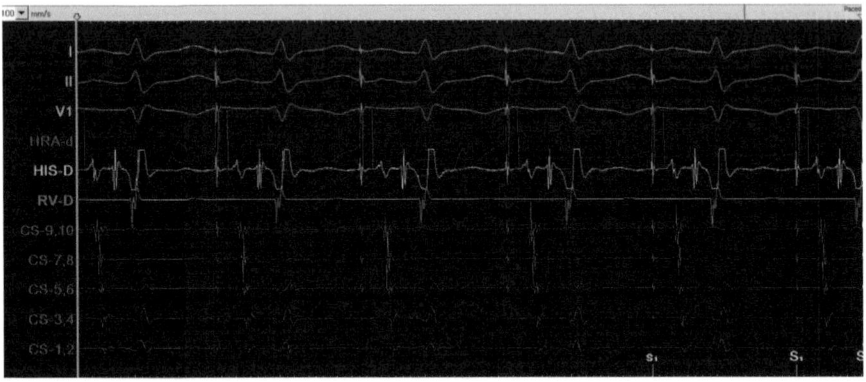

Fig. 15.6 No evidence of accessory pathway with atrial stimulation after ablation

Discussion

The first time, in 1938, nodoventricular fibers were described by Dr. Mahaim as fibers that connected from nodal region to the ventricular region by bypassing the His system. It was only a histologic description without any physiologic importance, but in early 1980, antidromic reciprocating tachycardias due to slowly conduction atrioventricular and atriofascicular accessory pathways were described and eponym of Mahaim was adopted for such fibers contributing in such arrhythmia [1–3].

These fibers are long, insulated fibers with decremental conduction properties that connect atrium directly to the distal part of His purkinje system. This structure is very similar to the nodal system with decremental conduction properties. Except for a single report of the left side Mahaim pathway, these pathways are almost always located at the right side, along the lateral part of the tricuspid annulus.

These pathways are associated with unique tachyarrhythmia using the accessory pathway as the antegrade limb and AV node as the retrograde limb, resulting in antidromic AV reciprocating tachycardia with LBBB morphology [4–6].

They can only conduct antegrade, and are mostly right-sided, giving rise to an antidromic AVRT with LBBB type morphology, which is sensitive to adenosine and verapamil. Similar to the AV node, there are some reports of ducal conduction properties in such accessory pathways [7].

Maximally preexcited QRS, during rapid atrial pacing or during antidromic tachycardia, is very similar to typical LBBB, without broad R wave in V1, with mid precordial R were transition (beyond V4), and an R wave in lead I. QRS duration during tachycardia is less than 150 ms, because atriofascicular pathway allows for more rapid activation to the His-Purkinje system. The distal insertion of atriofascicular pathways is at the distal part of the right bundle in the anterior free wall of the right ventricle. Similar to the AV node, decremental conduction in the atriofascicular pathways occur in the proximal portion, between the atrial insertion and the M potential. Initiation of the tachycardia could be done by atrial or ventricular stimulation.

In the atrial stimulation initiation of the tachycardia may be more easily done by atrial stimulation near the AV node, such as proximal of coronary sinus stimulation, because it may allow more time for AV node for recover and facilitate retrograde conduction. Because initiation of tachycardia by atrial stimulation requires AV nodal block for conduction through the accessory pathway, and because these accessory pathways cannot conduct retrogradely, ventricular stimulation can almost always initiate the tachycardia [8].

Ventricular stimulation when could result in sufficiently short retrograde V-H interval, or sufficient delay on retrograde HPS activation because of retrograde RBBB could result in the initiation of the tachycardia. The AV interval during antidromic tachycardia is often more than 150 ms. Direct insertion of the pathways to the distal RBB or fascicle results in the rapid simultaneous activation of His and ventricular with a very short V-H interval the V-H interval during tachycardia is shorter than V-H interval during sinus rhythm, because of the simultaneous activation of the His and the ventricular via right bundle [9, 10].

In the setting of the retrograde RBBB, V-H, and V-A interval may be prolonged and in this situation, the tachycardia cycle length increase, because the conduction occurs across interventricular septum via myocardium and then up to system via left bundle to reach to the His bundle and then to the atrium. In the absence of retrograde RBBB, rapid retrograde conduction over the right bundle to the His may allow for antegrade left ventricular activation via left anterior fascicule, resulting in a narrower QRS with the inferior axis.

A late PAC, could preexcite the tachycardia and advance or delay the following ventricular activation without affecting the septal atrial activation, and reset the tachycardia. Cycle length oscillation following extrastimulus is common and is characteristic for such pathways. Mapping of the atriofascicular accessory pathway is done by locating to the M (Mahaim) potential along the tricuspid ring during atrial stimulation or during antidromic tachycardia.

The site of successful ablation is defined by simultaneous of the A, M, and RV potential in the lateral part of the tricuspid annulus [11].

In some situations ablation of the atrial insertion of the accessory pathway is done that can be achieved by recording the shortest stimulus to the fully preexcited ventricular electrogram, or by mapping the tricuspid annulus during antidromic AVRT. The second one could be done by mapping of the site where the latest PAC could reset the tachycardia cycle length without activating the atrial tissue near the AV node.

Radiofrequency ablation of atriofascicular pathways has a success rate of about 90–100%.

References

1. Gallagher JJ, Smith WM, Kasell J, et al. Role of Mahaim fibers in cardiac arrhythmias in man. Circulation. 1981;64:176–89.
2. Ellenbogen KA, O'Callaghan WG, Colavita PG, Packer DL, Gilbert MR, German LD. Catheter atrioventricular junction ablation for recurrent supraventricular tachycardia with nodoventricular fibers. Am J Cardiol. 1985;55:1227–9.
3. Bardy OH, German LD, Packer DL, Coitorti F, Gallagher JJ. Mechanism of tachycardia using a nodofascicular Mahaim fiber. Am J Cardiol. 1984;54:1140–1.
4. Gillette PC, Garson A Jr, Cooley DA, McNamara DG. Prolonged and decremental antegrade conduction properties in right anterior accessory connections: wide QRS antidromic tachycardia of left bundle branch block pattern without Wolff-Parkinson-White configuration in sinus rhythm. Am Heart J. 1982;103:66–74.
5. Tchou P, Lehmann MH, Jazayeri M, Akhtar M. Atriofascicular connection or a nodoventricular Mahaim fiber electrophysiologic elucidation of the pathway and associated reentrant circuit. Circulation. 1988;77:837–48.
6. Klein GJ, Guiraudon GM, Kerr CR, et al. Nodoventricular accessory pathway: evidence for a distinct accessory atrioventricular pathway with atrioventricular node-like properties. J Am Coll Cardiol. 1988;11:1035–40.
7. Kent AFS. A conducting path between the right auricle and the external wall of the right ventricle in the heart of the mammal. J Physiol. 1914;48:57.
8. Hluchy J, Schickel S, Jörger U. Electrophysiologic characteristics and radiofrequency ablation of concealed nodofascicular and left anterograde atriofascicular pathways. J Cardiovasc Electrophysiol. 2000;11(2):211–7.
9. Johnson CT, Brooks C, Jaramillo J, et al. A left free-wall, decrementally conducting, atrioventricular (Mahaim) fiber: diagnosis at electrophysiological study and radiofrequency catheter ablation guided by direct recording of a Mahaim potential. Pacing Clin Electrophysiol. 1997;20:2486–8.
10. Tada H, Nogami A, Naito S, et al. Left posteroseptal Mahaim fiber associated with marked longitudinal dissociation. Pacing Clin Electrophysiol. 1999;22:1696–9.
11. Francia P, Pittalis M, Ali H, Cappato R. Electrophysiological study and catheter ablation of a Mahaim fibre located at the mitral annulus-aorta junction. J Interv Card Electrophysiol. 2008;23:153–7.

Chapter 16
An Unusual Location of Accessory Pathway Anteromedial Side of the Mitral Annulus

Shabnam Madadi

Abstract This brief case presents a patient with frequent episodes of palpitations and electrocardiographic abnormality consistent with preexcitation and multiple episodes of tachyarrhythmia such as atrioventricular reciprocating tachycardia and preexcited AF, with an unusual location of accessory pathway.

This patient was a 42-year-old female. Her 12 lead ECG showed evidence of preexcitation with positive delta wave in V1, and II, III, aVF, and negative delta wave in I, aVL, and aVR. During electrophysiologic study, an orthodromic atrioventricular reciprocating tachycardia was induced and the earliest site of retrograde atrial depolarization was recorded at the proximal site of the coronary sinus, of course not so fused.

Meticulous mapping via septostomy and during tachycardia showed the local VA fusion in the anteromedial mitral annulus and radiofrequency application in this area resulted in the termination of tachycardia and elimination of accessory pathway.

Case History

A 42-year-old woman with a 20 year history of paroxysmal supraventricular tachycardia was referred for intracardiac electrophysiologic study.

A 12 lead ECG showed ventricular preexcitation (that was manifest during AF) with positive delta wave in V1 and inferior leads and negative delta wave in lead I and aVL and aVR, during electrophysiology study patient demonstrated antidromic AVRT (Fig. 16.1).

S. Madadi (✉)
Rajaie Cardiovascular Medical and Research Center, Iran University of Medical Sciences, Tehran, Iran
e-mail: madadi@rhc.ac.ir

M. Maleki, A. Alizadehasl (eds.), *Case-Based Clinical Cardiology*,
https://doi.org/10.1007/978-1-4471-7496-7_16

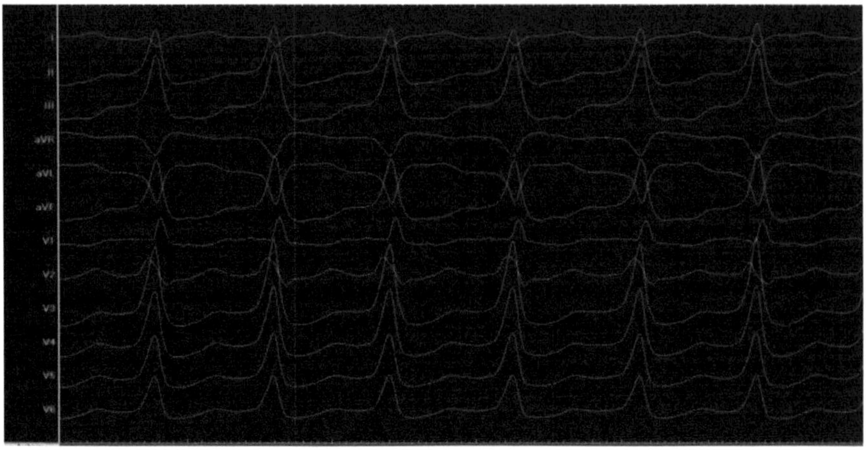

Fig. 16.1 Antidromic AVRT, positive concordance, negative aVL, Iso-Negative I

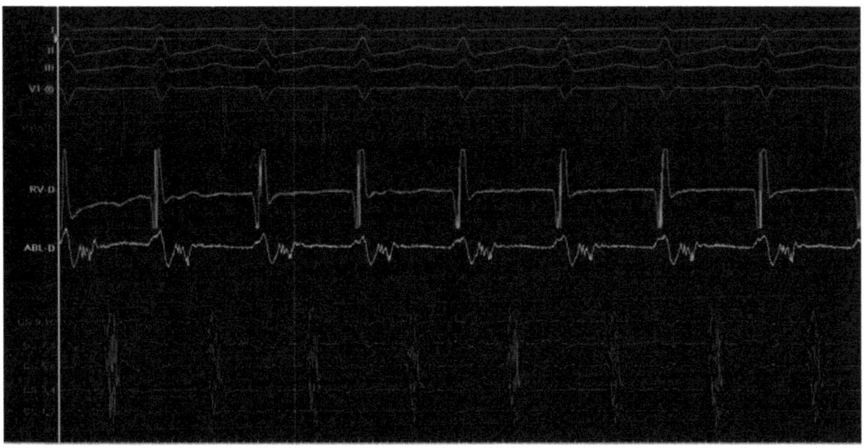

Fig. 16.2 Narrow QRS tachycardia with earliest atrial activation in CS 9–10

With standard percutaneous techniques, intracardiac multipolar electrode catheter was placed in the high right atrium, right ventricular apex, his bundle region, and coronary sinus.

During electrophysiology study, AF was induced and demonstrated with positive QRS complex in lead V1 and negative delta and QRS complexes in leads I and aVL and aVR.

With programmed electrical stimulation a narrow QRS tachycardia consistent with orthodromic atrioventricular reciprocating tachycardia was induced with the earliest site of atrial activation in the proximal part of the coronary sinus, but not so fused signal (Fig. 16.2).

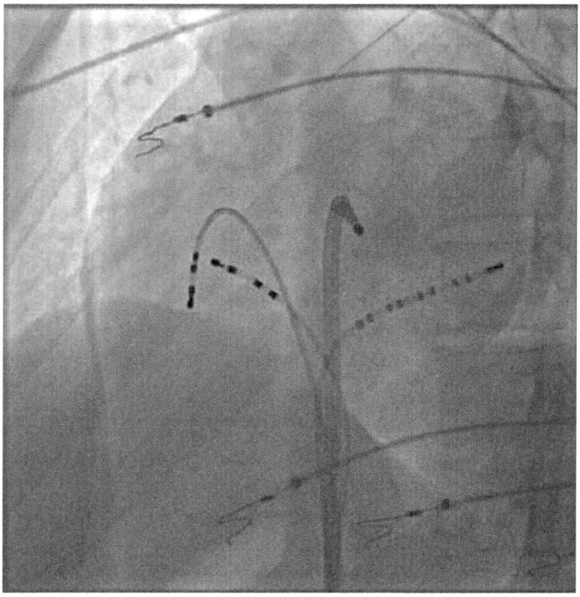

Fig. 16.3 Success site of ablation in aortomitral continuity

Septostomy was done and meticulous mapping of the left atrioventricular ring during tachyarrhythmia showed the most fused VA signal in the anteromedial mitral annulus (Fig. 16.3).

Radiofrequency application in this area resulted in the termination of tachycardia with VA dissociation and elimination of delta wave during antegrade conduction.

Discussion

The aortomitral continuity is a fibrous body that couples the mitral and aortic valves together as these two structures originate in widely separated parts of the early embryonic heart tube. Accessory atrioventricular pathway located at or near the anteromedial mitral annulus has rarely been reported [1–5].

In one report, Reginal Liew reported two cases of accessory pathway at aortomitral continuity with positive delta waves and QRS polarities in the inferior leads and negative delta waves and QRS polarities in leads aVL and aVR [6].

In some reports para-Hisian accessory pathways were ablated via coronary cusps and in all of them, aVL was positive [7–10].

Compared with the ablation at the right anteroseptal area, RF delivered at the aortic cusps had a higher immediate success, lower complication rate, and good long-term outcome [11–13].

In this case surface, ECG analysis according to previous algorithms was concordant with left lateral accessory pathway, but during sinus rhythm with the proper position of coronary sinus catheter and during atrial pacing for manifest preexcitation, distal coronary sinus electrodes showed no fused AV potentials [14, 15].

During orthodromic atrioventricular reciprocating tachycardia, the earliest site of atrial activation was at the proximal part of coronary sinus without fused VA signal.

During preexcited AF a pattern like aortomitral continuity PVC was seen with qR like potential in V1 and positive delta wave in the inferior leads and negative delta in leads I and aVL.

Mapping of the left atrioventricular ring via septostomy showed no evidence of a fused signal in the lateral and anterior portions of the ring consistent with that seen in the surface ECG.

There was no history of prior ablation and suspected iatrogenic isthmus block.

Mapping of the aortomitral continuity showed the most fused signal during tachyarrhythmia and radiofrequency ablation in this area was successful.

Mapping and success signal at this unusual location showed an uncommon site for left-sided accessory pathway.

There were few reports of the accessory pathway in this location, one concealed form of the accessory pathway at this location was reported in 1996 by WuTj and colleagues.

In summary, we present a case of an accessory pathway in the anteromedial mitral annulus with both antegrade and retrograde conduction properties.

References

1. Iturralde P, Araya-Gomez V, Colin L, et al. A new ECG algorithm for the localization of accessory pathways using only the polarity of the QRS complex. J Electrocardiol. 1996;29:289–99.
2. Xie B, Heald SC, Bashir Y, et al. Localization of accessory pathways from the 12-lead electrocardiogram using a new algorithm. Am J Cardiol. 1994;74:161–5.
3. Arruda MS, McClelland JH, Wang X, et al. Development and validation of an ECG algorithm for identifying accessory pathway ablation site in Wolff-Parkinson-White syndrome. J Cardiovasc Electrophysiol. 1998;9:2–12.
4. Chiang CE, Chen SA, Teo WS, et al. An accurate stepwise electrocardiographic algorithm for localization of accessory pathways in patients with Wolff-Parkinson-White syndrome from a comprehensive analysis of delta waves and R/S ratio during sinus rhythm. Am J Cardiol. 1995;76:40–6.
5. Fitzpatrick AP, Gonzales RP, Lesh MD, et al. New algorithm for the localization of accessory atrioventricular connections using a baseline electrocardiogram. J Am Coll Cardiol. 1994;23:107–16.
6. Liew R, Ward D. Two cases of accessory pathways located at the aortomitral continuity: clues from the 12-lead ECG where the algorithms have failed. Heart Rhythm. 2008;5(8):1206–9.
7. Godin B, Guiot A, Savoure A, Anselme F. The left coronary cusp as an unusual location for accessory pathway ablation. Heart Rhythm. 2011;8(11):1769–72.
8. Oloriz T, Gulletta S, Della Bella P. Successful radiofrequency ablation of an anteroseptal accessory pathway from the right coronary cusp. Europace. 2014;16(8):1204. https://doi.org/10.1093/europace/euu157.

9. Guo XG, Sun QI, Ma J, Liu XU, Zhou GB, Yang JD, Zhang S. Electrophysiological characteristics and radiofrequency catheter ablation of accessory pathway connecting the right atrial appendage and the right ventricle. J Cardiovasc Electrophysiol. 2015;26(8):845–52. https://doi.org/10.1111/jce.12693.
10. Han B, Li XJ, Hsia HH. Catheter ablation of arrhythmia from the aortic sinus cusp: the presence of a dead-end tract of the conduction system. Europace. 2013;15(10):1515. https://doi.org/10.1093/europace/eut069.
11. Laranjo S, Oliveira M, Trigo C. Successful catheter ablation of a left anterior accessory pathway from the non-coronary cusp of the aortic valve. Cardiol Young. 2015;25(6):1200–2. https://doi.org/10.1017/S1047951114001589.
12. Hindricks G, Kottkamp H, Xu C, Willems S, Haverkamp W, Shenasa M, Günter B, Borggrefe M. Localization and radiofrequency catheter ablation of left-sided accessory pathways during atrial fibrillation Feasibility and electrogram criteria for identification of appropriate target sites. J Am College Cardiol. 1995;25(2). https://doi.org/10.1016/0735-1097(94)00363-U
13. Jackman WM, Wang X, Friday KJ, Roman CA, Moulton KP, Beckman KJ, McClelland JH, Twidale N, Hazlitt HA, Prior MI, Margolis PD, Calame JD, Edward RN, Overholt D, Lazzara R. Catheter ablation of accessory atrioventricular pathways (Wolff–Parkinson–White Syndrome) by radiofrequency current. N Engl J Med. 1991;324:1605–11. https://doi.org/10.1056/NEJM199106063242301.
14. Langberg JJ, Man KC, Vorperian VR, Kalbfleisch SJ, Strickberger A, Hummel JD, Morady F. Recognition and catheter ablation of subepicardial accessory pathways. J Am Coll Cardiol. 1993;22(4):1100–4.
15. Kobza R, Kottkamp H, Piorkowski C, Tanner H, Schirdewahn P, Dorszewski A, Wetzel U, Gerds-Li JH, Arya A, Hindricks G. Radiofrequency ablation of accessory pathways. Contemporary success rates and complications in 323 patients. Z Kardiol. 2005;94(3):193–9.

Chapter 17
Epicardial Left Anterolateral Wall AP

Shabnam Madadi

Abstract PI was a 39-year-old man, with some episodes of palpitation, but not documented ECG during arrhythmia; Family history of SCD was present in his young brother without any evaluation.

PI was a 39-year-old man, with some episodes of palpitation, but not documented ECG during arrhythmia; Family history of SCD was present in his young brother without any evaluation.

Twelve lead surface ECG showed evidence of minimal preexcitation with short PR interval with positive delta wave in V1 and negative delta wave in aVL (Fig. 17.1).

Echocardiography revealed normal ventricular size and function without any structural abnormality.

Because of atypical chest pain, coronary angiography was done elsewhere and was normal (NECA).

Because of the family history of SCD, we decided to evaluate the accessory pathway characteristics. So EPS was done, using two quadripolar catheters In HRA (High right atrium) and RV (right ventricle) and a decapolar catheter in CS (coronary sinus).

With HRA pacing, manifest preexcitation was revealed with a negative QRS complex in I, aVL, and positive concordance in V1–V6 and positive QRS in II, III, aVF, all consistent with a left anterolateral accessory pathway (Fig. 17.2).

Any attempt for the right positioning of the CS was difficult and CS was positioned in a CS branch, so there was not any fused AV potential in CS. EPR (Effective refractory period) of the AP (accessory pathway) was about 250 ms, we tried to do septostomy for transseptal mapping and ablation of the accessory pathway. The best earliest ventricular signal was in the anterolateral portion of the ring, around the base of the LAA (Fig. 17.3).

Any attempt for ablation there was unsuccessful so we changed our approach, and unfortunately, it was very difficult to position the catheter in the anterolateral of

S. Madadi (✉)
Rajaie Cardiovascular Medical and Research Center, Iran University of Medical Sciences, Tehran, Iran
e-mail: madadi@rhc.ac.ir

M. Maleki, A. Alizadehasl (eds.), *Case-Based Clinical Cardiology*,
https://doi.org/10.1007/978-1-4471-7496-7_17

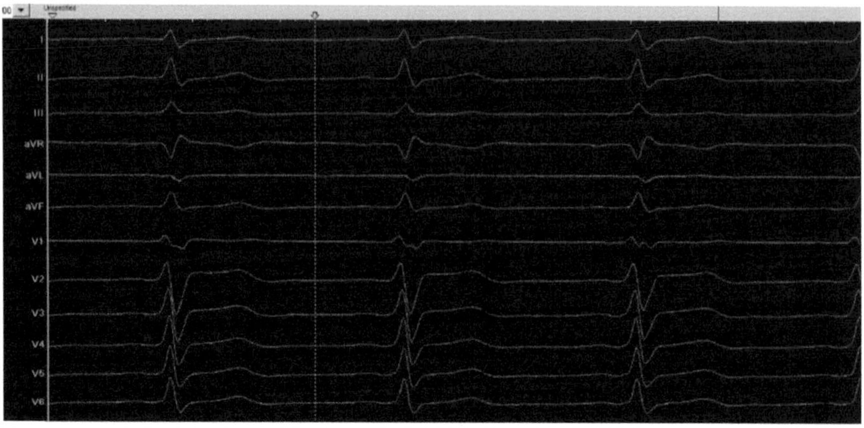

Fig. 17.1 Short PR with positive delta wave in V1, Ang negative delta in aVL

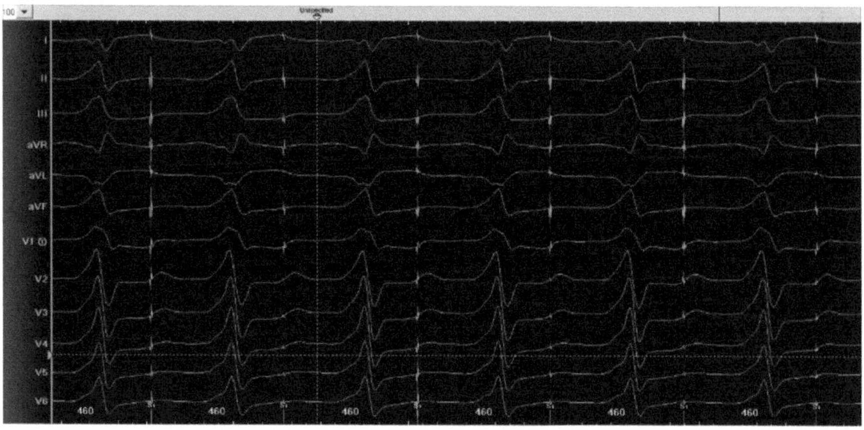

Fig. 17.2 HRA pacing demonstrated manifest preexcitation as negative delta in I, aVL, and positive delta in V1

MV (Mitral valve) ring with this approach so we came back so the right side. Then we decided to remap the coronary sinus and great cardiac vein.

Unbelievably there is was a very nice and early ventricular signal in the anterolateral part of CS (Fig. 17.4) and RFA with irrigated tip catheter with power 20 W and target temperature 43 °C resulted in immediate disappearance of the delta wave (Fig. 17.5).

It was very uncommon, so we did coronary sinus venography and there was an amazing pattern of CS anatomy (Fig. 17.6).

Adenosine injection 30 min after ablation showed no evidence of accessory pathway and ablation was terminated successfully (Fig. 17.7).

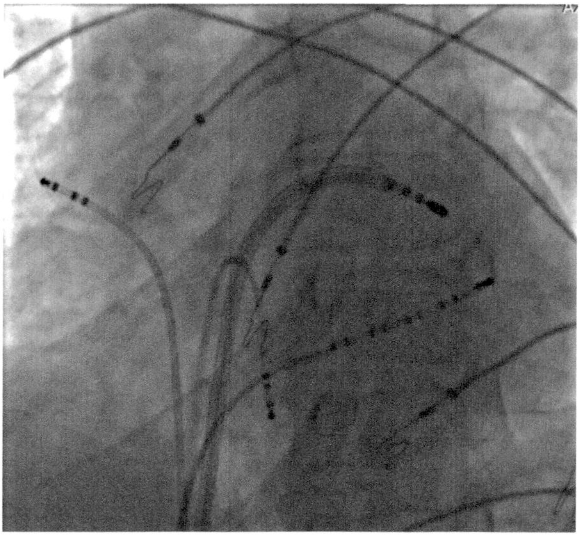

Fig. 17.3 The site of best signal in the base of LAA

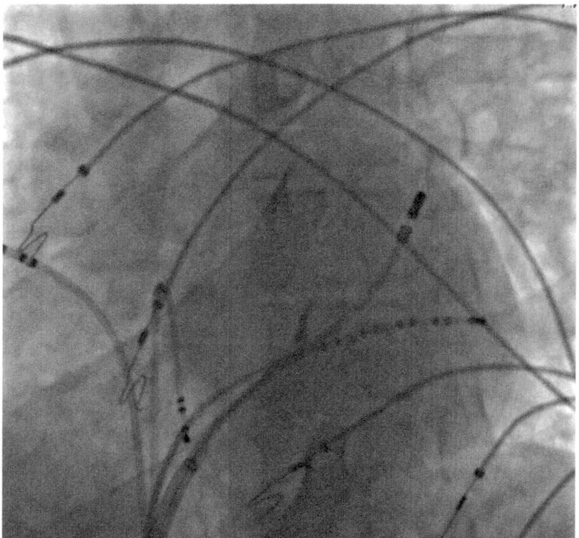

Fig. 17.4 Site of the success signal in CS

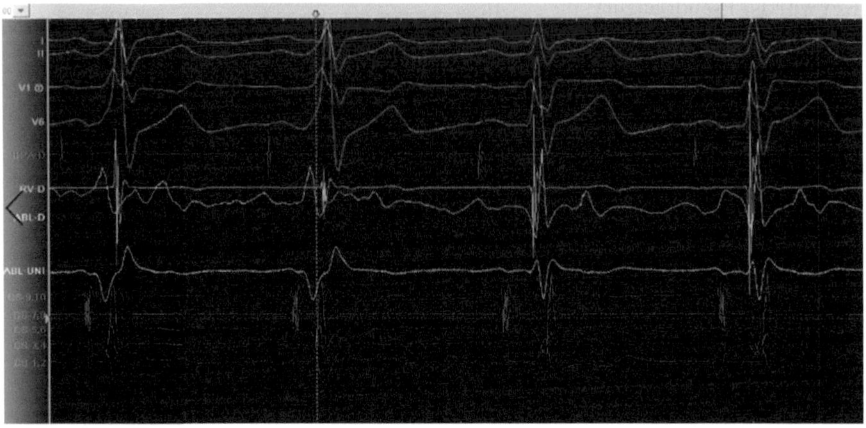

Fig. 17.5 Delta wave disappearance during RFA

Fig. 17.6 Interesting pattern of CS anatomy

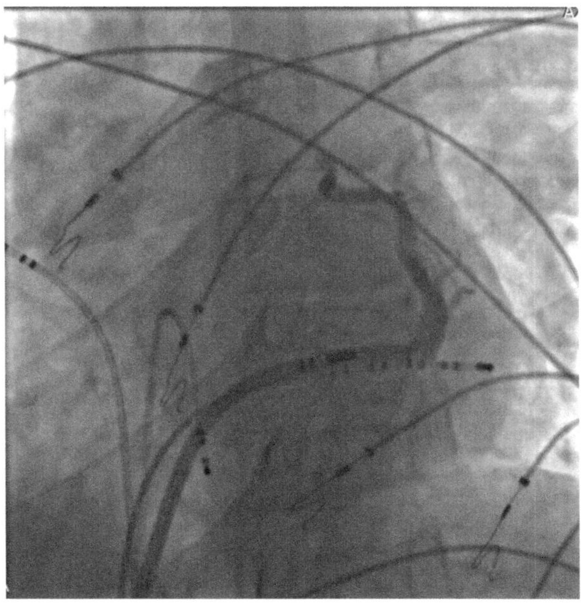

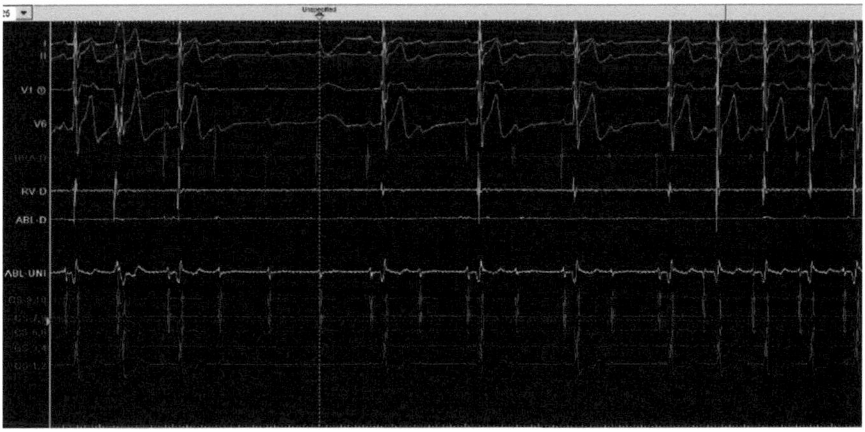

Fig. 17.7 Absence of accessory pathway conduction during Adenosine injection

Discussion

Left free wall accessory pathway is the most common type of all APs and accounts for about 50–60% of all of them. Epicardial APs account for 4% of all left free wall accessory pathways and are more frequent in the cases of failed ablation [1].

If manifest preexcitation was present, all left free wall APs should have positive delta wave in V1, with R wave greater than the S wave in leads V1 or V2. Mapping and ablation of the left free wall APs could be done via transseptal or retrograde approaches. If the ratio of the dominant amplitude in limb lead II was more than III, the pathway is likely anterior [2, 3].

A negative delta in I, aVL is infavor of the left lateral accessory pathway.

In the retrograde approach via aorta, the target is an accessory pathway ventricular insertion site.

It is often difficult to achieve a good position in the lateral and mitral annulus via retrograde approach. In the transseptal approach, the target is the atrial side of the annulus, the ability to maneuver the catheter is greater with the transseptal approach. The target sites for ablation in the left free wall accessory pathways are delta-VEGM difference less than 0 s and AEGM-VEGM ≤40 ms and atrial ECG EGM amplitude should be more than 0.4 mV. In unipolar electrogram, the maximum negative d*v*/d*t* reflects local ventricular activation. The AV intervals for left lateral APs are less than other free wall APs [4, 5].

In the cases of failed endocardial ablation, ablation could be done successfully via CS. For irrigated catheters, maximal power of 20–30 W and target temperature about 50 °C is recommended.

Cryoablation in the CS has also been used safely and effectively.

Coronary sinus muscular connections to the ventricle are mostly mapped in the MCV (middle cardiac vein) or posterior cardiac vein. Ablation within the CS or venous tributaries could be done safely by cryoablation, followed by irrigated tip

RFA and finally noncooled RFA. Epicardial approach through percutaneous pericardial access provides another approach for mapping and ablating such pathway [6–8].

In our patient, there was no evidence of ECG manifestations of epicardial AP according to the previously known characterization of epicardial accessory pathways such as negative delta wave in lead II or steep positive delta wave in aVR, but because of failed endocardial attempts for ablation, we changed to epicardial approach via CS.

Although it is recommended to do coronary angiography prior to ablation in the CS because of the proximity of RCA (Right coronary artery) to MCV (Middle cardiac vein) and LAD (Left anterior descending artery) and LCX (Left circumflex artery) to great Cardiac vein (GCV), we did not do coronary angiography in this case [9].

References

1. Shinbane JS, Lesh MD, Stevenson WG, et al. Anatomic and electrophysiologic relation between the coronary sinus and mitral annulus: implications for ablation of left-sided accessory pathways. Am Heart J. 1998;135:93–8.
2. Katsouras CS, Greakas GF, Goudevenos JA, et al. Localization of accessory pathways by the electrocardiogram. Pacing Clin Electrophysiol. 2004;27:189–93.
3. Hwang C, Peter CT, Chen P-S. Radiofrequency ablation of accessory pathways guided by the location of the ligament of Marshall. J Cardiovasc Electrophysiol. 2003;14:616–20.
4. Madadi S, Emkanjoo Z, Sharifi M, et al. An unusual location of the accessory pathway on the anteromedial side of the mitral annulus. Iranian Heart J. 2019;2:75–8.
5. Chen S-A, Tai C-T. Ablation of atrioventricular accessory pathways:current technique-state of the art. Pacing Clin Electrophysiol. 2001;24:1795–809.
6. Chen XU, Borggrefe M, Shenasa M, Haverkamp W, Hindricks G, Breithardt G. Characteristics of local electrogram predicting successful transcatheter radiofrequency ablation of left-sided accessory pathways. J Am Coll Cardiol. 1992;20:656–65.
7. Chauvin M, Shah DC, Haïssaguerre M, et al. The anatomic basis of connections between the coronary sinus musculature and the left atrium in humans. Circulation. 2000;101:647–52.
8. Sun Y, Arruda M, Otomo K, et al. Coronary sinus-ventricular accessory connections producing posteroseptal and left posterior accessory pathways: incidence and electrophysiological identification. Circulation. 2002;106:1362–7.
9. Kosinski D, Burket M, Durzinsky D. Occlusion of the left main coronary artery during radiofrequency ablation for the Wolff-Parkinson-White syndrome. Eur J Card Pacing Electrophysiol. 1993;3:63–6.

Chapter 18
Fascicular VT

Shabnam Madadi

Abstract In any young patient without structural heart disease and wide QRS tachycardia with RBBB morphology be aware of fascicular VT.

A 19 y/o patient, presented with frequent episodes of palpitation and wide QRS tachycardia with RBBB pattern and inferior axis, positive QRS in I, aVL, small S wave in V5–V6.

Echo findings: Normal LVEF, Normal LV size, no significant valvular disease.

HR during tachycardia about 198/min. EPS was done; with retrograde aortic approach and mapping was done using a 3D Navx precision system; a tachycardia similar to the clinical one was induced with HRA pacing, and showed negative HV, all findings in favor of fascicular left posteroseptal VT. RFA was done and resulted in terminated of the arrhythmia during ablation and noninducibility with and without Isuprel.

Methods

Patient was brought to the EP lab in NSR and good general condition. Conscious sedation was started for him. Invasive hemodynamic monitoring was done and the RV and coronary sinus catheter were introduced via the left femoral vein and right femoral artery access was archived for retrograde aortic approach.

The patient had documented wide QRS tachycardia with RBBB pattern and superior axis; positive QRS in I, aVL, and small S wave in V5–V6.

Atrial programed extra stimulation with protocol 300–280–240 ms with Isuprel resulted in initial of wide QRS tachycardia similar to the patient's clinical arrhythmia (Fig. 18.1). Flexibility ablation catheter was introduced via the femoral artery and via retrograde approach and inserted in the LV cavity by looping in the level of

S. Madadi (✉)
Rajaie Cardiovascular Medical and Research Center, Iran University of Medical Sciences, Tehran, Iran
e-mail: madadi@rhc.ac.ir

M. Maleki, A. Alizadehasl (eds.), *Case-Based Clinical Cardiology*,
https://doi.org/10.1007/978-1-4471-7496-7_18

valsalva sinus. Heparin administrated with dose 100 IU/kg and ACT was checked every 20% with a target ACT about 300 ms.

Because of the history of Verapamil sensitivity of the arrhythmia and because the arrhythmia was inducible with atrial programed stimulation, so Fascicular VT was considered for the patient and because of the axis of the arrhythmia, left posteroseptal fascicular VT was the first diagnosis. So we tried to find diastolic potentials during VT in the apical third of the septum, but it was not so easy to find them, then we found and ablated Purkinje potentials but arrhythmia also inducible with PES and Isuprel yet.

Then we tried to ablate more proximal sites and RFA in more proximal sites resulted in the termination of the VT and noninducibility with Isuprel and PES. During sinus rhythm, there was also late potential suggesting unidirectional block to the diseased myocardium (Fig. 18.2).

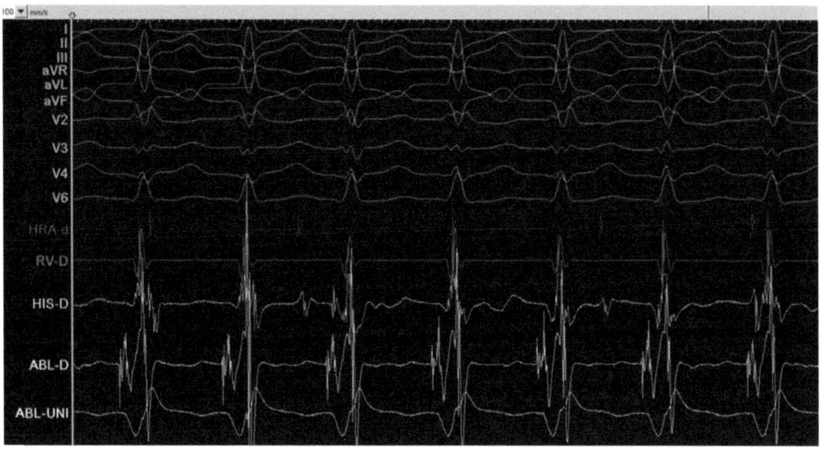

Fig. 18.1 Wide QRS tachycardia, RBBB pattern, superior axis, AV diss

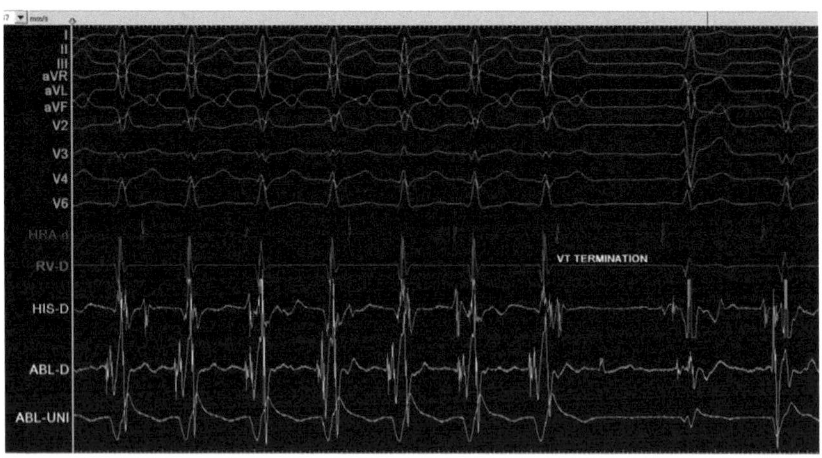

Fig. 18.2 VT termination during RFA in the more proximal portion

Discussion

Verapamil-sensitive fascicular VT is one of the most popular forms of the idiopathic VTs and was recognized by Zipes et al. in 1979 with RBBB morphology and left axis deviation and normal hearts.

In 1981 Belhassen et al. demonstrated the verapamil sensitivity of the tachycardia. RBBB, inf axis and then an upper septal variant of this arrhythmia were reported by 2016; and three forms of this tachycardia were known as:

1. LPF-VT pattern and super axis
2. LAF-VT with RBBB morphology and inferior axis and
3. Upper septal variant with narrow QRS and normal or right axis duration

The most common type was LPF-VT and the least common type was upper septal variant [1–4].

Recently Nogami et al. reported a distinct subtype of verapamil-sensitive fascicular VTs as papillary muscle fascicular VT.

The mechanism of these VTs is reentry because it can be induced, entrained, and terminated by programed electrical stimulation. The circuit of LPF-VT is a P1 represents the activation potential in the distal part of the Purkinje tissue, with verapamil sensitivity and decremented conduction (and is a slow conductive pathway of the arrhythmia) [5–7].

P2 is the activation of the left posterior fascicle or Purkinje fibers near the left posterior fascicle and is a bystander in VT.

Arrhythmia circus in VT is antergrade conduction via P1 and retrograde conduction via left ventricle septal muscle.

During sinus rhythm, the activation is from P2 to P1 (activation via left posterior fascicle to the distal Purkinje system), but arrhythmia circulation is from P1 to P2 during VT and P1 is buried in ventricular activation during VT.

So during arrhythmia P1 as a mid-diastolic potential could be appeared and P2 could be seen just before of the QRS.

Because the mechanism of the arrhythmia is reentry any lesion in the arrhythmia circulation could terminate arrhythmia but it is not so easy to do it. Nakagawa ablation sites were at the apical inferior septum of the LV, but Tsuchiya's et al., recommend to ablate at the basal regions close to the main LBBB trunk [8, 9].

In this care; we finally used Tsuchiya's approach for arrhythmia termination and noninducibility.

Two differential diagnosis for our patient and such patients is present:

1. Posterior papillary muscle fascicular VT, was ruled out with the absence of superior right axis deviation (extreme axis).
2. Non-reentrant posterior fascicle VT: That is a VT that could be induced by exercise and catecholamine and cannot be induced or terminated by programed ventricular stimulation and also is not responsive to verapamil. Fascicular VT can be slowed or terminated by verapamil but is unresponsive to the beta-blockers. Class Ia and Ic antiarrhythmic drugs may be effective. If the arrhythmia shows catecholamine dependency adenosine responsiveness may occur.

The success and recurrence rate for the ablation of LPT-VT HF is reported about 97% and 4% respectively and for LAF-VT about 90% and 11% respectively. For upper septal VT, success rate is about 100% and the recurrence rate about 2.5% [10, 11].

Left posterior fascicle in contrast with the upper septal variant is not a part of the arrhythmia circuit so left posterior hemiblock induction could not result in termination of arrhythmia.

The only predictor for recurrence after arrhythmia is the rate of the tachycardia and may be because of the catheter instability in the rapid heart rates, shorter CL of the arrhythmia could predict the arrhythmia recurrence [12].

References

1. Talib AK, Nogami A, Nishiuchi S, et al. Verapamil-sensitive upper septal idiopathic left ventricular tachycardia: prevalence, mechanism, and electrophysiological characteristics. J Am Coll Cardiol EP. 2015;1:369–80.
2. Nishiuchi S, Nogami A, Naito S. A case with occurrence of antidromic tachycardia after ablation of idiopathic left fascicular tachycardia: mechanism of left upper septal ventricular tachycardia. J Cardiovasc Electrophysiol. 2013;24:825–7.
3. Komatsu Y, Nogami A, Kurosaki K, et al. Fascicular ventricular tachycardia originating from papillary muscles: Purkinje network involvement in the reentrant circuit. Circ Arrhythm Electrophysiol. 2017;10. pii:e004549.
4. Gallagher JJ, Selle JG, Svenson RH, et al. Surgical treatment of arrhythmias. Am J Cardiol. 1988;61:27A–44A.
5. Suwa M, Yoneda Y, Nagao H, et al. Surgical correction of idiopathic paroxysmal ventricular tachycardia possibly related to left ventricular false tendon. Am J Cardiol. 1989;64:1217–20.
6. Maruyama M, Terada T, Miyamoto S, Ino T. Demonstration of the reentrant circuit of verapamil-sensitive idiopathic left ventricular tachycardia: direct evidence for macroreentry as the underlying mechanism. J Cardiovasc Electrophysiol. 2001;12:968–72.
7. Lin FC, Wen MS, Wang CC, et al. Left ventricular fibromuscular band is not a specific substrate for idiopathic left ventricular tachycardia. Circulation. 1996;93:525–7.
8. Haïssaguerre M, Vigmond E, Stuyvers B, et al. Ventricular arrhythmias and the His-Purkinje system. Nat Rev Cardiol. 2016;13:155–66.
9. Nogami A, Naito S, Tada H, et al. Demonstration of diastolic and presystolic Purkinje potential as critical potentials on a macroreentry circuit of verapamil-sensitive idiopathic left ventricular tachycardia. J Am Coll Cardiol. 2000;36:811–23.
10. Kuo JY, Tai CT, Chiang CE, et al. Is the fascicle of left bundle branch involved in the reentrant circuit of verapamil-sensitive idiopathic left ventricular tachycardia. Pacing Clin Electrophysiol. 2003;26:1986–92.
11. Morishima I, Nogami A, Tsuboi H, Sone T. Negative participation of the left posterior fascicle in the reentry circuit of verapamil-sensitive idiopathic left ventricular tachycardia. Heart Rhythm. 2012;23:556–9.
12. Maeda S, Yokoyama Y, Nogami A, et al. First case of left posterior fascicle in a bystander circuit of idiopathic left ventricular tachycardia. Can J Cardiol. 2014;30:e11–3.

Chapter 19
Left Posteroseptal PVC

Shabnam Madadi

Abstract Left posteroseptal area is in close proximity to cardiac crux, if there is any finding in ECG in favour of epicardial origin this may be misleading. In this case, we had similar problem and after epicardial mapping of crux, we ablated the PVC in left posteroseptal area.

A 55 years old Patient; with Hx of inferior STEMI and fibrinolytic therapy elsewhere, and coronary angiography 6 months ago, which revealed ectatic coronary arteries without significant stenosis.

The patient was referred to because of frequent PVCs and palpitation, LVEF: 40%.

PVCs were LBBB like pattern; with the rapid transition in V2 (breakthrough) and rS in V5–V6 (Fig. 19.1).

We planned for ablation, and EPS and ablation were started using one quadripolar catheter in RV; one decapolar catheter in CS, and one vein for ablation. Using 3D precision mapping system with meticulous mapping in the right posteroseptal area there was no proper signal, so we attempted for middle cardiac vein mapping, mapping in the proximal part of the middle cardiac vein showed earliest about 20–24 ms, but ablation in that area was not successful (Fig. 19.2).

So we decided to do epicardial approach for mapping the apical crux. We did not do the left side approach before the epicardial approach because of the risk of bleeding (due to heparin administration). So the epicardial anterior approach was done.

Short steerable catheter (Agillis) was introduced and meticulous epicardial mapping in the basal and apical crux was done but there was not an appropriate signal.

So we decided to do an arterial approach. Using retrograde arterial approach and posteroseptal mapping, these were an early signal in the left posteroseptal area and RF application in this area immediately eliminated PVCs (Fig. 19.3).

Triamcinolone 1 mg/kg was injected in the epicardial space then Agillis extracted. 30 min waiting showed no recurrence of PVC, and the Patient discharged 1 day later with the good general condition; without PVC.

S. Madadi (✉)
Rajaie Cardiovascular Medical and Research Center, Iran University of Medical Sciences, Tehran, Iran
e-mail: madadi@rhc.ac.ir

M. Maleki, A. Alizadehasl (eds.), *Case-Based Clinical Cardiology*,
https://doi.org/10.1007/978-1-4471-7496-7_19

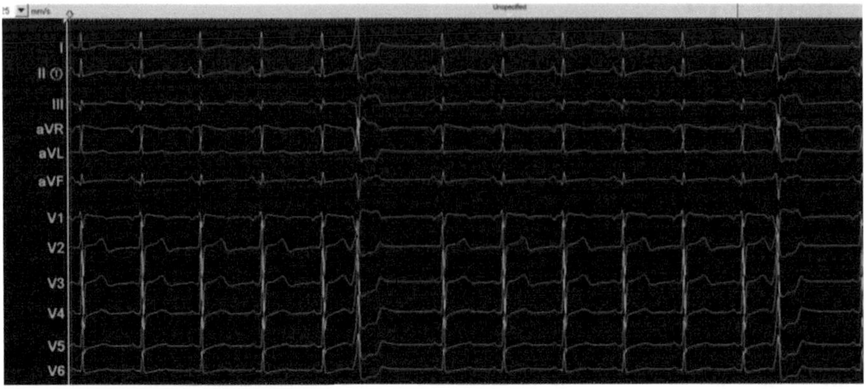

Fig. 19.1 Positive QRS in lead II and negative in III, aVF, positive in lead I and aVL, breakthrough in V2

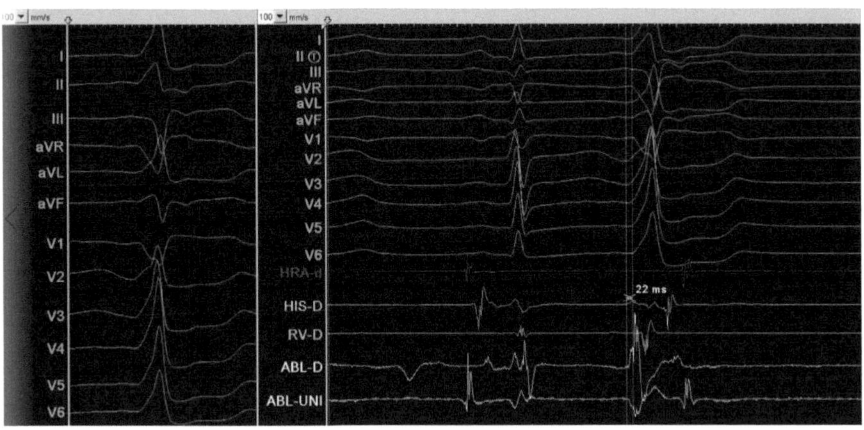

Fig. 19.2 MCV (middle cardiac vein) signal in PVC

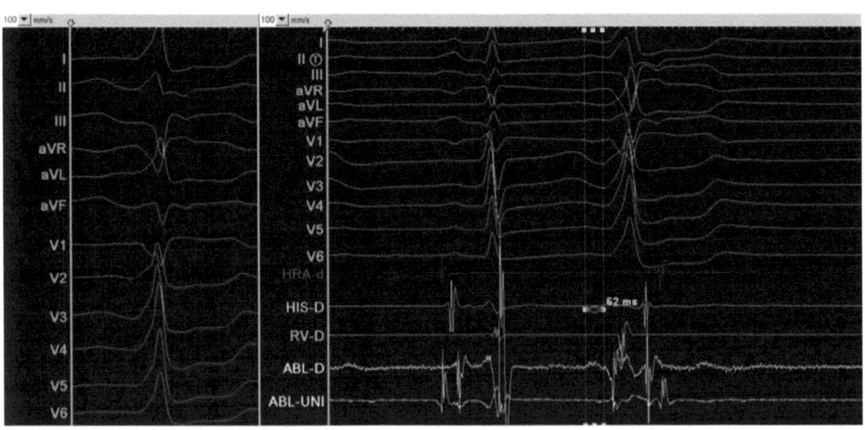

Fig. 19.3 Site of success signal

Discussion

In about 1.8% of idiopathic PVC, the origin of PVC is the crux of the heart. In one report about 80% of these patients had sustained monomorphic VT and syncope and for some of those ICD was implanted. Basal curx PVCs could be ablated from the middle cardiac vein within 2 cm of the middle cardiac vein ostium [1, 2].

The ECG pattern of crux PVC, is a superior axis PVC with QS pattern in III and aVF and epicardial pattern morphologies, with maximal deflection index ≥55%, Pseudo delta wave >34 ms; and $R \geq S$ in V2 [3–5].

Those with LBBB pattern have an early transition in V2 with a late transition to an rS or qS in V6.

In patients with apical crux PVCs, the ECG morphology could be changed to RBBB or vice vera.

Basal curx PVCs have either negative or isoelectric potential in V1, positive potential in V6, and an early transition in V2. An algorithm to predict the precise focus of the crux PVCs was introduced by Kawamura et al. in 2014 and suggested that if there was an RBBB pattern PVCs; with $R > S$ in V6; the apical crux is suspected; otherwise basal crux could be the origin of the PVC.

Our patient had LBBB like morphologie with $R > S$ in V2 and $R < S$ in V6, maximal deflection index was more than 55% and pseudodelta wave was present; so strongly suggested epicardial origin but middle cardiac vein mapping showed no good signal so the epicardial approach was done and at the end; endocardial approach via LV in the left posteroseptal area resulted in the elimination of PVCs, this site was very adjacent to the sites with the earliest signal in electroanatomical mapping (Navx precision) in both right site and epicardial site [2].

In posteroseptal MV ring PVC, there is a precordial transition before V2 and negative QRS polarity in the inferior leads; posteroseptal VTs have a negative QRS component in V1, and the amplitude ratio of lead III to lead II is greater than posterior PVSs.

Anterior and anteromedial VTs arising from the aortomitral continuity exhibit an absence of S wave in lead V6, and RBBB or LBBB with an early transition and inferior axis. In posterior and posterolateral mitral ring PVCs there is a notching in the late phase of the QRS complex in the inferior leads that may result from phased excitation from the LV free wall to the RV.

According to all finding and relatively higher frequency of MV ring PVCs than crux PVCs; MV posteroseptal origin was a suspected region in mind from the beginning of the procedure; but because of the need to anticoagulation during retrograde approach and risk of bleeding, we performed epicardial approach before retrograde aortic approach.

We did the anterior epicardial approach, because it is recommended to puncture at the site further from the desired region of mapping to avoid "U" turns around the target area [6, 7].

A 17 gauge Curved tipped needle (Tuohy) was used then Agillis's introduced and with an open irrigated tip catheter epicardial mapping was done using 3D precision. At the end; endocardial LV posteroseptal site mapping and ablation resulted in the elimination of PVCs.

References

1. Kawamura M, Gerstenfeld EP, Vedantham V, et al. Idiopathic ventricular arrhythmia originating from the cardiac crux or inferior septum: epicardial idiopathic ventricular arrhythmia. Circ Arrhythm Electrophysiol. 2014;7:1152–8.
2. Kawamura M, Hsu JC, Vedantham V, et al. Clinical and electrocardiographic characteristics of idiopathic ventricular arrhythmias with right bundle branch block and superior axis: comparison of apical crux area and posterior septal left ventricle. Heart Rhythm. 2015;12:1137–44.
3. Yui Y, Sekiguchi Y, Nogami A, et al. Electrophysiological characteristics and radiofrequency catheter ablation treatment of idiopathic ventricular arrhythmias successfully ablated from the ostium of the coronary sinus. Circ J. 2017;81(12):1807–15.
4. Doppalapudi H, Yamada T, Ramaswamy K, et al. Idiopathic focal epicardial ventricular tachycardia originating from the crux of the heart. Heart Rhythm. 2009;6:44–50.
5. Daniels DV, Lu YY, Morton JB, et al. Idiopathic epicardial left ventricular tachycardia originating remote from the sinus of Valsalva: electrophysiological characteristics, catheter ablation, and identification from the 12-lead electrocardiogram. Circulation. 2006;113:1659–66.
6. Sosa E, Scanavacca M, d'Avila A, Pilleggi F. A new technique to perform epicardial mapping in the electrophysiology laboratory. J Cardiovasc Electrophysiol. 1996;7:531–6.
7. Stevenson WG, Wilber DJ, Natale A, et al. Irrigated radiofrequency catheter ablation guided by electroanatomic mapping for recurrent ventricular tachycardia after myocardial infarction: the multicenter thermocool ventricular tachycardia ablation trial. Circulation. 2008;118:2773–82.

Chapter 20
GCV (Great Cardiac Vein) PVC

Shabnam Madadi

Abstract LV summit PVCs are not infrequent and sometimes could be ablated via coronary sinus in the great cardiac vein.

The patient was a 44-year-old man, with complaints of palpitation, and dyspnea on exertion. Frequent PVCs were determined in ECG; with an inferior axis; LBBB pattern with the early precordial transition, and breakthrough pattern in precordial leads (Fig. 20.1).

In ECG Holter monitoring there was about 20% PVC count. LVEF by echocardiography was about 40%. Ablation recommended.

EPS and ablation was done; using quadripolar catheter for RV potential recording and pacing; one decapolar catheter for CS; and an arterial line for retrograde aortic approach; and another vein for GCV mapping via CS.

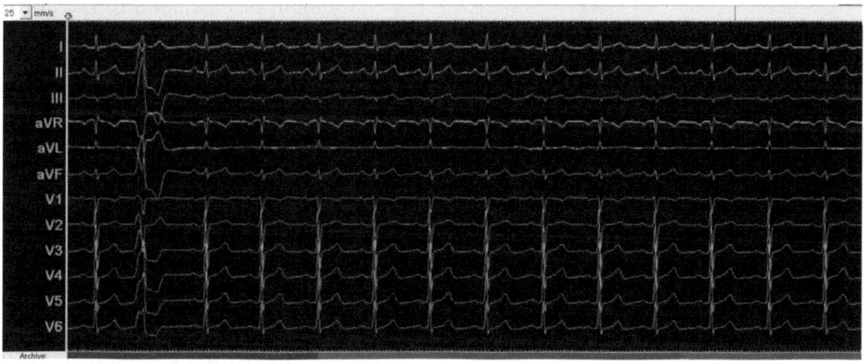

Fig. 20.1 PVC with breakthrough in V2, inferior axis, iso-neg in I, negative in aVL

S. Madadi (✉)
Rajaie Cardiovascular Medical and Research Center, Iran University of Medical Sciences, Tehran, Iran
e-mail: madadi@rhc.ac.ir

M. Maleki, A. Alizadehasl (eds.), *Case-Based Clinical Cardiology*,
https://doi.org/10.1007/978-1-4471-7496-7_20

The procedure was done during conscious sedation using 3D Carto mapping (CARTO; Biosense Webster) (Fig. 20.2). A 3.5 mm open irrigation tip catheter was used. With the retrograde mapping of the aortic cusp, the earliest site of activation was an LCC with about 30 ms earliest signal but ablation in that area was unsuccessful.

So RVOT (right ventricular outflow tract) and GCV (Great cardiac vein) mapping was done. The earliest signal in GCV was found and was about 34 ms earlier than surface ECG (Fig. 20.3); and RF ablation in that area with 20 W and target temperature 43 °C resulted in the elimination of the PVCs abruptly, but because of the impedance rise in the coronary sinus, ablation was interrupted; and intermittent titrated RF currents were applied. PVCs were eliminated without recurrence after 30 min waiting period.

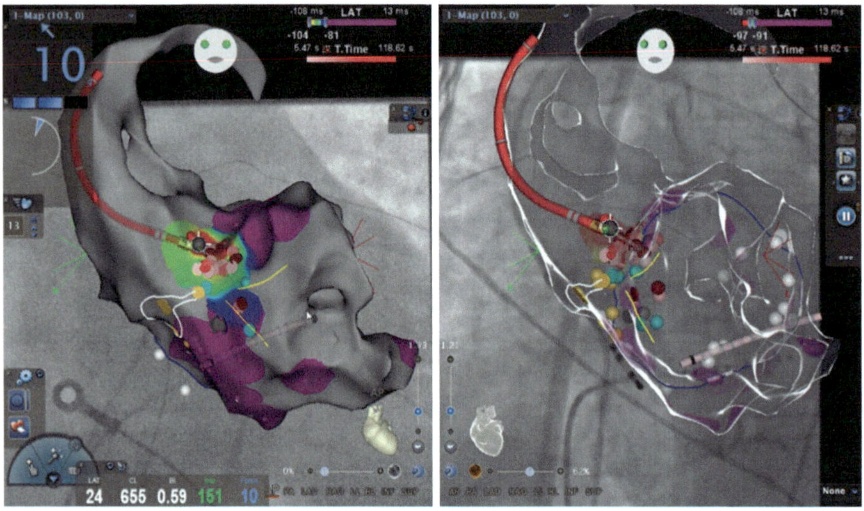

Fig. 20.2 CARTO mapping of PVCs (a left aortic cusp ablation was not successful)

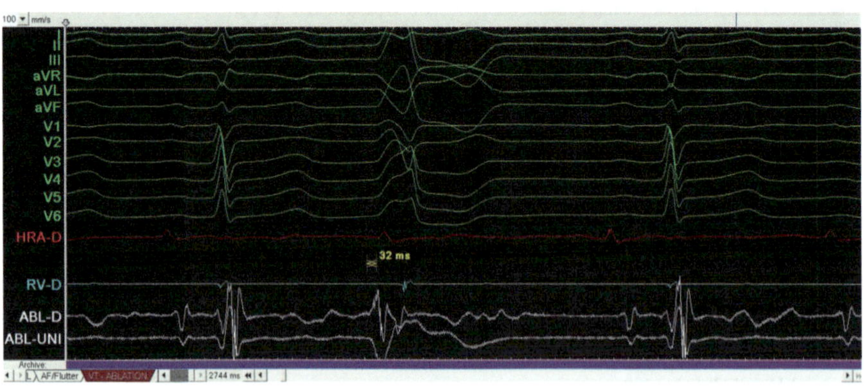

Fig. 20.3 Earliest signal about 32 ms (in GCV)

Discussion

The most common site of idiopathic PVCs is in right and left ventricular outflow tract. Patients with a high PVC burden could develop a reversible from of LV cardiomyopathy. So PVC ablation could reverse the process of cardiomyopathy and cardiomyopathy could regress after PVC ablation [1, 2].

The classic ECG profile of outflow tract PVC is LBBB pattern and tall R waves in leads II, III, aVF, and QS pattern in aVR and aVL.

Idiopathic PVC could be ablated from aortic cusps. ECG criteria for RCC (right coronary cusp) PVC is a QS or rS pattern in lead V1, but LCC (left coronary cusp) PVC overall has multiphasic components with a positive complex in V1 [3, 4].

Target site for ablation in LCC is a site with very small presystolic up to 80 ms earlier than QRS onset with isoelectric segment before QRS and a delayed signal in NSR which reverse during PVC and a QS pattern in unipolar ablation recording, with an M or W shaped QRS complex. In RCC PVCs there is a QS or rS pattern in V1 and in right–left junction the potential in V1 has a notching on downstroke or a QS pattern [5, 6].

AMC (Aortomitral continuity) PVCs have RBBB, inferior axis, and q R pattern in V1. The LV summit is a triangular portion of the LVOT epicardium between LAD and LCX bifurcation. Epicardial LV summit PVC, have a maximum deflection index in the precordial leads. LVS is dissected by GCV into the basal and apical portion of the triangle [7–9].

In this PVCs, there is a QS pattern in lead I about 30%, and early precordial R wave transition in 70%. Intrinsicoid deflection time is also prolonged. LV summit arrhythmia could be ablated via GCV or via the epicardial approach [9].

Epicardial approach is only successful for ablation of the PVCs arising from the basal and lateral aspects of the LV summit, because of proximity to coronary vessels.

Because of epicardial fat, basal, and apical LV summit epicardial ablation is mostly unsuccessful.

ECG criteria predictive for the basal or lateral summit are: Q wave ratio >1.8 in aVL/aVR, $R/S > 2$ in lead V1 and absence of q wave in lead V1 [9].

Ablation with irrigated tip catheter in the cusps and GCV should be done with caution and start with 10–15 W and increase slowly to 30 W.

In PVCs originating for GCV, coronary angiography should be done before an attempt for ablation.

The acute success rate of ablation in idiopathic PVC is about 80 and 70% with and without antiarrhythmic drugs, respectively.

Complications during ablation consist of the development of bundle branch block or AV block, or aortic regurgitation or pulmonic regurgitation or coronary damage.

Sometimes the origin of the PVC is midmyocardial and longer duration lesions are required.

Bipolar ablation could be done for eliminating mid myocardial foci.

References

1. Yamashina Y, Yagi T, Namekawa A, et al. Clinical and electrophysiological difference between idiopathic right ventricular outflow tract arrhythmias and pulmonary artery arrhythmias. J Cardiovasc Electrophysiol. 2010;21:163–9.
2. Storey J, Iwasa A, Feld GK. Left ventricular outflow tract tachycardia originating from the right coronary cusp: identification of location of origin by endocardial noncontact activation mapping from the right ventricular outflow tract. J Cardiovasc Electrophysiol. 2002;13:1050–3.
3. Kanagaratnam L, Tomassoni G, Schweikert R, et al. Ventricular tachycardias arising from the aortic sinus of valsalva: an under-recognized variant of left outflow tract ventricular tachycardia. J Am Coll Cardiol. 2001;37:1408–14.
4. Ouyang F, Fotuhi P, Ho SY, et al. Repetitive monomorphic ventricular tachycardia originating from the aortic sinus cusp: electrocardiographic characterization for guiding catheter ablation. J Am Coll Cardiol. 2002;39:500–8.
5. Lin D, Ilkhanoff L, Gerstenfeld E, et al. Twelve-lead electrocardiographic characteristics of the aortic cusp region guided by intracardiac echocardiography and electroanatomic mapping. Heart Rhythm. 2008;5:663–9.
6. Bala R, Garcia FC, Hutchinson MD, et al. Electrocardiographic and electrophysiologic features of ventricular arrhythmias originating from the right/left coronary cusp commissure. Heart Rhythm. 2010;7:312–22.
7. Maeda S, Chik WW, Han Y, et al. Effects of age-related aortic root anatomic changes on left ventricular outflow tract pace-mapping morphologies: a cardiac magnetic resonance imaging validation study. J Cardiovasc Electrophysiol. 2015;20.
8. Yamada T, McElderry HT, Doppalapudi H, et al. Idiopathic ventricular arrhythmias originating from the left ventricular summit: anatomic concepts relevant to ablation. Circ Arrhythm Electrophysiol. 2010;3:616–23.
9. Santangeli P, Marchlinski FE, Zado ES, et al. Percutaneous epicardial ablation of ventricular arrhythmias arising from the left ventricular summit: outcomes and electrocardiogram correlates of success. Circ ArrhythmElectrophysiol. 2015;8:337–43.

Chapter 21
AS and HCM

Shabnam Madadi

Abstract LVH (left ventricular hypertrophy) is one of the most common presentations in aortic stenosis and sometimes it would be missed to evaluate for other causes of the LVH in the presence of AS. Combination of AS and hypertrophic CMP is not common too. In this case of such combination, HCM was missed until presentation with VT and apical aneurysm.

A 36-year-old man with history of aortic valve replacement (AVR) 8 years ago because of severe aortic stenosis (AS) and bicuspid aortic valve (BAV) presented with palpitation and cold sweating with hemodynamically compromised state and wide QRS tachycardia to the Emergency room (ER). Electrocardiography showed a wide QRS tachycardia with RBBB pattern and transition in V2, and superior axis, considering VT with left ventricular (LV) origin (Fig. 21.1, ER ECG was inaccessible so we used the figure of the 12 lead ECG of the induced VT in EP lab).

QRS Synchronized electrical cardioversion was done in the ER with 100 J and resulted in the termination of arrhythmia 0.12 lead ECG revealed LVH in normal sinus rhythm state (NSR).

Echocardiography was done by cardiology assistant and showed LVH with normal functioning prosthetic valve without significant valvular gradient. CMR was recommended because of the discrepancy between LVH and normal function of the prosthetic valve without significant size mismatch. CMR was done with 1.5 Tesla Aventus Siemens device and showed LVH with apical aneurysm and diffuse LGE with mid-cavity gradient, all findings infavour of HCM (Fig. 21.2a, b).

Because of history of sustained monomorphic VT (SMMVT), electrophysiological study (EPS) and mapping was done, using transseptal approach because of the prosthetic aortic valve. Substrate mapping during NSR revealed large low voltage

S. Madadi (✉)
Rajaie Cardiovascular Medical and Research Center, Iran University of Medical Sciences, Tehran, Iran
e-mail: madadi@rhc.ac.ir

M. Maleki, A. Alizadehasl (eds.), *Case-Based Clinical Cardiology*,
https://doi.org/10.1007/978-1-4471-7496-7_21

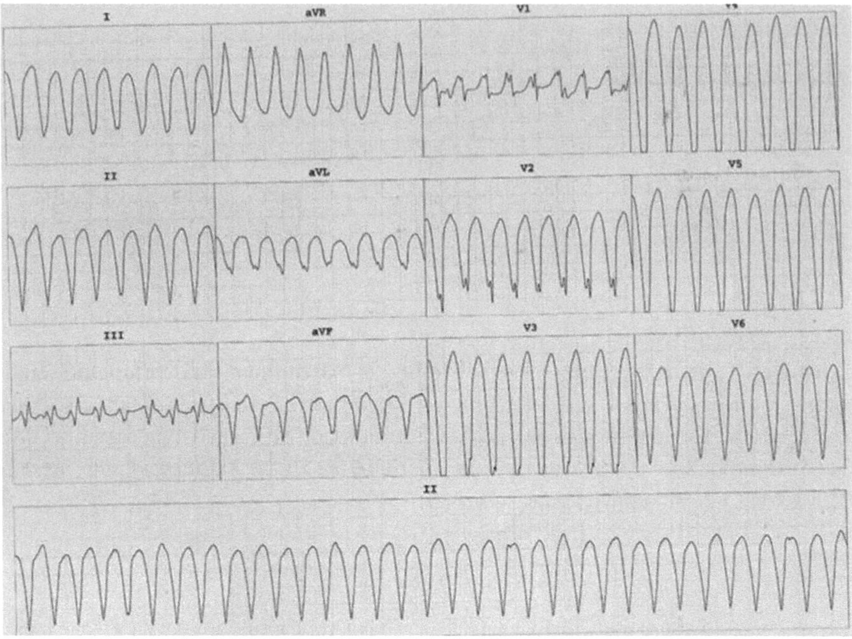

Fig. 21.1 VT with RBBB pattern, transition in V2, superior axis

apical area and activation mapping after VT induction showed reentrant VT around the apical aneurysm.

Radiofrequency ablation (RFA), using a cooled tip catheter with 30 W and 43 °C was done and the apical aneurysm was isolated (Fig. 21.3).

At the end of the procedure, VT was non-inducible. Then because of high-risk features of the patient, ICD was inserted.

Discussion

The coincidence of BAV and HCM was already described by Brown in 1990 in four adult patients [1–5]. The coincidence of HCM with other cardiomyopathies such as left ventricular noncompaction (LVNC) has been previously reported in some studies [6]. Also echocardiography remains now as a gold standard in examination of patients with HCM heart morphology, weak points of echocardiography are the anterolateral segments of the LV, Papillary muscles, Some Portions of the right ventricle (RV) and apex [7, 8]. CMR using gadolinium can reveal areas of fibrosis and also better clarify missing points of echocardiography. However, necrosis can be found in half of the patients suffering from hypertrophy of LV as a consequence of aortic stenosis or arterial hypertension but diffuse fibrosis with an apical aneurysm are seldom findings of BAV and AS, and strongly suggest HCM [9].

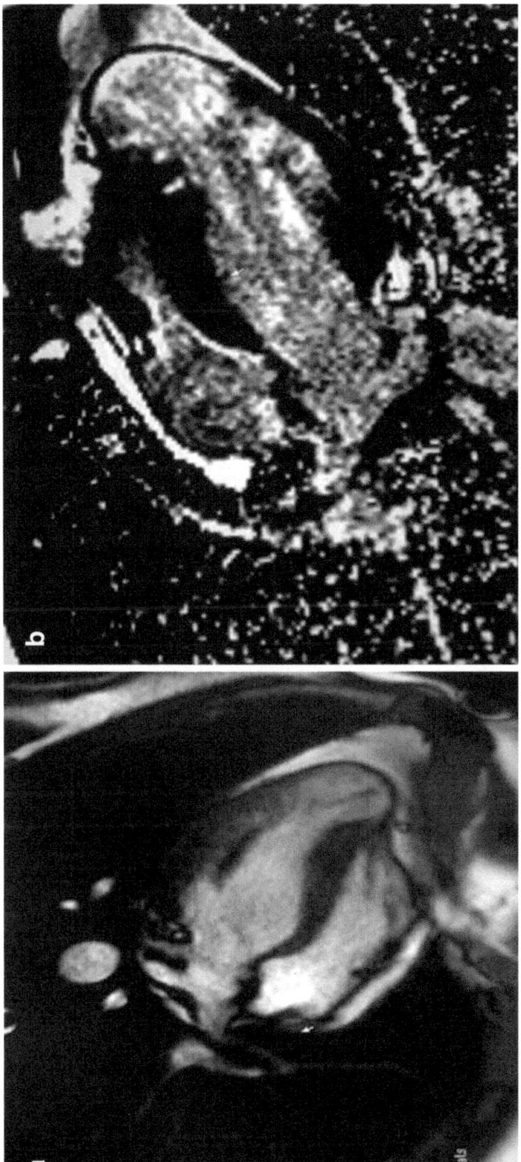

Fig. 21.2 (**a**, **b**) LV apical aneurysm with LGE

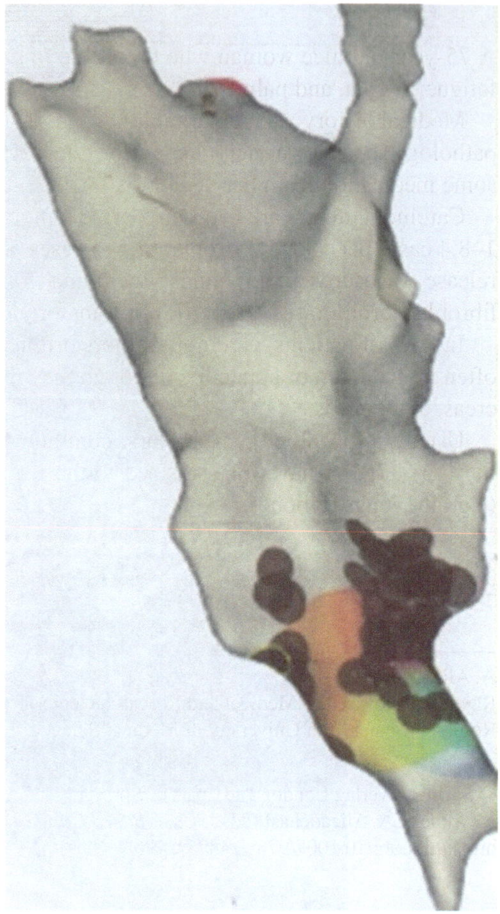

Fig. 21.3 Apical aneurysm core isolation using 3D Navx system

Late gadolinium enhancement in CMR in many studies has been suggested to be a high-risk predicting factor [9].

LV apical aneurysm is also a high-risk factor for arrhythmia.

In this patient despite arrhythmia ablation, ICD was implanted, because of high-risk features for sudden cardiac death [10].

References

1. Maron BJ, Gardin JM, Flack JM, Gidding SS, Kurosaki TT, Bild DE. Prevalence of hypertrophic cardiomyopathy in a general population of young adults. Echocardiographic analysis of 4111 subjects in the CARDIA study. Coronary artery risk development in (young) adults. Circulation. 1995;92:785–9.

2. Maron BJ, Ommen SR, Semsarian C, Spirito P, Olivotto I, Maron MS. Hypertrophic cardiomyopathy: present and future, with translation into contemporary cardiovascular medicine. Am Coll Cardiol. 2014;64:83–99.
3. Somerville J, McDonald Congenital L. Anomalies in the heart with hypertrophic cardiomyopathy. Br Heart J. 1968;30:713–22.
4. Obžut B, Blaško P, Porzer M. Coincidence of bicuspid aortic valve presence and hypertrophic cardiomyopathy, and significance of magnetic resonance in its diagnostics. Cor Vasa. 2013;55(3):e271–6.
5. Padang R, Gersh BJ, Ommen SR, Geske JB. Prevalence and impact of coexistent bicuspid aortic valve in hypertrophic cardiomyopathy. Heart Lung Circ. 2018;27(1):33–40. https://doi.org/10.1016/j.hlc.2017.01.020.
6. Alizadeh-Sani Z, Madadi S, Sadeghpour A, Khajali Z, Golnari P, Kiavar M. Cardiac MRI in a patient with coincident left ventricular non-compaction and hypertrophic cardiomyopathy. J Tehran Heart Cent. 2011;6(4):214–6.
7. Rudolph A, Abdel-Aty H, Bohl S, et al. Noninvasive detection of fibrosis applying contrast-enhanced cardiac magnetic resonance in different forms of left ventricular hypertrophy relation to remodeling. J Am Coll Cardiol. 2009;53:284–2913.
8. Naeini SJ, Parsaee M, Madadi S, Hosseini Z. Is there concordance between CMR and echocardiography in assessing aortic stenosis severity? Iranian Heart J. 2016;17(2):38–43.
9. Kyavar M, Mohammadi S, Madadi S. Relationship between syncope and sudden cardiac death in patients with hypertrophic cardiomyopathy and left ventricular mass index calculated by cardiac MRI. Iranian Heart J. 2015;16(1):12–9.
10. Madadi S, Emkanjoo Z, Aliakbar HP, Ahmadpour H. LV apical aneurysm and ventricular tachycardia in a patient with bicuspid aortic valve and hypertrophic cardiomyopathy. Iranian Heart J. 2018.

Chapter 22
Air Embolism During Septostomy

Shabnam Madadi

Abstract Systemic and coronary air embolism is one the complications in left heart catheterizations and also could be seen during septostomy. In this case we had it in a patient with left side accessory pathway during septostomy.

A 30-year-old female with a history of frequent episodes of supraventricular tachycardia presented with ECG manifestations of minimal left side accessory pathway and WPW syndrome.

An electrophysiologic study was performed in conscious sedation status, and diagnostic catheters were introduced via the left and right femoral vein.

Intracardiac electrograms were recorded using the Bard (Boston scientific) electrophysiology system.

The evaluation of the conduction system revealed the most fused AV signal in the left lateral side of the coronary sinus (CS) (Fig. 22.1).

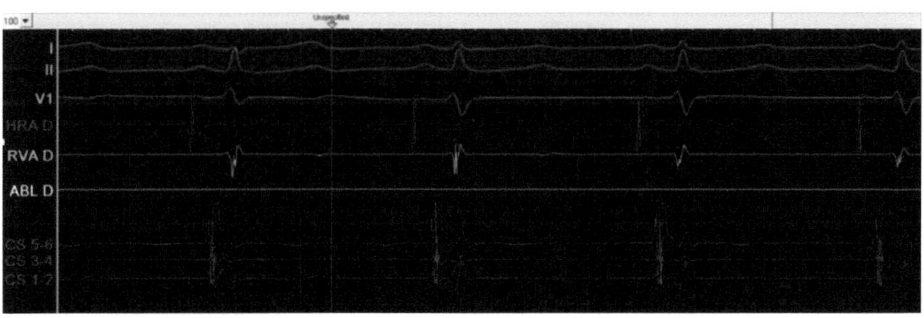

Fig. 22.1 The most fused AV signal in the left lateral side of the coronary sinus

S. Madadi (✉)
Rajaie Cardiovascular Medical and Research Center, Iran University of Medical Sciences, Tehran, Iran
e-mail: madadi@rhc.ac.ir

M. Maleki, A. Alizadehasl (eds.), *Case-Based Clinical Cardiology*,
https://doi.org/10.1007/978-1-4471-7496-7_22

The retrograde conduction pattern was also eccentric and the earliest retrograde atrial signal was recorded in the distal part of the CS during RV pacing.

A narrow QRS tachycardia was reproducibly inducible with programmed atrial and ventricular stimulation.

We attempted to do septostomy with Agillis long sheet (Agillis NxT™ Steerable Introducer, St. Jude Medical).

Needle was proceeded into the left atrium without the need for puncture of the interatrial septum.

Immediately after septostomy, we observed air bubbles in the left ventricular apex (Fig. 22.2).

Immediately 100% oxygen was administrated. Right femoral artery was cannulated and a pigtail catheter (Dawson–Mueller Drainage Catheter) was introduced via femoral artery with a retrograde approach into the left ventricular cavity and suction was done.

During suction ST elevation in the inferior leads was appeared with sinus bradycardia and manifest accessory pathway conduction infavor of AV block (Fig. 22.3).

Rapid RV pacing was done, 100% Oxygen was administrated and Inotrope was injected too. ST elevation was resolved in about 1–2 min.

The procedure was terminated without any attempt for ablation.

Propofol injection was omitted, after consciousness, the patient was alert and awake with obey to orders but with left side hemiparesis without left central hemifacial weakness.

Brain CT scan was done and was normal. The distal force of left upper extremity was resolved in about 1 h but yet the proximal force of the left arm and total force of the left leg was compromised. The neurologic consult was done and heparin drip and dexamethasone were recommended by the neurologist.

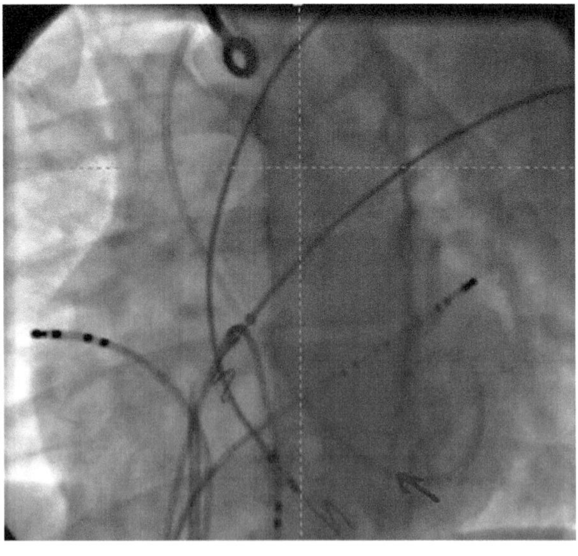

Fig. 22.2 Air bubbles in the left ventricular apex

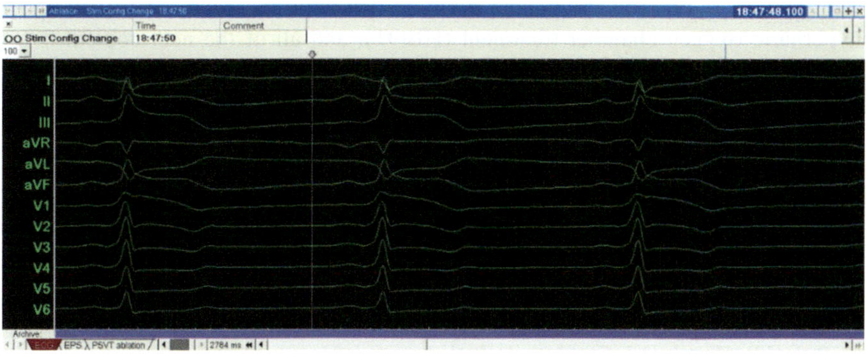

Fig. 22.3 Manifest AP with bradycardia and inferior ST elevation

After 24 h of procedure, all forces returned to normal status and after 72 h patient was discharged with the good general condition without any problem.

Follow-up of the patient showed no any problem and redo procedure was done 14 days later and the accessory pathway was successfully ablated via a retrograde approach.

Transesophageal echocardiography in the second admission revealed a patent foramen oval (PFO)with size about 2 × 5 mm and right to left shunt.

Discussion

RFA for WPW syndrome could be done via retrograde or transseptal approach. Retrograde approach may be associated with the risk of prolonged catheter manipulation and potential arrhythmogenic ventricular lesions created during ablation [1–3].

Potential risks can be avoided using transseptal atrial insertion. This approach was developed in 1950s and nowadays is on the most useful approaches for the ablation of the left-sided targets in electrophysiology studies [4].

Lesh et al. reported one case of coronary air embolism complicating transseptal radiofrequency ablation of the left lateral accessory pathway during catheter exchange and recommended continuous flushing with heparinized saline during catheter exchange.

Khurram et al. in 2016 reported a case of catastrophic coronary air embolism during AF ablation with massive air embolism into the RCA leading to the hemodynamic collapse and successful management with catheter-based coronary aspiration [3].

Murat Tulmac et al. reported a case of massive systemic air embolism during aortic root angiography in 2012, with the collapse of the patient and pulseless electrical activity. The patient became electrically stable shortly after cardiopulmonary resuscitation but she had a garbled speech and left hemiplegia with partial weakness and paresthesia in the right leg and arm. The brain CT was of the patient was normal such as our patient and the patient was transferred to the center with facility of hyperbaric oxygen chamber treatment (HBOT), and all of the neurological functions were normal after 1 day.

We do not have facility of HBOT but we administered 100% O_2 and after 24 h everything was normal and the patient was discharged after 72 h without any residual defect.

References

1. Park C-B, Hwang H-J, Cho J-M, Jo B-H, Kim C-J. Massive right coronary air embolism in the right coronary artery during left coronary angiography: a case report. Exp Ther Med. 2013;5(4):1073–4.
2. Voci P, Yang Y, Greco C, Nigri A, Critelli G. Coronary air embolism complicating accessory pathway catheter ablation: detection by echocardiography. J Am Soc Echocardiogr. 1994;7:312–4.
3. Ahmad K, Asirvatham S, Kamath S, Peck S, Liu X. Successful interventional management of catastrophic coronary arterial air embolism during atrial fibrillation ablation. Heart Rhythm Case Rep. 2016;2(2):153–6.
4. Khan M, Schmidt DH, Bajwa T, Shalev Y. Coronary air embolism: incidence, severity, and suggested approaches to treatment. Catheter Cardiovasc Diagn. 1995;36:313–8.

Chapter 23
Case 12: A 56 y/o Man, with Typical AFL

Shabnam Madadi

Abstract Any atrial flutter which is cavotricuspid isthmus dependent is typical AFL and creation a line of RFA in CTI is the ablation strategy.

Patient was a 56 y/o man, with Hx of PCI on LAD years ago, presented with two episodes of palpitation and documented ECG in favor of typical AFL.

LVEF about 50%, no significant valvular disease.

ECG: inverted saw tooth F wave in the inferior leads, low amplitude biphasic F wave in I, aVL, upright F wave in V1, and negative F wave in V6.

EPS

Activation mapping was done using multielectrode catheters introduced via right and left femoral vein.

Quadripolar catheters were positioned in HRA and RV and a decapolar catheter was positioned in CS. Some time we position a duo-decapolar catheter (Halo) in the right atrium around tricuspid valve annulus.

Patient was present to the EP lab in sinus rhythm, so induction of AFL was done by atrial programmed stimulation. A narrow QRS tachycardia with CL 280 ms was induced by electrical stimulation (Fig. 23.1).

The initial atrial activation was recorded at CS ostium for confirmation of the typical AFL using cavotricuspid isthmus entrainment mapping was done with pacing in the CTI and concealed entrainment revealed typical AFL with PPI and TCL difference less than 30 ms (Fig. 23.2).

S. Madadi (✉)
Rajaie Cardiovascular Medical and Research Center, Iran University of Medical Sciences, Tehran, Iran
e-mail: madadi@rhc.ac.ir

M. Maleki, A. Alizadehasl (eds.), *Case-Based Clinical Cardiology*,
https://doi.org/10.1007/978-1-4471-7496-7_23

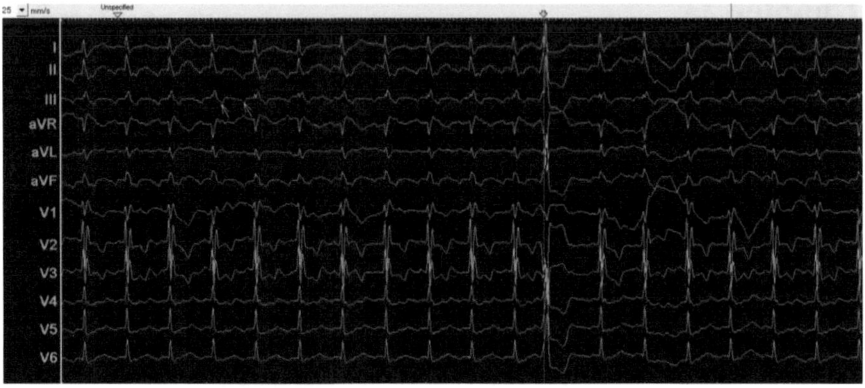

Fig. 23.1 Sawtooth F waves without isoelectric interval, negative in the inferior leads, positive in V1

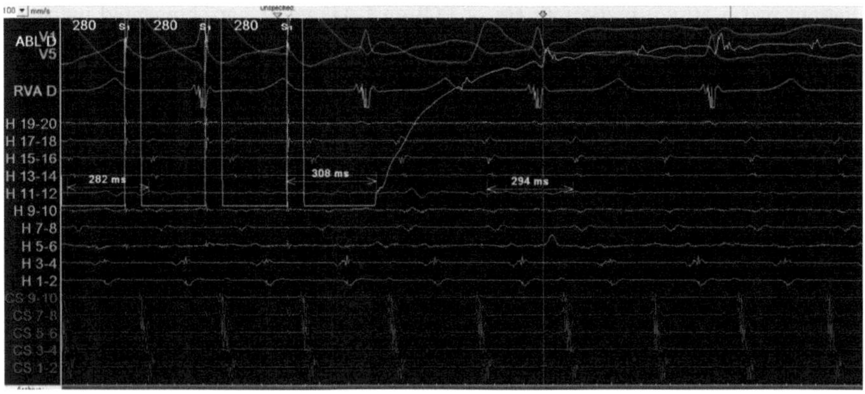

Fig. 23.2 Entrainment via ablation catheter positioned in CTI showed that arrhythmia is CTI dependent

Stimulus-to-F wave and stimulus-to-reference EGM interval and pacing EGM to F wave were the same during AFL and pacing.

For ablation of the CTI-dependent AFL, a line of RF ablation was created across the CTI and then bidirectional conduction block was checked across the CTI.

We usually use an external irrigated ablation catheter for ablation using a long steerable deflectable sheet (Agillis).

We commonly target the central isthmus for ablation, because is the narrowest site of CTI and also has a lower risk for AV block compared with the medial isthmus. In the case of the pouch in this site, lateral isthmus ablation is done, although it is thicker than central isthmus.

We usually use a maximal power of 35 W with a max temperature of 48 °C. Impedance drop about 10 Ω is acceptable (Fig. 23.3).

After the termination of flutter, bidirectional CTI block was checked, because of the persistence of CTI conduction, we tried to create a new line of RF ablation (Fig. 23.4 a, b).

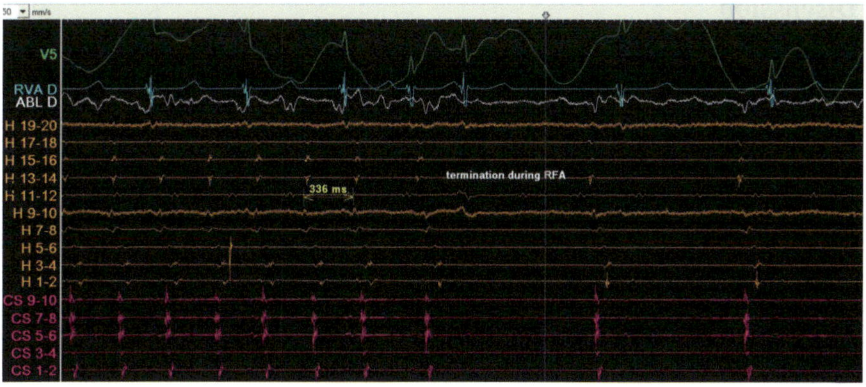

Fig. 23.3 Arrhythmia termination during RFA

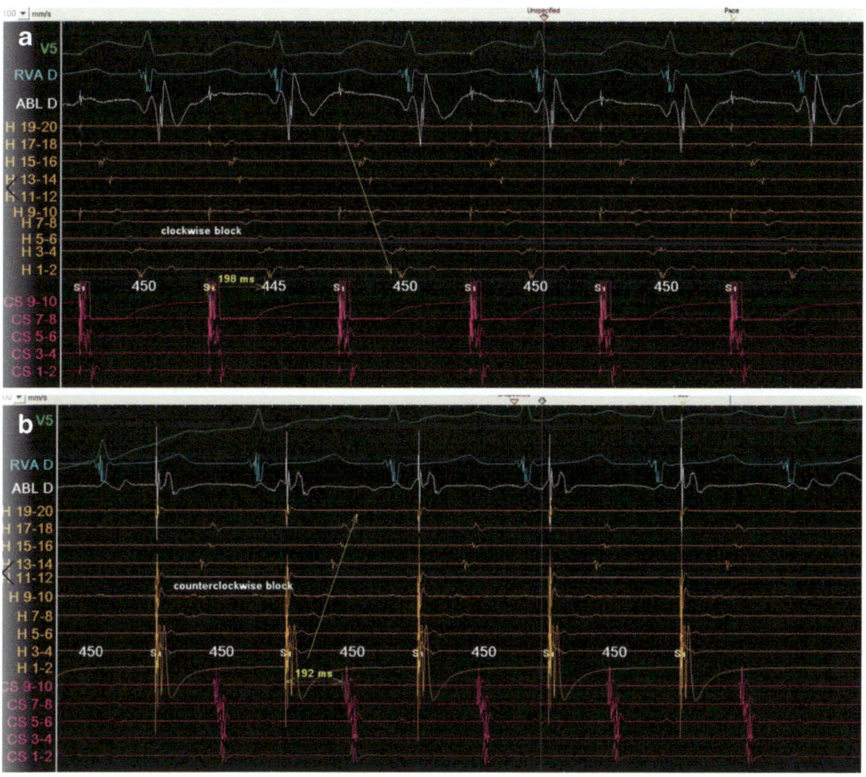

Fig. 23.4 (**a**, **b**) Bidirectional block across isthmus after ablation

Discussion

CTI-dependent atrial flatter is a common arrhythmia that often occurs in structural normal hearts. This arrhythmia often causes by a macro reentry in the right atrium around the tricuspid valve annulus and the slow conduction area at the lower posterior right atrium [1–3].

CTI is a portion of the right atrium between the TVA (tricuspid valve annulus) and IVC (inferior vena cava) and is anatomically bounded by the IVC and Eustachian ridge posteriorly and TVA anteriorly [3].

In about 80% of the patients, there is an inferior pouch in the CTI (sub-Eustachian pouch or sinus of Keith).

The posterior portion of the CTI is membranous part, near the IVC; the mid part is trabeculated portion and the anterior portion near the tricuspid valve is called vestibular (muscular portion) [3].

In the LAO view, CTI is divided into three portions: medical isthmus at 5 o'clock; central isthmus at 6 o'clock and lateral isthmus that is positioned at 7 o'clock. The central isthmus is the narrowest part and easy for ablation, but sometimes because of the presence of the pouches it may be difficult to do ablate at this site and lateral and then medial isthmus if need could be tried for ablation [2, 3].

There are three other macro reentrant tachycardias in this area:

Lower loop reentry, partial isthmus flutter, and intra-isthmus reentry.

Lower loop reentry is also isthmus dependent and in which the circuit is essentially around the ostium of the IVC in the right atrium and the direction of rotation may be clockwise or counterclockwise [4–7].

In this reentry caudal to cranial activation in the right atrium crosses over gaps in the crista terminalis in the low RA to middle RA. There is a collision in the lateral RA that results in a decrease in the inferior forces. In lower loop reentry there is evidence of concealed entrainment in the CTI and also inferior-posterior of the RA.

In partial isthmus flutter, reentrant wave short circuits through the Eustachian ridge to pass between the IVC and CS ostium. In this type of AFL, concealed entrainment is present in the lateral isthmus but not medical isthmus. There is also early activation of the CS ostium and collision in the medical CTI. Intra-isthmus reentry is a micro reentry localized within the septal region of the CTI.

We used a maximal power of 35 W with max temperature of 48 °C. Impedance drop about 10 Ω was acceptable [8].

References

1. Saoudi N, Cosio F, Waldo A, et al. Classification of atrial flutter and regular atrial tachycardia according to electrophysiologic mechanism and anatomic bases: a statement from a joint expert group from the working group of arrhythmias of the European Society of Cardiology and the North American Society of Pacing and Electrophysiology. J Cardiovasc Electrophysiol. 2001;12:852–66.

2. Feld GK, Fleck RP, Chen PS, et al. Radiofrequency catheter ablation for the treatment of human type 1 atrial flutter: identification of a critical zone in the re-entrant circuit by endocardial mapping techniques. Circulation. 1992;86:1233–40.
3. Cosio FG, Lopez-Gil M, Goicolea A, et al. Radiofrequency ablation of the inferior vena cava-tricuspid valve isthmus in common atrial flutter. Am J Cardiol. 1993;71:705–9.
4. Jais P, Haissaguerre M, Shah DC, et al. Successful irrigated-tip catheter ablation of atrial flutter resistant to conventional radiofrequency ablation. Circulation. 1998;98:835–8.
5. Atiga WL, Worley SJ, Hummel J, et al. Prospective randomized comparison of cooled radiofrequency versus standard radiofrequency energy for ablation of typical atrial flutter. Pacing Clin Electrophysiol. 2002;25:1172–8.
6. Scavee C, Jais P, Hsu LF, et al. Prospective randomized comparison of irrigated-tip and large-tip catheter ablation of cavotricuspid isthmus-dependent atrial flutter. Eur Heart J. 2004;25:963–9.
7. Calkins H. Catheter ablation of atrial flutter: do outcomes of catheter ablation with "large-tip" versus "cooled-tip" catheters really differ. J Cardiovasc Electrophysiol. 2004;15:1131–2.
8. Matsuo S, Yamane T, Tokuda M, et al. Prospective randomized comparison of a steerable versus a non-steerable sheath for typical atrial flutter ablation. Europace. 2010;12:402–9.

Chapter 24
An Atypical Roof Dependent AFL

Shabnam Madadi

Abstract A case of valvular heart disease presented with frequent episodes of palpitations and atypical AFL in ECG, EPS was done and entrainment study showed that the isthmus of the arrhythmia was in LA roof and ablation in that area resulted in termination of the arrhythmia.

Introduction

Patient was a 58 y/o man, with moderate MS and moderate MR, presented with frequent episodes of palpitations, not responsive to medical treatment, and candidated for ablation.

ECG showed a narrow QRS tachycardia with 2:1 AV association and AFL appearance and positive F waves in the inferior leads and V1 and positive F waves n V6 also. EPS was done using a halo catheter in RA, one quadripolar catheter in RV, and A decapolar catheter in CS.

EPS demonstrated a narrow QRS tachycardia with 2:1 AV conduction; CS activation was distal to proximal, arrhythmia CL was about 250 ms.

EPS

Using halo catheter in RA there was evidence of early septal activation in RA and fusion of wavefronts in the RA lateral wall. RA mapping should <50% of tachycardia cycle length.

Entrainment mapping in multiple cites of RA resulted in post-pacing interval more than 30 ms, all of findings were infavor of left side atrial macro reentrant

S. Madadi (✉)
Rajaie Cardiovascular Medical and Research Center, Iran University of Medical Sciences, Tehran, Iran
e-mail: madadi@rhc.ac.ir

M. Maleki, A. Alizadehasl (eds.), *Case-Based Clinical Cardiology*,
https://doi.org/10.1007/978-1-4471-7496-7_24

tachycardia and there was a distal to proximal CS activity; all of above findings were infavor of left side AFL.

After septostomy, entrainment mapping of the multiple sites in LA was done. CS proximal and distal entrainment showed manifest fusion and PPI–TCL > 30 ms, so perimetral reentry was ruled out and other sites in LA were mapped and entrainment was done in other sites.

In 3D mapping using the Navx velocity system, there was the presence of areas of early activation adjacent to late regions.

During mapping of the LA roof there were low voltage areas and entrainment study in the roof demonstrated concealed fusion with very short PPI–TCL difference so, RFA was done using irrigated tip catheter with power 20 W and target temperature 43 °C and resulted in tachycardia cycle length prolongation and termination of the arrhythmia (Figs. 24.1 and 24.2).

Roof line RFA (radiofrequency ablation) from left to right superior pulmonary veins was completed and pacing in the anterior and posterior walls showed bidirectional block and no evidence of conduction recurrence after 30 min.

Discussion

Macroreentrant circuits not dependent on the cavotricuspid isthmus are called atypical atrial flutter. Atypical flutter in contrast with typical AFL mostly occurs in organic heart disease [1–3].

In the ECG, in focal atrial tachycardia P wave durations are shorter and isoelectric interval are longer than macroreentrant atrial tachycardia.

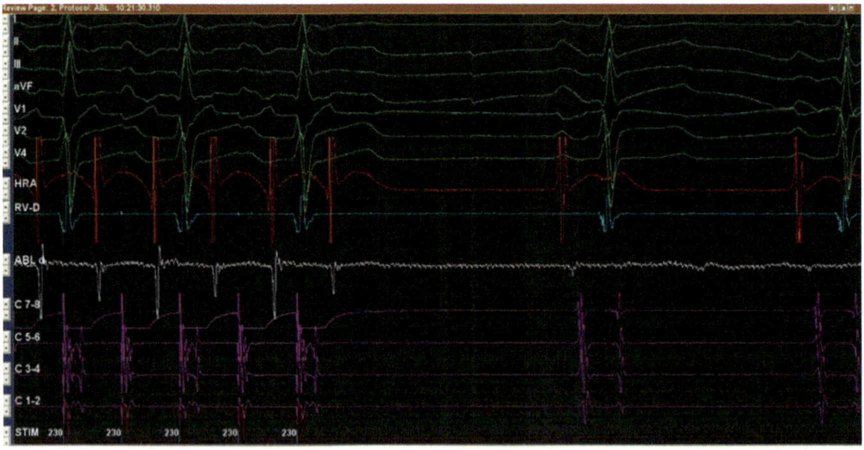

Fig. 24.1 Entrainment maneuver in LA roof, terminated the arrhythmia infavor of protected isthmus site of arrhythmia

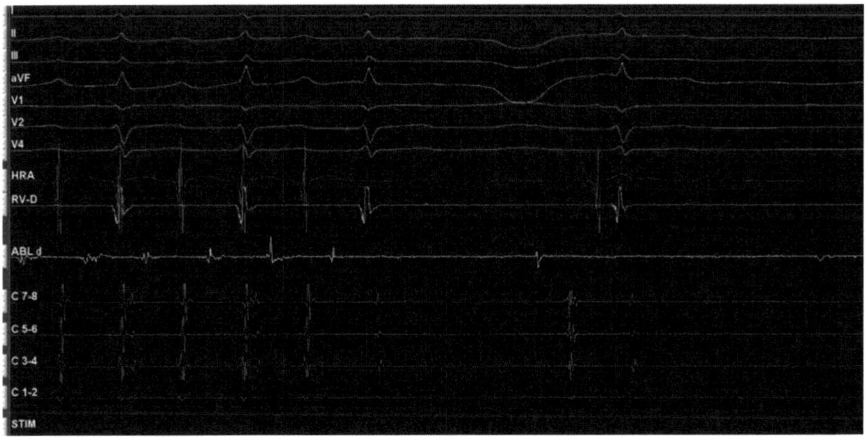

Fig. 24.2 Termination of the arrhythmia with ablation

Flutter waves arising from RA are predominantly negative in V1, but broad positive F waves in V1 without any isoelectric or negative initial component arise from LA mostly [4].

In circuit entrainment, from anterior and posterior LA demonstrates roof dependent LA reentry. Distal to proximal CS activity is strongly infavor of LA reentry, although proximal to distal CS activity may be seen in both RA and LA macroreentrant tachycardia.

Mostly, in roof dependent LA marcoreentry Chevron and reverse Chevron patterns occur.

Chevron pattern occurs when LA activation is done via descending a wavefront from posterior walls then propagating in both septal and lateral dimensions [5].

The reverse chevron occurs when wavefronts descend the anterior LA wall and then propagate to the posterior LA wall.

In this patient, although there was a roof dependent AFL absence of Chevron or reverse Chevron pattern may be due to accelerated conduction via Backmann's bundle.

According to the concealed entrainment in the LA roof and successful ablation in that area, the mechanism of the arrhythmia was strongly considered to be roof dependent AFL.

There are multiple variants of non-isthmus-dependent AFL such as upper loop reentry, right atrial free wall reentry, and dual loop reentry in the right atrium and perimitral annulus reentry, roof dependent reentry and periseptal reentry in the left atrium.

In addition, lesion tachycardia can occur on each side of atrial fibrosis following atriotomy or after Maze surgery [6].

So the first step for an approach to such arrhythmia is to confirm the mechanism of the arrhythmia that is reentry or not. Then entrainment maneuvers should be done in CTI for rule/out of typical AFL.

Then entrainment mapping in lateral septal sides in RA and proximal and distal CS, then anterior and posterior LA, could demonstrate the position of the reentrant circuit [7].

Electroanatomical mapping with mapping of the >90% of the tachycardia cycle length, could be helpful. A hallmark of macroreentrant arrhythmia in 3D mapping is the presence of the areas that earliest meets the latest [8, 9].

It should be noted that very low voltage areas can be the critical components of the tachycardia circuits. RFA with irrigated tip catheter and impendence drop of 10 Ω could be more effective than nonirrigated tip areas [10].

References

1. Saoudi N, Cosio F, Waldo A, et al. Classification of atrial flutter and regular atrial tachycardia according to electrophysiologic mechanism and anatomic bases: a statement from a joint expert group from the working group of arrhythmias of the European Society of Cardiology and the North American Society of Pacing and Electrophysiology. J Cardiovasc Electrophysiol. 2001;12:852–66.
2. Shah D. ECG manifestations of left atrial flutter. Curr Opin Cardiol. 2009;24:35–41.
3. Fukamizu S, Sakurada H, Hayashi T, et al. Macroreentrant atrial tachycardia in patients without previous atrial surgery or catheter ablation: clinical and electrophysiological characteristics of scar-related left atrial anterior wall reentry. J Cardiovasc Electrophysiol. 2013;24:404–12.
4. Pap R, Kohari M, Makai A, et al. Surgical technique and the mechanism of atrial tachycardia late after open heart surgery. J Interv Card Electrophysiol. 2012;35:127–35.
5. Brown JP, Krummen DE, Feld GK, Narayan SM. Using electrocardiographic activation time and diastolic intervals to separate focal from macro- re-entrant atrial tachycardias. J Am Coll Cardiol. 2007;49:1965–73.
6. Yokokawa M, Latchamsetty R, Ghanbari H, et al. Characteristics of atrial tachycardia because of small vs large reentrant circuits after ablation of persistent atrial fibrillation. Heart Rhythm. 2013;10:469–76.
7. Yang Y, Cheng J, Bochoeyer A, et al. Atypical right atrial flutter patterns. Circulation. 2001;103:3092–8.
8. Kall JG, Rubenstein DS, Kopp DE, et al. Atypical atrial flutter originating in the right atrial free wall. Circulation. 2000;101:270–9.
9. Almendral J. Resetting and entrainment of reentrant arrhythmias: part II: informative content and practical use of these responses. Pacing Clin Electrophysiol. 2013;36:641–61.
10. Barbhaiya CR, Kumar S, Ng J, et al. Avoiding tachycardia alteration or termination during attempted entrainment mapping of atrial tachycardia related to atrial fibrillation ablation. Heart Rhythm. 2015;12:32–5.

Chapter 25
AF Cryoballoon: Pulmonary Vein Isolation in a Patient with Amplatzer ASD Closure Device

Shabnam Madadi

Abstract Patient with Hx of ASD closure with Amplatzer, presented with AF rhythm and pulmonary vein isolation was done with cryoablation.

A 50 y/o man, with Hx of ASD closure (Amlatzer), with frequent episodes of palpitation, no one last more than 24 h, without any history of CAD risk factor, presented with AF rhythm, and with the diagnosis of paroxysmal AF; non responding to anti-arrhythmic drugs, referred for pulmonary vein isolation. After talk with patient about pros and cons of the two most available ablation strategies for AF (Cryoballoon and radiofrequency), the patient selected cryoballoon ablation so she was scheduled for cryoballoon ablation.

EPS was started with introducing one decapolar catheter and another quadripolar catheter for recording and stimulation of the CS and RV potentials, respectively.

Electrophysiology study for AF trigger was done and there was no evidence of any promoting arrhythmia. AF was induced reproducibly by AES and converted to sinus rhythm by cardioversion (Fig. 25.1).

So we started for cryoballoon ablation, after septostomy and introducing Flexcath catheter, which has 12 F line diameter and 14.5 F outer diameter. It was challenging because of Amplatzer device (Fig. 25.2).

Heparin was administered with target ACT about 300–350 ms.

In contrast with other septostomies for left lateral accessory pathway ablation and other types of the left side arrhythmia, a recommended approach for transseptal puncture in AF cryoballoon PVI (Pulmonary Vein Isolation) is a low and anterior transseptal puncture, at the lower limbs of the septum. We used second-generation cryoballoon, Arctic front advance, 28 mm, for our patient.

S. Madadi (✉)
Rajaie Cardiovascular Medical and Research Center, Iran University of Medical Sciences, Tehran, Iran
e-mail: madadi@rhc.ac.ir

M. Maleki, A. Alizadehasl (eds.), *Case-Based Clinical Cardiology*,
https://doi.org/10.1007/978-1-4471-7496-7_25

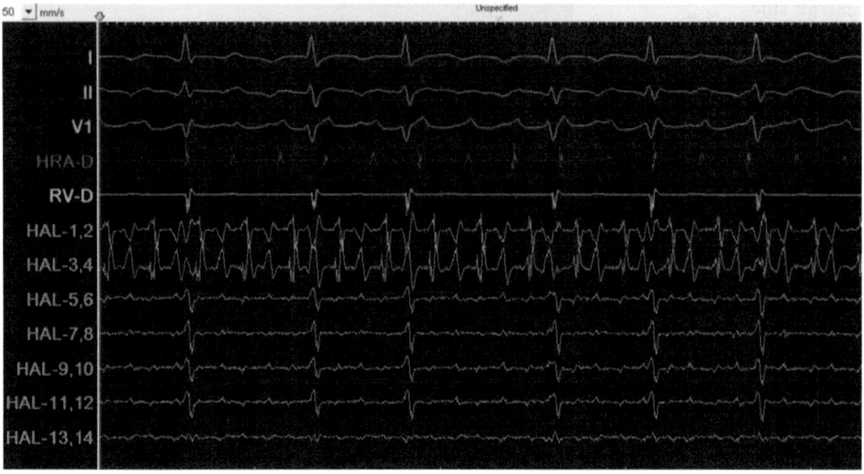

Fig. 25.1 AF induction during EPS

Fig. 25.2 Septostomy was done after several attempts. Dye staining in the septum of previous tries is present

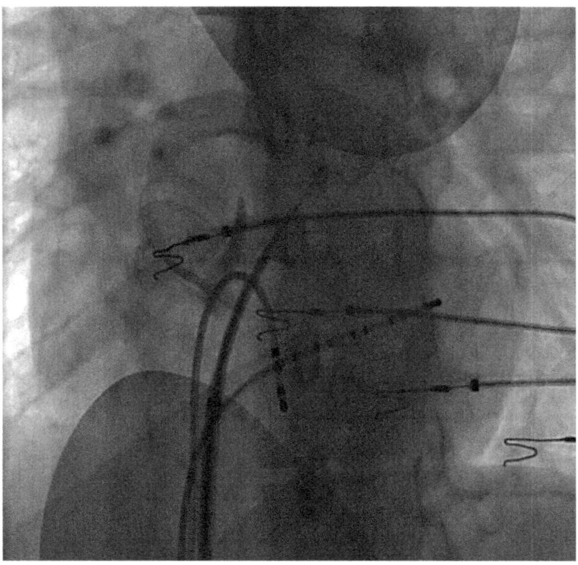

After introducing cryoballoon via catheter sheet, we accessed the PVs using achieve catheter, then the cryoballoon was inflated in the left atrium and engaged the PV antrum, and if the PV occlusion was confirmed with contrast injection, ablation was started by proximal seal method.

In the proximal seal method, ablation initiates for approximately 3 s to allow for cryoballoon expansion, then the balloon advances toward the antrum (Figs. 25.3, 25.4, 25.5 and 25.6).

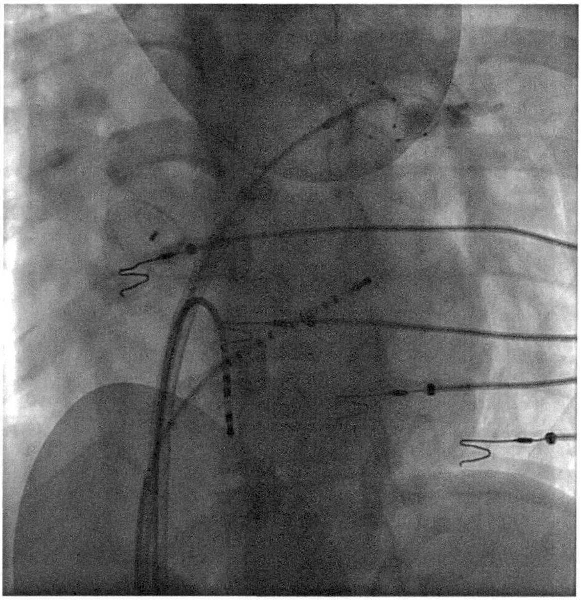

Fig. 25.3 Complete occlusion of LUPV with cryoballoon, before freezing

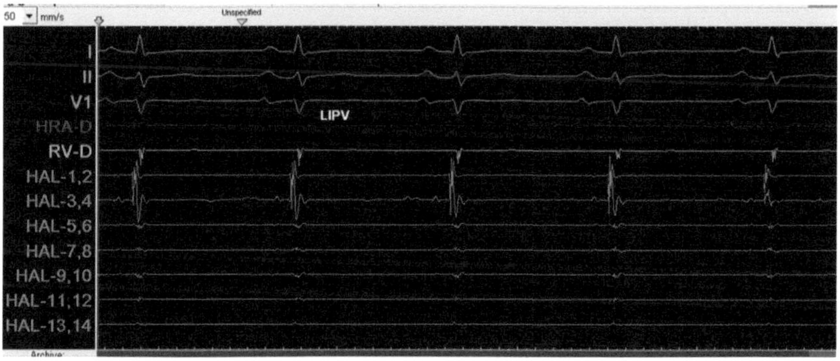

Fig. 25.4 Silent LUPV after ablation

Regarding TIT (Tissue to Isolation), ablation was continued for 180 s or 240 s, in each PV. Phrenic nerve reservation was checked in the right PVs, during ablation. PV potentials were disappeared after ablation.

Ablation was terminated without any major and minor complications.

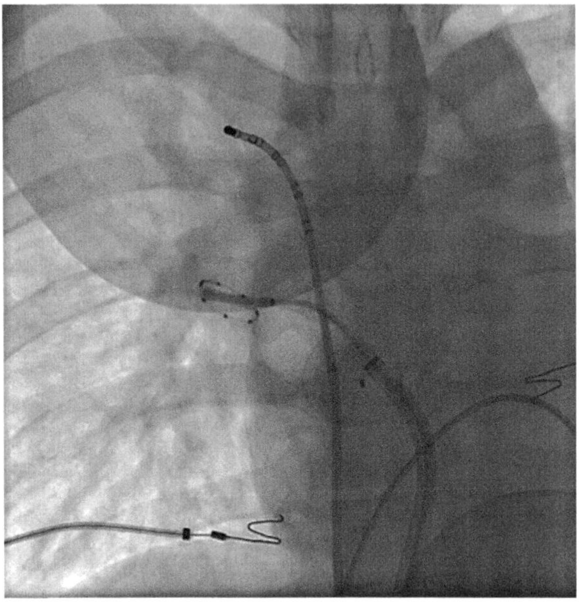

Fig. 25.5 RUPV cryoablation

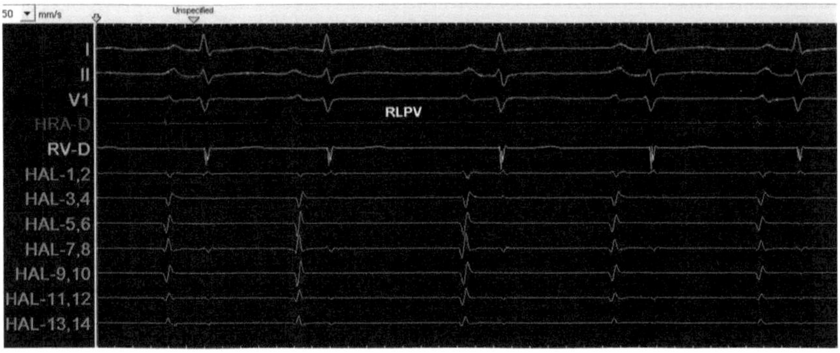

Fig. 25.6 Silent RUPV after ablation

Discussion

According to the 2014 H ACC/AHA/AHRS guidelines and 2017 (HRS/EHRA) expert consensus, there is a class I indication for catheter ablation of drug refractory, symptomatic paroxysmal AF and a class IIa indication for persistent AF that is drug refractory and symptomatic [1].

AF affected more than 33 million people worldwide. AF with less than 7 days duration is defined as paroxysmal AF and early persistent AF is now defined as sustaining for less than 3 months but more than 7 days [1–3].

In 1998, Haissaguerre et al., published that PV triggers, often initiate AF and reported that elimination of these potentials may eliminated AF in some patients. Now, pulmonary vein isolation is the cornerstone of AF ablation and could be done by electrical isolation via antral PV modification [4, 5].

Unlike traditional focal ablation, cryoballoon ablation achieves wide, homogenous, and large antral modification.

Rate of complications such as pulmonary vein stenosis, atrial-esophageal fistula, stroke, and death with cryoballoon ablation is reported but are less than traditional radiofrequency ablation [6–8].

In conclusion, cryoballoon ablation is a safe and more predictable toolset for a reliable large area PV antral modification, for the treatment of AF [8].

References

1. Calkins H, Kuck KH, Cappato R, et al. Heart rhythm society task force on catheter and surgical ablation of atrial fibrillation. 2012HRS/EHRA/ECAS expert consensus statement on catheter and surgical ablation of atrial fibrillation: recommendations for patient selection, procedural techniques, patient management and follow-up, definitions, endpoints, and research trial design: a report of the Heart Rhythm Society (HRS) Task Force on Catheter and Surgical Ablation of Atrial Fibrillation. Developed in partnership with the European Heart Rhythm Association (EHRA), a registered branch of the European Society of Cardiology (ESC) and the European Cardiac Arrhythmia Society (ECAS); and in collaboration with the American College of Cardiology (ACC), American Heart Association (AHA), the Asia Pacific Heart Rhythm Society (APHRS), and the Society of Thoracic Surgeons (STS). Endorsed by the governing bodies of the American College of Cardiology Foundation, the American Heart Association, the European Cardiac Arrhythmia Society, the European Heart Rhythm Association, the Society of Thoracic Surgeons, the Asia Pacific Heart Rhythm Society, and the Heart Rhythm Society. Heart Rhythm. 2012;9(4):632–96.
2. Haïssaguerre M, Jaïs P, Shah DC, et al. Spontaneous initiation of atrial fibrillation by ectopic beats originating in the pulmonary veins. N Engl J Med. 1998;339(10):659–66.
3. Avitall B, Urboniene D, Rozmus G, et al. New cryotechnology for electrical isolation of the pulmonary veins. J Cardiovasc Electrophysiol. 2003;14(3):281–186.
4. Van Belle Y, Janse P, Rivero-Ayerza MJ, et al. Pulmonary vein isolation using an occluding cryoballoon for circumferential ablation: feasibility, complications, and short-term outcome. Eur Heart J. 2007;28(18):2231–7.
5. Packer DL, Kowal RC, Wheelan KR, STOP AF Cryoablation Investigators, et al. Cryoballoon ablation of pulmonary veins for paroxysmal atrial fibrillation: first results of the North American Arctic Front (STOP AF) pivotal trial. J Am Coll Cardiol. 2013;61(16):1713–23.
6. Schmidt M, Dorwarth U, Andresen D, et al. Cryoballoon versus RF ablationin paroxysmal atrial fibrillation: results from the German ablation registry. J Cardiovasc Electrophysiol. 2014;25(1):1–7.
7. Okumura K, et al. Safety and efficacy of cryoballoon ablation for paroxysmal atrial fibrillation in Japan – results from the Japanese prospective post-market surveillance study. Circ J. 2016;80(8):1744–9.
8. Kuck KH, et al. Cryoballoon or radiofrequency ablation for symptomatic paroxysmal atrial fibrillation: reintervention, rehospitalization, and quality-of-life outcomes in the FIRE AND ICE trial. Eur Heart J. 2016;37(38):2235–45.

Chapter 26
AF Radiofrequency Ablation Using CARTO 3D System

Shabnam Madadi

Abstract Radiofrequency ablation of paroxysmal AF is Class I indication for drug refractory, symptomatic cases. In this case we did it for a highly symptomatic lady using CARTO 3D mapping system.

A 56 y/o lady presented with four episodes of palpitation and documented paroxysmal AF, nonresponsive to medical therapy, referred for pulmonary veins isolation.

Methods

PV isolation is the cornerstone of catheter ablation of AF.

Haussaguerre et al. first time demonstrated that focal discharges from pulmonary veins could be triggers for initiation of AF and ablation of the sources of such discharges could diminish paroxysmal AF episodes [1–3].

In patients with symptomatic paroxysmal AF who have failed treatment with optimal antiarrhythmic drugs, pulmonary vein isolation is a class I indication. All patients with paroxysmal AF, who are candidate for PV isolation should discontinue antiarrhythmic drugs for at least 3–5 half-lives for evaluation about AF triggers [4–6].

In case of Amiodarone, it is recommended to discontinue the drug for 4–6 months before ablation. We usually use Warfarin or factor Xa inhibitors in the preablation setting.

After vascular access obtaining we administer Heparin (100 IU/kg up to 10,000 IU for warfarin and up to 12,000–15,000 IU with factor Xa inhibitors [7–9].

The target ACT is about 350–400 s. PV triggers are the dominant mechanism of initiation of AF.

S. Madadi (✉)
Rajaie Cardiovascular Medical and Research Center, Iran University of Medical Sciences, Tehran, Iran
e-mail: madadi@rhc.ac.ir

M. Maleki, A. Alizadehasl (eds.), *Case-Based Clinical Cardiology*,
https://doi.org/10.1007/978-1-4471-7496-7_26

Our approach to PVI is wide antral ablation. Almost always we use 3-Dimentional electroanatomical system such as Precision Navx or CARTO mapping [10–13].

Sometimes we do double septostomy but often we use sequential mapping and ablation of the PV potentials [14, 15].

We use open irrigated catheters with Max power of 23 W for the posterior wall and 25 W for anterior walls.

The end point of PVI is the entrance and exit block in PVs. In this case, we used CARTO mapping system (Fig. 26.1a, b).

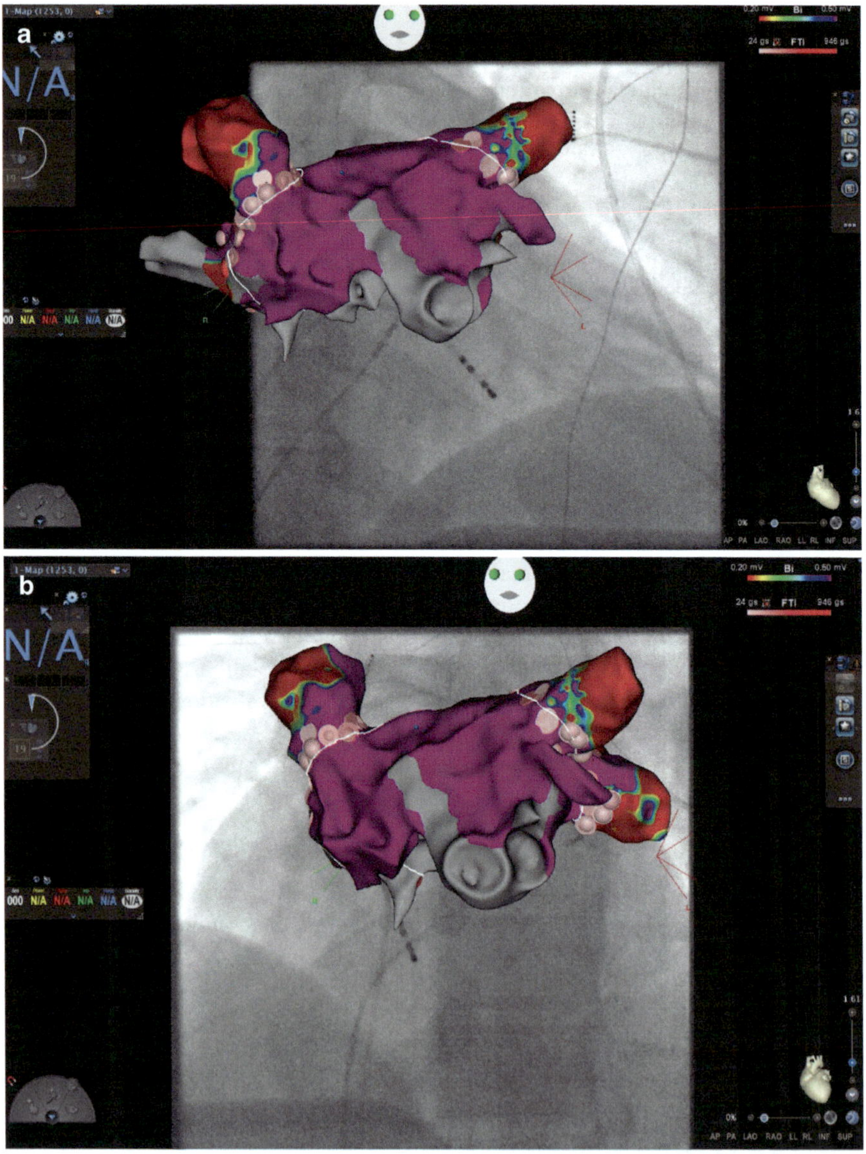

Fig. 26.1 (**a**, **b**) PVI using CARTO mapping system

Discussion

We used 3D CARTO mapping system in this case. After deep anesthesia and vascular and left atrial access, we ablated a wide antral region of four PVs sequentially and checked entrance and exit block in each PV.

Optimal anticoagulation using Heparin with ACT 350–400 s was achieved during the procedure.

Sometimes we do double septostomy and use circular mapping catheters for recording of PV potentials, but in this case, we did only single septostomy and sequentially checked for PV potentials.

After isolation of all PVs, we checked for reconnection (without Isuprel) and the procedure terminated successfully.

References

1. Wazni OM, Marrouche NF, Martin DO, et al. Radiofrequency ablation vs antiarrhythmic drugs as first-line treatment of symptomatic atrial fibrillation: a randomized trial. JAMA. 2005;293:2634–40.
2. Jaïs P, Cauchemez B, Macle L, et al. Catheter ablation versus antiarrhythmic drugs for atrial fibrillation: the A4 study. Circulation. 2008;118:2498–505.
3. Wilber DJ, Neuzil P, De Paola A, et al. Comparison of antiarrhythmic drug therapy and radiofrequency catheter ablation in patients with paroxysmal atrial fibrillation. J Am Med Assoc. 2013;303:333–40.
4. Haïssaguerre M, Jaïs P, Shah DC, et al. Spontaneous initiation of atrial fibrillation by ectopic beats originating in the pulmonary veins. N Engl J Med. 1998;339(10):659–66.
5. Calkins H, Hindricks G, Cappato R, et al. 2017 HRS/EHRA/ECAS/APHRS/SOLAECE expert consensus statement on catheter and surgical ablation of atrial fibrillation. Heart Rhythm. 2017;14(10):e275–444. https://doi.org/10.1016/j.hrthm.2017.05.012.
6. January CT, Wann LS, Alpert JS, et al. 2014 AHA/ACC/HRS guideline for the management of patients with atrial fibrillation. J Am Coll Cardiol. 2014;64:e1–76.
7. Kirchhof P, Benussi S, Kotecha D, et al. 2016 ESC guidelines for the management of atrial fibrillation developed in collaboration with EACTS. Europace. 2016;18(11):1609–78.
8. Di Biase L, Conti S, Mohanty P, et al. General anesthesia reduces the prevalence of pulmonary vein reconnection during repeat ablation when compared with conscious sedation: results from a randomized study. Heart Rhythm. 2011;8:368–72.
9. Hutchinson MD, Garcia FC, Mandel JE, et al. Efforts to enhance catheter stability improve atrial fibrillation ablation outcome. Heart Rhythm. 2013;10:347–53.
10. Cosedis Nielsen J, Johannessen A, Raatikainen P, et al. Radiofrequency ablation as initial therapy in paroxysmal atrial fibrillation. N Engl J Med. 2012;367:1587–95.
11. Morillo CA, Verma A, Connolly SJ, et al. Radiofrequency ablation vs antiarrhythmic drugs as first-line treatment of paroxysmal atrial fibrillation (RAAFT-2). JAMA. 2014;311:692.
12. Mohanty S, Di Biase L, Mohanty P, et al. Effect of periprocedural amiodarone on procedure outcome in patients with longstanding persistent atrial fibrillation undergoing extended pulmonary vein antrum isolation: results from a randomized study (SPECULATE). Heart Rhythm. 2015;12:477–83.
13. Di Biase L, Burkhardt JD, Santangeli P, et al. Periprocedural stroke and bleeding complications in patients undergoing catheter ablation of atrial fibrillation with different anticoagulation management: results from the role of Coumadin in preventing thromboembolism in

atrial fibrillation (AF) patients undergoing catheter ablation (COMPARE) randomized trial. Circulation. 2014;129(25):2638–44.
14. Cappato R, Marchlinski FE, Hohnloser SH, et al. Uninterrupted rivaroxaban vs. uninterrupted vitamin K antagonists for catheter ablation in non-valvular atrial fibrillation. Eur Heart J. 2015;36:1805–18011.
15. Calkins H, Willems S, Gerstenfeld EP, et al. Uninterrupted dabigatran versus warfarin for ablation in atrial fibrillation. N Engl J Med. 2017;376:1627–36.

Chapter 27
Epicardial Approach for VT Ablation in an ARVC Case

Shabnam Madadi

Abstract A young old man, with frequent episodes of VT, referred for ablation suspected for sarcoidosis and ARVC in CMR, after ICD implantation presented with VT storm, without any endocardial scar and with extensive epicardial scar in voltage mapping, so epicardial VT ablation was done.

Patient was a 36 y/o man, referred from elsewhere with diagnosis of RVOT–VT and hemodynamic compromise and termination of the arrhythmia with D/C shock. Echocardiography revealed moderate RV dysfunction and mild LV dysfunction, so cardiac MRI was recommended for patient.

Cardiac MRI revealed patchy areas of Late gadolinium enhancement (LGE) suggesting fibrosis in the RV inflow and outflow tract and another site of LGE in the mid posterolateral wall of LV with LVEF about 45%, and moderate RV dysfunction.

Patient was infertile.

The first diagnosis in cardiac MRI was Sarcoidosis and ARVC was recommended as the second diagnosis (Fig. 27.1a, b).

ICD was implanted for patients.

He refused ablation so was referred for Rheumatology consult.

Three weeks later he presented with VT storm.

S. Madadi (✉)
Rajaie Cardiovascular Medical and Research Center, Iran University of Medical Sciences, Tehran, Iran
e-mail: madadi@rhc.ac.ir

M. Maleki, A. Alizadehasl (eds.), *Case-Based Clinical Cardiology*,
https://doi.org/10.1007/978-1-4471-7496-7_27

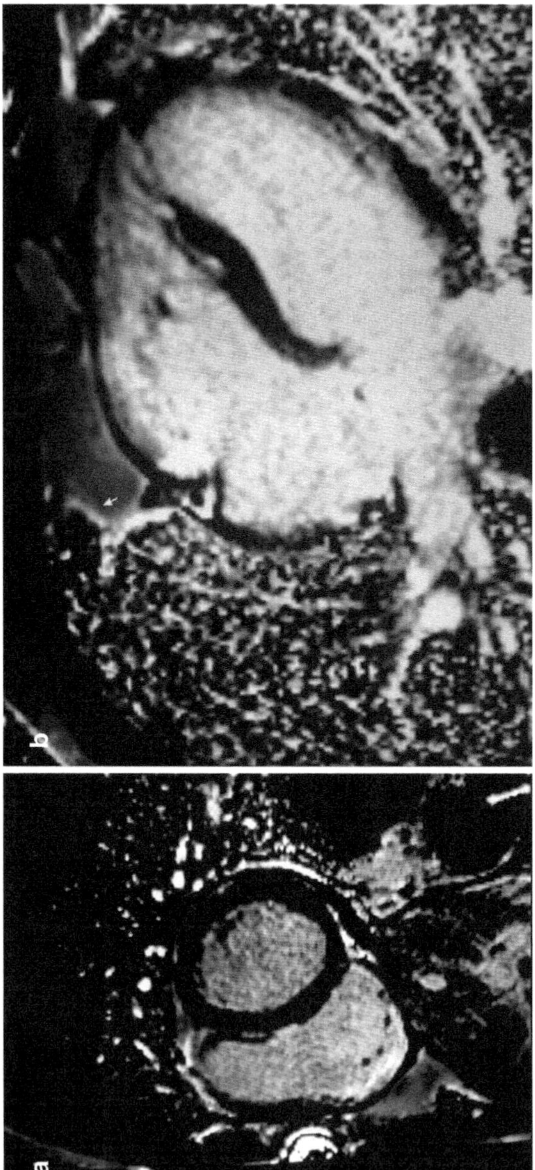

Fig. 27.1 (**a**, **b**) LGE in CMR in the septum, RV free wall and a small portion in the LV posterolateral are

Ablation

We tried to do endocardial biopsy using guide of 3D voltage mapping, but interestingly there was not any low voltage area in bipolar voltage mapping, but unipolar mapping revealed large scar burden, so ARVC with RV epicardial involvement was considered for him.

We did not do an endocardial biopsy because of the absence of any site of the endocardial scar.

So we tried to do an epicardial approach for VT ablation.

Subxiphoid puncture was done and 3D electroanatomical mapping of the epicardium revealed multiple sites of patchy scars in the RVOT and RV inflow areas.

Because of hemodynamic deterioration with VTs (Figs. 27.2 and 27.3), substrate modification was done for patients (Fig. 27.4a, b).

Before ablation coronary angiography was done determination of the position of the coronary arteries (Fig. 27.5).

We ablated all of the entrance conducting channels and late potentials in the RVOT and RV inflow (Figs. 27.6 and 27.7).

No arrhythmia was inducible after ablation with three ventricular extrastimuluses and Isuprel infusion (Fig. 27.8), so ablation was terminated and no arrhythmia was present in the 1 and 3 months follow-ups later.

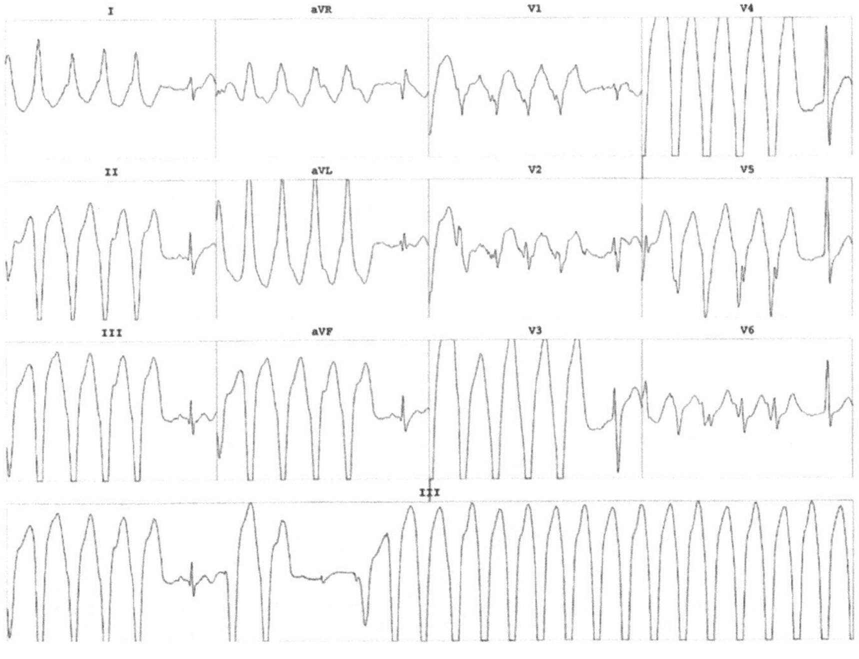

Fig. 27.2 VT1, Induced by VES (ventricular extra stimulation), the superior axis with negative concordance and positive I, aVL

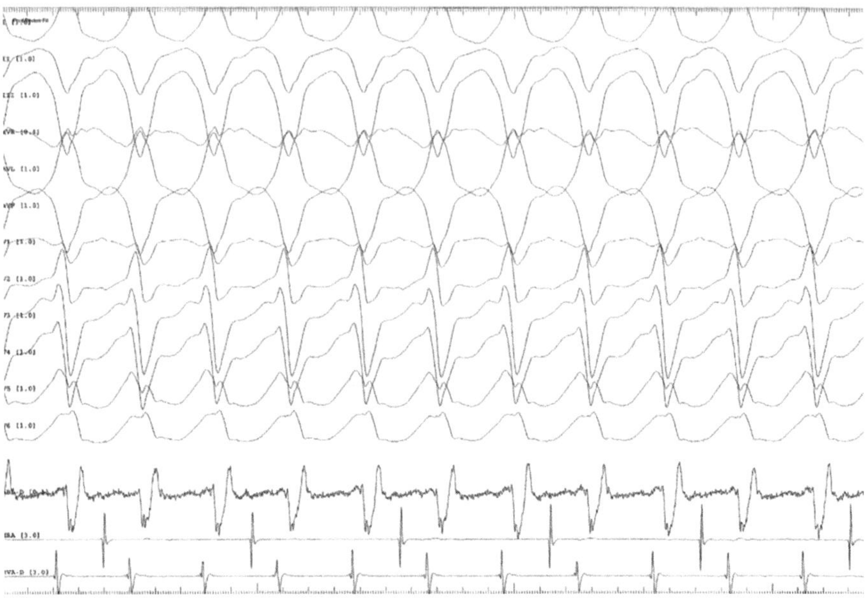

Fig. 27.3 VT2. Superior axis, breakthrough in V2, positive I, aVL

Discussion

Scar distribution patterns in cardiac MRI may be helpful by indicating disease-specific patterns of fibrosis on LGE images. Cardiac Sarcoidosis is a diagnostic challenge and work up for it requires biopsy [1–3].

A scar pattern of basal septal RV involvement may be infavor of Sarcoidosis, but does not prove it.

In ARVC, the disease process starts in the epicardial RV where fibrofatty tissue replaces myocardial tissue.

In about 50% of the patients with ARVC, for cardiac MRI and voltage mapping was done, endocardial voltage mapping failed to detect areas of scar, especially in the inferobasal part of RV [4–6].

Involvement of LV is present in up to ¾ of the ARVC patients [7–9].

An epicardial approach is often necessary to eliminate VT in ARCV patients. The presence of epicardial scar could be assessed by unipolar mapping.

Low amplitude electrograms in bipolar mapping are defined in the endocardium by less than 1.5 mv voltage and in the epicardium by less than 1 mv voltage.

Endocardial unipolar signals suggesting midmyocardial or epicardial substrates are defined as less than 5.5 mv in RV and 8.3 mv in LV [10, 11].

In this patient we did scar dechanneling with ablation of the conducting channels entrance sites within scar, characterized by earliest late potentials following global ventricular activation and end point of the ablation was the elimination of all conducting channels into scar. Following targeted ablation at entrance sites and

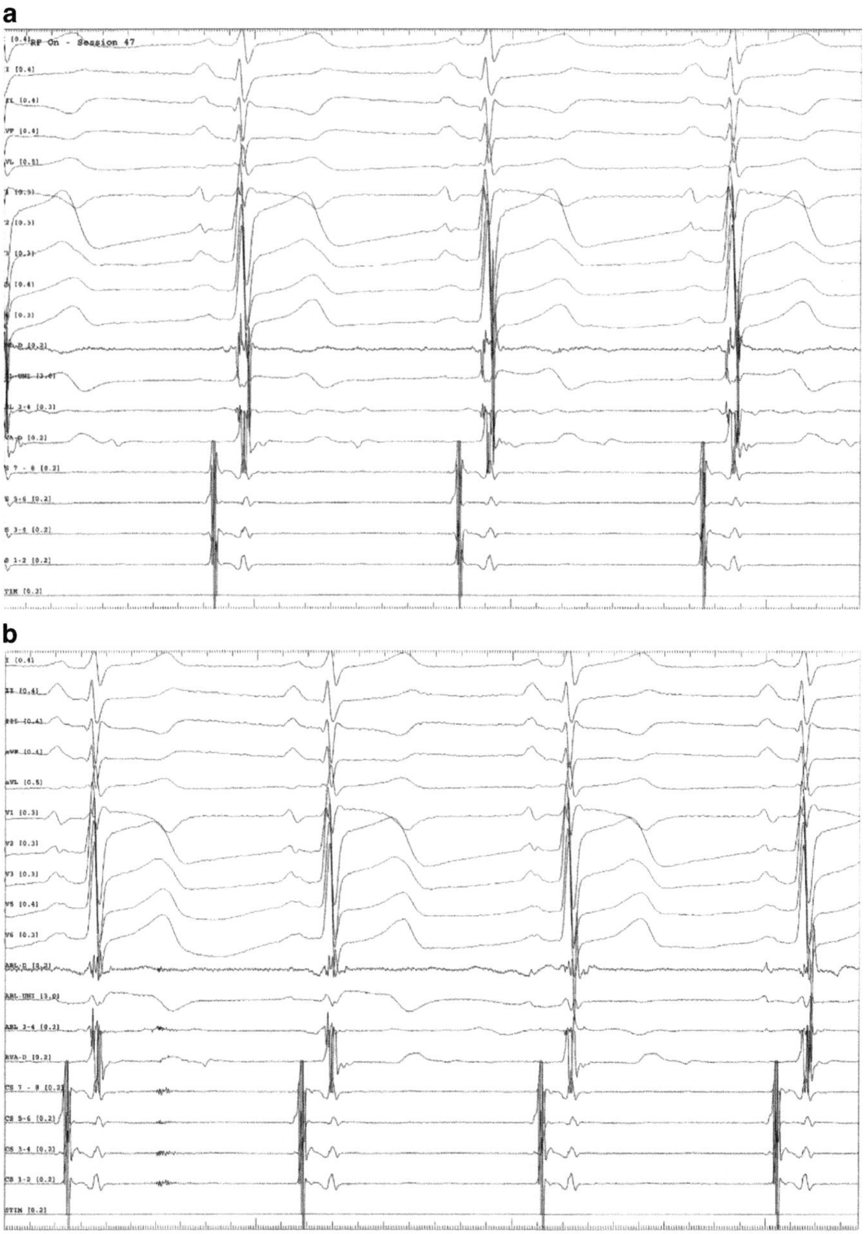

Fig. 27.4 (**a**) LAVAs (Local abnormal ventricular activity) in RV epicardium. (**b**) Disappearance of late potentials (LPs) after ablation

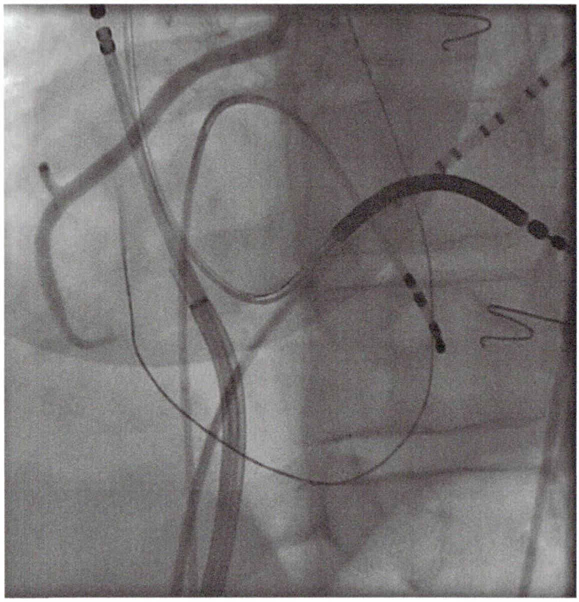

Fig. 27.5 Coronary angiography before epicardial RFA, epicardial ablation catheter is present

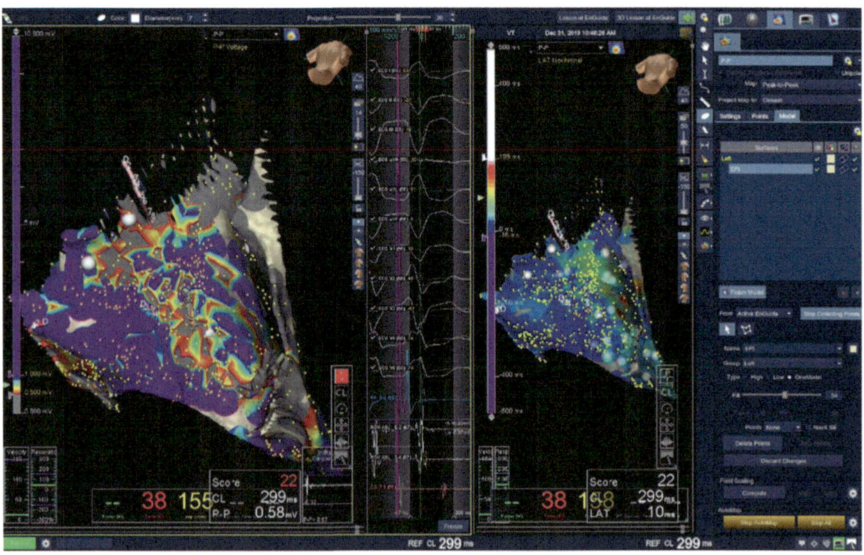

Fig. 27.6 Extensive ablation of RV epicardium, targeted entrance conducting channels, using LAT of late potentials

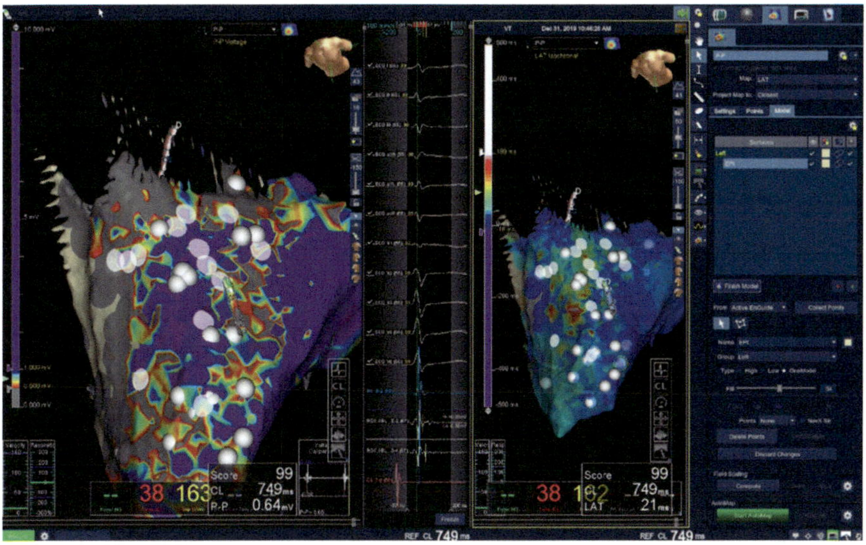

Fig. 27.7 Extensive ablation of RV epicardium, targeted entrance conducting channels, using LAT of late potentials

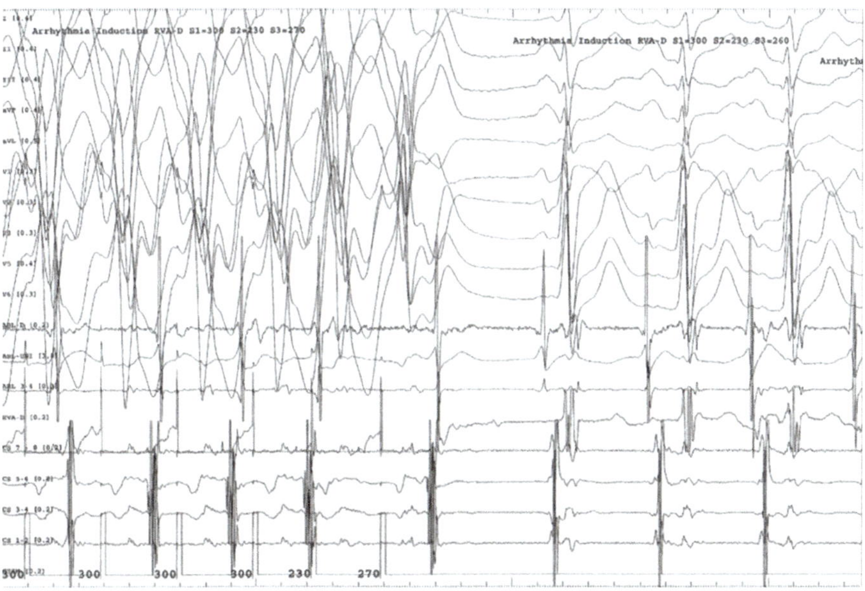

Fig. 27.8 No inducible arrhythmia post-ablation with VES

noninducibility of VT with three ventricular extrastimuluses with and without Isuprel infusion.

IN this patient ablation was successfully terminated, and intrapericardial triamcinolone was administered before long sheet withdrawn. Procedure was done without any complication [12, 13].

References

1. Cesario DA, Vaseghi M, Boyle NG, et al. Value of high-density endocardial and epicardial mapping for catheter ablation of hemodynamically unstable ventricular tachycardia. Heart Rhythm. 2006;3:1–10.
2. Garcia FC, Bazan V, Zado ES, Ren JF, Marchlinski FE. Epicardial substrate and outcome with epicardial ablation of ventricular tachycardia in arrhythmogenic right ventricular cardiomyopathy/dysplasia. Circulation. 2009;120:366–75.
3. Bai R, Di Biase L, Shivkumar K, et al. Ablation of ventricular arrhythmias in arrhythmogenic right ventricular dysplasia/cardiomyopathy: arrhythmia – free survival after endo-epicardial substrate based mapping and ablation. Circ Arrhythm Electrophysiol. 2011;4:478–85.
4. Santangeli P, Di Biase L, Lakkireddy D, et al. Radiofrequency catheter ablation of ventricular arrhythmias in patients with hypertrophic cardiomyopathy: safety and feasibility. Heart Rhythm. 2010;7:1036–42.
5. Dukkipati SR, d'Avila A, Soejima K, et al. Long-term outcomes of combined epicardial and endocardial ablation of monomorphic ventricular tachycardia related to hypertrophic cardiomyopathy. Circ Arrhythm Electrophysiol. 2011;4:185–94.
6. Sosa E, Scanavacca M, D'Avila A, Bellotti G, Pilleggi F. Radiofrequency catheter ablation of ventricular tachycardia guided by nonsurgical epicardial mapping in chronic Chagasic heart disease. Pacing Clin Electrophysiol. 1999;22:128–30.
7. Sosa E, Scanavacca M, d'Avila A. Transthoracic epicardial catheter ablation to treat recurrent ventricular tachycardia. Curr Cardiol Rep. 2001;3:451–8.
8. Reimer KA, Lowe JE, Rasmussen MM, Jennings RB. The wavefront phenomenon of ischemic cell death. 1. Myocardial infarct size vs duration of coronary occlusion in dogs. Circulation. 1977;56:786–94.
9. Jincun G, Faguang Z, Weibin H, Yan W, Kang D, Tung R. Outside-in subepicardial dissection during percutaneous epicardial ventricular tachycardia ablation. Circ Arrhythm Electrophysiol. 2016;9.
10. Valles E, Bazan V, Marchlinski FE. ECG criteria to identify epicardial ventricular tachycardia in nonischemic cardiomyopathy. Circ Arrhythm Electrophysiol. 2010;3:63–71.
11. Berruezo A, Fernández-Armenta J, Andreu D, et al. Scar dechanneling: new method for scar-related left ventricular tachycardia substrate ablation. Circ Arrhythm Electrophysiol. 2015;8:326–36.
12. Kuck KH, Schaumann A, Eckardt L, Willems S, Ventura R, Delacrétaz E, Pitschner HF, Kautzner J, Schumacher B, Hansen PS, VTACH Study Group. Catheter ablation of stable ventricular tachycardia before defibrillator implantation in patients with coronary heart disease (VTACH): a multicentre randomised controlled trial. Lancet. 2010;375:31–40.
13. Shani MM, Haghjoo M, Vasheghani A, Madadi S, Hashemi SN, Shabani R, Taraghi N. Evaluation of diagnostic characteristics and predictors of appropriate ICD therapy in patients with arrhythmogenic right ventricular cardiomyopathy. IHJ. 2016.

Chapter 28
ST-Segment Myocardial Infarction in Patient with Heavily Calcified Lesion

Mohammad Javad Alemzadeh-Ansari

Abstract An 83-year-old woman presented in our hospital with acute inferior ST-segment myocardial infarction. The fluoroscopy and angiogram revealed severe diffused coronary artery calcification (CAC) with diffused significant lesions. Also, subtotal and calcified thrombotic lesion was seen in the mid part of the right coronary artery (RCA). The primary percutaneous coronary intervention (PCI) was done very difficult because the presence of a heavily calcified lesion. Finally, stenting was done successfully. CAC is highly prevalent in patients with coronary heart disease and is associated with a higher rate of major adverse cardiovascular events in short and long-term follow-up.

History and Clinical Presentation

An 83-year-old woman presented in our hospital with acute chest pain from 2 hours ago. She was coming to our center with EMS (247 code system). She directly was transmitted in the cath lab. Past medical history was positive for chronic hypertension. At the time of presentation, the physical examination showed: blood pressure (100/60 mmHg), heart rate (70 bpm), respiratory rate (26 bpm), and temperature (37 °C).

Para-Clinic Assessment

The first electrocardiogram showed ST-segment elevation in inferior leads (lead III > lead II) and also T-wave inversion in lateral and anterior leads (Fig. 28.1).

M. J. Alemzadeh-Ansari (✉)
Cardiovascular Intervention Research Center, Cardio-Oncology Research Center, Rajaie Cardiovascular Medical and Research Center, Iran University of Medical Sciences, Tehran, Iran

M. Maleki, A. Alizadehasl (eds.), *Case-Based Clinical Cardiology*,
https://doi.org/10.1007/978-1-4471-7496-7_28

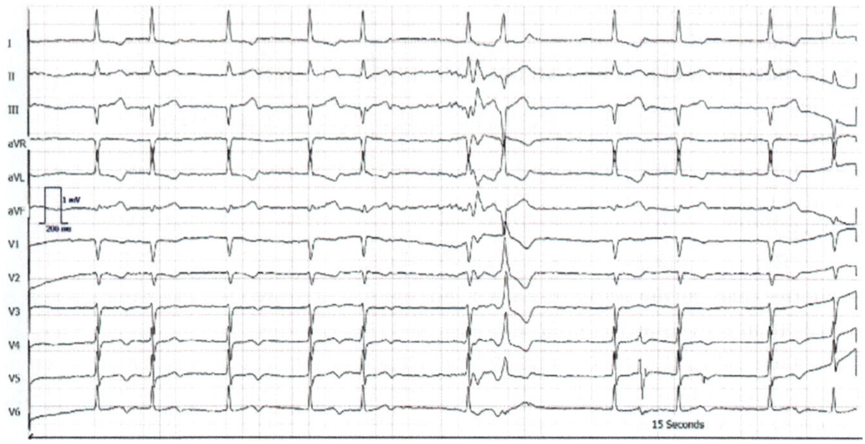

Fig. 28.1 The first electrocardiogram showed ST-segment elevation in inferior leads and also T-wave inversion in lateral and anterior leads

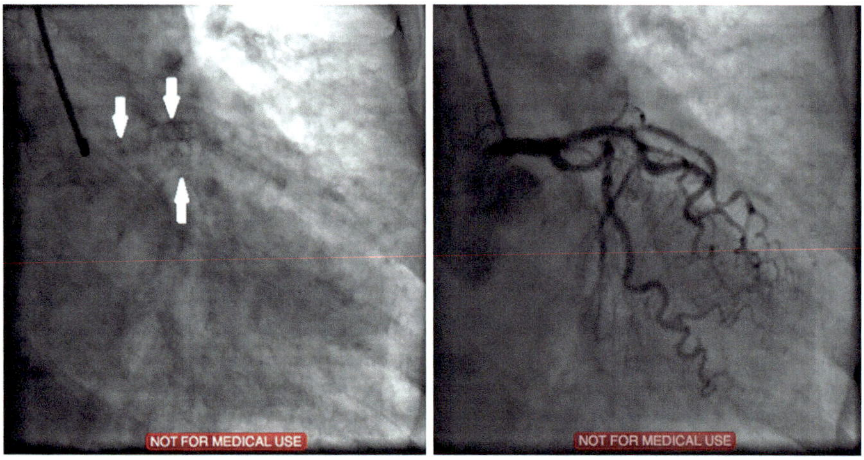

Fig. 28.2 The fluoroscopy showed diffused calcification (white arrow) in left main and proximal to mid part of left anterior descending (LAD) and circumflex (Cx) arteries (left figure). The angiogram in right anterior oblique (RAO) caudal view revealed significant lesion in mid part of LAD, proximal to mid part of diagonal, and proximal segment of Cx arteries (right figure)

Managements

The patient with a diagnosis of acute inferior ST-segment myocardial infraction underwent coronary angiography via right radial artery access. The fluoroscopy and angiogram revealed severe diffused coronary artery calcification (CAC) with diffused significant lesions (Figs. 28.2, 28.3, and 28.4). The angiogram in the left anterior oblique (LAO) view revealed subtotal and calcified thrombotic lesion in the mid

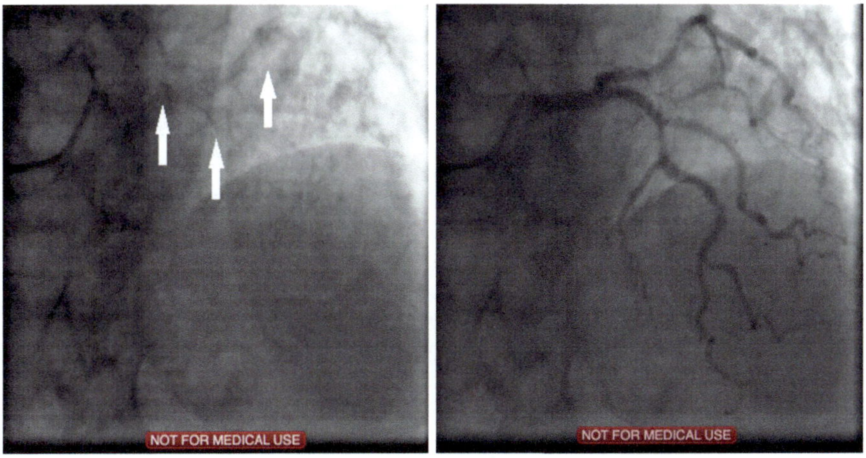

Fig. 28.3 The fluoroscopy showed diffused calcification (white arrow) in left main and proximal to mid part of left anterior descending (LAD) and circumflex (Cx) arteries (left figure). The angiogram in anterior cranial view revealed significant lesion in mid part of LAD, proximal to mid part of diagonal, and proximal segment of Cx arteries (right figure)

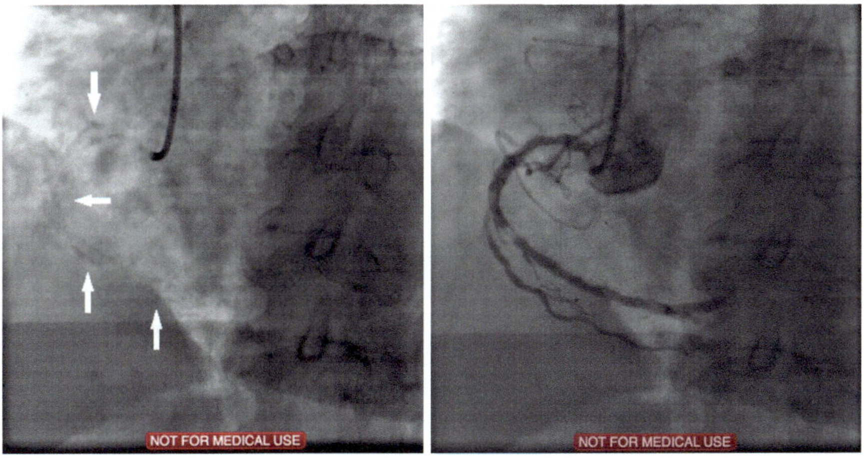

Fig. 28.4 The fluoroscopy showed diffused calcification (white arrow) in right coronary artery (RCA) (left figure). The angiogram in left anterior oblique (LAO) view revealed subtotal thrombotic lesion in mid part of RCA (right figure)

part of the right coronary artery (RCA). After RCA wiring, no balloon was passed from the lesion, even by support of the Guidion catheter. Finally, a 1.2 × 15 mm emerge balloon could be passed. After first balloon, no any balloon passed from the lesion. Interestedly, during attempts for passage the balloon, the drop-in heart rate and blood pressure occurred. It may because that the AV node artery which originated form posterolateral branch (PLB), one branch of dominant RCA, had no flow

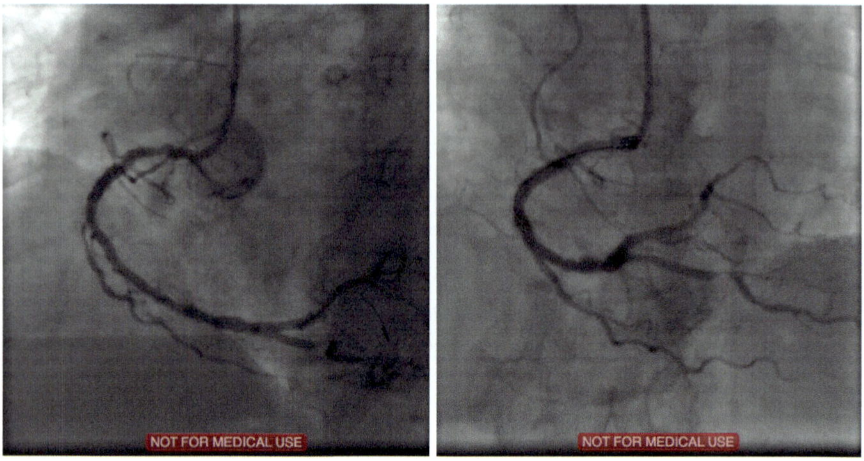

Fig. 28.5 After stenting

during occlusion the RCA with a balloon. So, another wire (BHW) was placed, and by support of Guidion catheter, other balloons (1.5 × 15 mm and 2.75 × 15 mm) were inflated. Finally, a 3.0 × 18 mm Xience Alpine stent was deployed, successfully (Fig. 28.5).

Conclusion

CAC is highly prevalent in patients with coronary heart disease and is associated with major adverse cardiovascular events. Interestedly, early detection of CAC in younger subjects has an important prognostic impact in terms of predicting future coronary heart disease risk [1]. The major factors associated with CAC are advanced age, renal disease, and diabetes [2]. Although CAC correlates with the extent of coronary artery disease. CAC is routinely underdiagnosed with fluoroscopy and angiography; and intravascular ultrasound (IVUS) studies have demonstrated that CAC is missed in nearly half of the cases with angiography alone [3].

Another modality that could be very good to illustrate the extension and pattern of CAC are computed tomography (CT). Detection of both the extent of calcification as well as its pattern has prognostic implications. Although the relationship of CAC to plaque instability is extremely complex and incompletely understood, but generally, spotty calcification is more commonly associated with unstable plaques and extensive calcification more so with stable plaques [4]. Also, serial intravascular ultrasound (IVUS) studies have reported that spotty calcification was associated with greater progression of plaque volume compared to noncalcified plaques, whereas heavily calcified plaques were resistant to change in plaque volume [5]. There are two distinct forms based on the location of calcification in the vessel (intima or medial layer). Medial calcification mostly affects the peripheral arteries of the lower extremities. In this arteries, loss of elasticity could be observed after affecting with medial calcification. On the other hand, intimal calcification is the dominant type of calcification seen in coronary arteries [4].

CAC is strongly associated with adverse outcomes in all the populations; also, treatment of these lesions is need to special attention. The previous studies showed that high intensive statin therapy has been associated with plaque volume reduction by serial IVUS imaging studies [6, 7]. Also, risk factor modification including treating hypertension, dyslipidemia, diabetes mellitus, as well as preventing the development of advanced kidney disease is recommended.

On the other hand, during the percutaneous coronary intervention (PCI), recognition of heavily calcified lesions allows appropriate utilization of ablative techniques for initial vessel preparation. In these patients, the major problems during the procedure include difficult to dilate adequately, failure to deliver a stent or balloon, impaired drug delivery and possible polymer disruption with drug-eluting stents, and stent underexpansion. Also, periprocedural complications such as coronary dissection or perforation, and also long-term complications such as in-stent thrombosis or restenosis are significantly increased in calcified lesions. Thus, optimal approach to calcified coronary lesions is mandatory. The options for treatment of these lesions during PCI include cutting and scoring balloons, rotational atherectomy, orbital atherectomy, and excimer laser coronary atherectomy [8]. Recently, shockwave Intravascular Lithotripsy as a novel balloon catheter-based device based on an established treatment strategy for kidney stones was introduced to modify circumferential calcium in the vessels by localized pulsatile sonic pressure waves. Optical coherence tomography demonstrated that the mechanism of this method is intraplaque calcium fracture in the majority of patients [9].

References

1. Carr JJ, Jacobs DR Jr, Terry JG, et al. Association of coronary artery calcium in adults aged 32 to 46 years with incident coronary heart disease and death. JAMA Cardiol. 2017;2:391–9.
2. Généreux P, Madhavan MV, Mintz GS, Maehara A, Palmerini T, LaSalle L, Xu K, McAndrew T, Kirtane A, Lansky AJ, Brener SJ, Mehran R, Stone GW. Ischemic outcomes after coronary intervention of calcified vessels in acute coronary syndromes. Pooled analysis from the HORIZONS-AMI (Harmonizing outcomes with revascularization and stents in acute myocardial infarction) and ACUITY (acute catheterization and urgent intervention triage strategy) TRIALS. J Am Coll Cardiol. 2014;63:1845–54.
3. Mintz GS, Popma JJ, Pichard AD, Kent KM, Satler LF, Chuang YC, Ditrano CJ, Leon MB. Patterns of calcification in coronary artery disease. A statistical analysis of intravascular ultrasound and coronary angiography in 1155 lesions. Circulation. 1995;91:1959–65.
4. Mori H, Torii S, Kutyna M, Sakamoto A, Finn AV, Virmani R. Coronary artery calcification and its progression: what does it really mean? JACC Cardiovasc Imaging. 2018;11(1):127–42.
5. Kataoka Y, Wolski K, Uno K, et al. Spotty calcification as a marker of accelerated progression of coronary atherosclerosis: insights from serial intravascular ultrasound. J Am Coll Cardiol. 2012;59:1592–7.

6. Okazaki S, Yokoyama T, Miyauchi K, et al. Early statin treatment in patients with acute coronary syndrome: demonstration of the beneficial effect on atherosclerotic lesions by serial volumetric intravascular ultrasound analysis during half a year after coronary event: the ESTABLISH study. Circulation. 2004;110:1061–8.
7. Banach M, Serban C, Sahebkar A, et al. Impact of statin therapy on coronary plaque composition: a systematic review and meta-analysis of virtual histology intravascular ultrasound studies. BMC Med. 2015;13:229.
8. Barbato E, Shlofmitz E, Milkas A, Shlofmitz R, Azzalini L, Colombo AJE. State of the art: evolving concepts in the treatment of heavily calcified and undilatable coronary stenoses-from debulking to plaque modification, a 40-year-long journey. EuroIntervention. 2017;13(6):696–705.
9. Ali ZA, Nef H, Escaned J, Werner N, Banning AP, Hill JM, et al. Safety and effectiveness of coronary intravascular lithotripsy for treatment of severely calcified coronary stenoses: the disrupt CAD II study. Am Heart Assoc. 2019;12(10):e008434.

Chapter 29
Myocardial Bridging

Mohammad Javad Alemzadeh-Ansari

Abstract A 56-year-old man presented in our emergency department with acute anterior ST-segment elevation myocardial infarction. The coronary angiogram showed that left anterior descending artery (LAD) was totally cut off at mid part. After LAD wiring, several manual thrombectomy was done. Final angiogram showed that there is dynamic systolic narrowing (myocardial bridging) of the mid one-third of the LAD. Myocardial bridging is a congenital anomaly in which an intramural segment of a major epicardial coronary artery (most frequently the middle segment of the LAD artery) overlies the segment of a coronary artery. This causes vessel compression in systole, resulting in hemodynamic changes that may be associated with ischemia symptoms and also progression of atherosclerosis.

History and Clinical Presentation

A 56-year-old man presented in our emergency department with acute chest pain from 2 hours ago. The electrocardiogram revealed ST-segment elevation in anterior leads.

Para-Clinic Assessment

Immediately the patient transferred to catheterization laboratory and selective coronary angiogram showed that the left anterior descending artery (LAD) was totally cut off at mid part (Fig. 29.1). After LAD wiring, several manual thrombectomy was done. Final angiogram showed that there is dynamic systolic narrowing (myocardial

M. J. Alemzadeh-Ansari (✉)
Cardiovascular Intervention Research Center, Cardio-Oncology Research Center, Rajaie Cardiovascular Medical and Research Center, Iran University of Medical Sciences, Tehran, Iran

M. Maleki, A. Alizadehasl (eds.), *Case-Based Clinical Cardiology*,
https://doi.org/10.1007/978-1-4471-7496-7_29

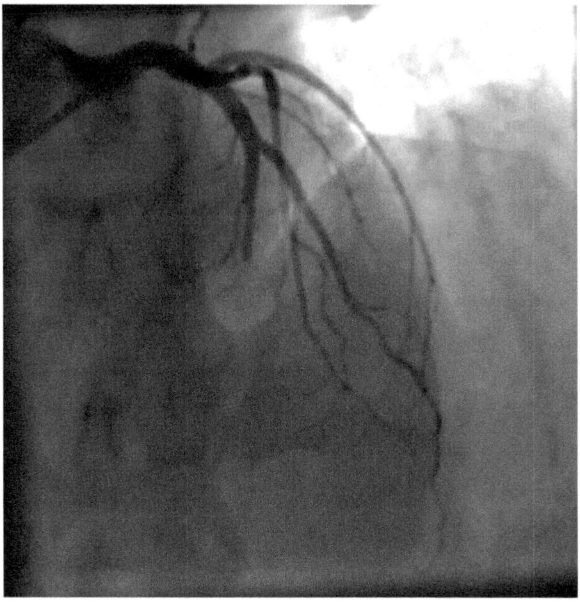

Fig. 29.1 The LAD was totally cut off in mid part segment

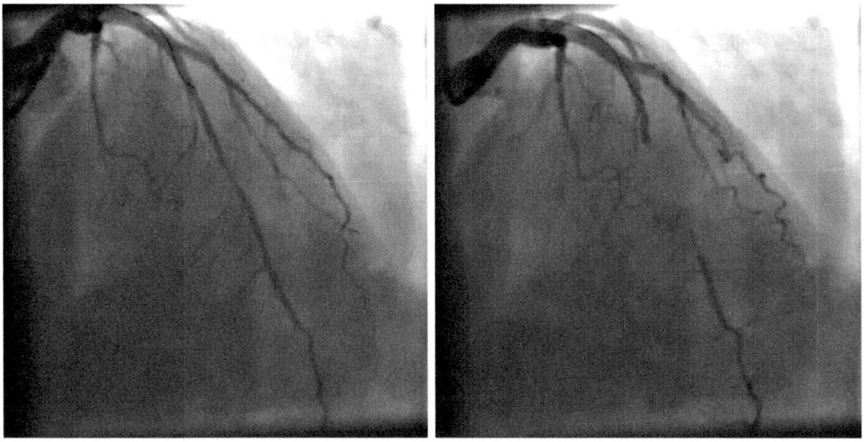

Fig. 29.2 After wiring and manual thrombectomy, angiogram showed that there is dynamic systolic narrowing (myocardial bridging) of the mid one-third of the LAD (Right: systolic phase; Left: diastolic phase), accomplished with a significant ulcerative plaque in mid part of myocardial bridge segment

bridging) of the mid one-third of the LAD, accomplished with a significant ulcerative plaque in the mid part of myocardial bridge segment (Fig. 29.2).

Interestedly, selective coronary angiography which was done for this patient 6 months later because of transient anterior ST-segment elevation in another center, showed myocardial bridging in the mid one-third of the LAD (with totally systolic compression) accomplished with nonsignificant plaque in mid part of myocardial bridge segment. Then, treatment with aspirin, beta-blocker, and statine was started for him. After the last admission, the patient was asymptomatic.

Managements

After partial revascularization, the echocardiogram revealed that LVEF: 45%, with no any mechanical complication. Because the presence of deep and long segment of bridge and also significant stenosis at the site of bridge, patients referred for coronary artery bypass graft surgery. 1 week after surgery, the patient was discharged with the good general condition.

Conclusion

Myocardial bridging is a congenital anomaly in which an intramural segment of a major epicardial coronary artery (most frequently the middle segment of the LAD artery) overlies the segment of a coronary artery [1]. Coronary arteries that tunnel through the myocardium are seen in as many as 40% to 80% of cases on autopsy; however, functional myocardial bridging is less commonly observed on angiography (0.5% to 16.0%) and can range from 4 to 80 mm in length [2]. This causes vessel compression in systole, resulting in hemodynamic changes that may be associated with ischemia symptoms. The hemodynamic impact of myocardial bridging depends on the thickness and length of the bridge, the presence of loose connective or adipose tissue around the bridged segment, and the orientation of the bridge relative to myocardial fibers [2].

Previous studies have shown that the intramural and distal segments of myocardial bridges remain free from atherosclerosis while the proximal segment of the vessel is prone to developing atherosclerosis [3, 4]. The wall shear stress (WSS) immediately proximal to myocardial bridges is low, where is structurally dysfunctional, flat, and polygonal endothelial cells; whereas endothelial cells lining bridged segments, where WSS is physiological or high, are structurally intact. The fluid dynamics model at end-systole of the LAD in a patient with a symptomatic myocardial bridge revealed that there is relatively low WSS proximal and distal to the bridge, whereas high WSS within the bridge [2]. Also, some showed that systolic vessel compression may persist into mid-to-late diastole [5]. Thus both systolic and diastolic flow impairment contribute to myocardial supply–demand imbalance in patients with myocardial bridging.

By increase in age, additional pathophysiological changes, especially by increasing hypertrophied muscle and negative remodeling of the vessel, can induce symptoms related to myocardial bridging in patients who were previously asymptomatic. Development in left ventricular diastolic dysfunction, hypertension, and coronary atherosclerosis can exacerbate the supply–demand imbalance imposed by the bridge segment. Increase in left ventricular hypertrophy can increase compression and reduce the reserve of coronary microvascular. The presence of coronary vasospasm, microvascular dysfunction, or endothelial dysfunction secondary to an increase in cardiovascular risk factors can exacerbate myocardial ischemia. Plaque development proximal to the bridge can augment coronary obstruction by the bridge. Finally, the negative remodeling within the bridge segment can reduce myocardial flow [2].

Although bridging is not thought to be of any hemodynamic significance in most cases, myocardial bridging has been associated with angina, acute coronary syndromes, arrhythmia (such as supraventricular tachycardia, ventricular tachycardia, or atrioventricular conduction block), depressed LV function, myocardial stunning, early death after cardiac transplantation, and syncope, or even sudden death [4]. The presence of previous factors that influence the pathophysiological changes can contribute to a varying degree to the development of symptoms in patients with myocardial bridging. For example, deep myocardial bridges over coronary arteries have been reported in association with sudden cardiac death occurring during strenuous exercise [6]. Also, increase in myocardial bridge thickness and length, as well as proximal vessel location, correlated with increased risk for myocardial infarction, proposed to result from the promotion of proximal atherosclerosis [1]. Interestedly, our patient presented with STEMI secondary to plaque rupture in the mid part of the myocardial bridging segment; that not commonplace for atherosclerotic plaque development.

Several modalities for diagnosis myocardial bridging and evaluation of physiological effects have been described. Multiple-slice computed tomography (MSCT) defines bridges as segments surrounded by myocardium. On angiography, a significant "milking effect" is present when there is more than 70% reduction in minimal luminal diameter during systole and persistent more than 35% reduction in minimal luminal diameter during mid-to-late diastole. Intracoronary injection of nitroglycerin can accentuate the systolic narrowing by vasodilating adjacent non-bridged coronary segments. On intravascular ultrasound the half-moon sign could be seen that is an echolucent area present only between the bridged coronary segment and epicardial tissue. A fractional flow reserve (FFR) less than 0.75 indicates hemodynamically significant stenoses of myocardial bridging. Although an FFR of 0.75 to 0.80 is a gray zone of ischemia, like other non-bridged coronary arteries [2].

The pharmacological therapy is the first treatment of symptomatic patients with myocardial bridging; and PCI and open surgery should be remained for those with refractory to maximal medical therapy. Beta-blockers and calcium channel blockers are the first treatment for these patients. Some believed that aggressive risk factor modification and antiplatelet therapy beginning should be considered, because they are at increased risk for developing atherosclerosis. Although others recommended antiplatelet therapy for those with evidences of atherosclerosis development based on MSCT or angiography. On the other hand, pure vasodilating agents such as nitroglycerin should be used cautiously in these patients [2].

Although PCI is an option for treatment in symptomatic patients, the rates of stent fracture, in-stent restenosis, and stent thrombosis are high in these patients. Another option for treatment is surgical intervention (supra-arterial myotomy or CABG). The major concern about myotomy is wall perforation, ventricular aneurysm formation, and postoperative bleeding, whereas major concern about CABG is graft failure especially in those without significant atherosclerotic stenosis. In cases of extensive (>25 mm) or deep (>5 mm) myocardial bridges or when the bridged coronary segment fails to decompress completely in diastole, CABG may be favored over myotomy [7, 8].

References

1. Lee MS, Chen C-H. Myocardial bridging: an up-to-date review. J Invasive Cardiol. 2015;27(11):521.
2. Corban MT, Hung OY, Eshtehardi P, Rasoul-Arzrumly E, McDaniel M, Mekonnen G, et al. Myocardial bridging: contemporary understanding of pathophysiology with implications for diagnostic and therapeutic strategies. J Am Coll Cardiol. 2014;63(22):2346–55.
3. Ge J, Jeremias A, Rupp A, Abels M, Baumgart D, Liu F, et al. New signs characteristic of myocardial bridging demonstrated by intracoronary ultrasound and Doppler. Eur Heart J. 1999;20(23):1707–16.
4. Ishikawa Y, Akasaka Y, Suzuki K, Fujiwara M, Ogawa T, Yamazaki K, et al. Anatomic properties of myocardial bridge predisposing to myocardial infarction. Circulation. 2009;120(5):376–83.
5. Bourassa MG, Butnaru A, Lespérance J, Tardif J-C. Symptomatic myocardial bridges: overview of ischemic mechanisms and current diagnostic and treatment strategies. J Am Coll Cardiol. 2003;41(3):351–9.
6. Tio RA, Van Gelder IC, Boonstra PW, Crijns H. Myocardial bridging in a survivor of sudden cardiac near-death: role of intracoronary Doppler flow measurements and angiography during dobutamine stress in the clinical evaluation. Heart. 1997;77(3):280–2.
7. Wu Q-Y, Xu Z-H. Surgical treatment of myocardial bridging: report of 31 cases. Chin Med J. 2007;120(19):1689–93.
8. Attaran S, Moscarelli M, Athanasiou T, Anderson J. Is coronary artery bypass grafting an acceptable alternative to myotomy for the treatment of myocardial bridging? Interact Cardiovasc Thorac Surg. 2012;16(3):347–9.

Chapter 30
Hypertrophic Cardiomyopathy and Deep Myocardial Bridge

Mohammad Javad Alemzadeh-Ansari

Abstract A 49-year-old woman presented in our hospital with Dyspnea and atypical chest pain from one year ago. The electrocardiogram revealed left ventricular (LV) hypertrophy and secondary ST-T changes. The echocardiogram showed normal LV cavity and systolic function (LVEF: 55-60%) with asymmetric left ventricular hypertrophy, and a significant dynamic left ventricular outflow obstruction, suggestive for hypertrophic cardiomyopathy. Also, moderate to severe mitral regurgitation accomplished with significant systolic anterior motion of the mitral valve touching the septum was seen in echocardiogram. The angiogram showed deep myocardial bridging in mid part of LAD; which during systole, the vessel was totally occulted.

History and Clinical Presentation

A 49-year-old woman presented in our hospital with Dyspnea NYHA function class III and atypical chest pain from 1 year ago. The electrocardiogram revealed left ventricular (LV) hypertrophy and secondary ST-T changes.

Para-Clinic Assessment

The echocardiogram showed normal LV cavity and systolic function (LVEF: 55–60%) with asymmetric left ventricular hypertrophy (septum, 36 mm; posterior wall, 12 mm), and a significant dynamic left ventricular outflow obstruction (a resting peak systolic gradient of 100 mmHg and mean gradient 56 mmHg) due to

M. J. Alemzadeh-Ansari (✉)
Cardiovascular Intervention Research Center, Cardio-Oncology Research Center, Rajaie Cardiovascular Medical and Research Center, Iran University of Medical Sciences, Tehran, Iran

M. Maleki, A. Alizadehasl (eds.), *Case-Based Clinical Cardiology*,
https://doi.org/10.1007/978-1-4471-7496-7_30

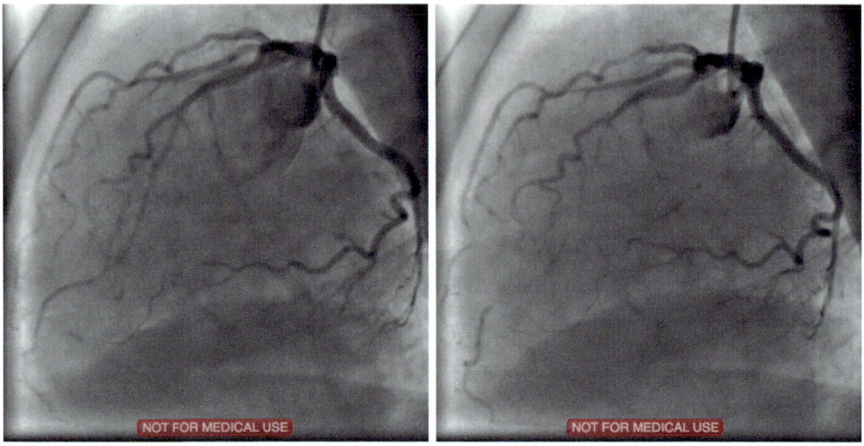

Fig. 30.1 Left coronary injection in lateral view showed dynamic systolic narrowing (deep myocardial bridging) of the mid one-third of the LAD (Right: systolic phase; Left: diastolic phase)

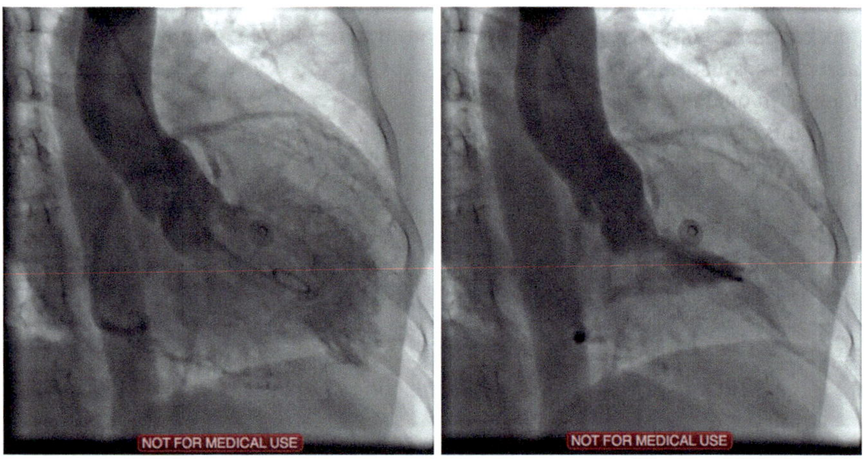

Fig. 30.2 Left ventriculography revealed good systolic function and left ventricle hypertrophy with spade-like left ventricular cavity during diastole (left) systole (right)

systolic anterior motion of the mitral valve. Also, moderate to severe mitral regurgitation accomplished with significant systolic anterior motion of the mitral valve touching the septum was seen in echocardiogram.

Then, the patient underwent coronary angiography. The angiogram showed deep myocardial bridging in the mid part of LAD; which during systole, the vessel was totally occulted (Fig. 30.1). The left ventriculography revealed good systolic function accomplished with left ventricle hypertrophy with a spade-like left ventricular cavity during diastole systole (Fig. 30.2).

Managements

The patient underwent full medical therapy for 3 months. But the patient was symptomatic, so she was referred to surgeon for myomectomy.

Conclusion

Hypertrophic cardiomyopathy (HCM), the most common of the genetic cardiovascular diseases, is characterized by a thickened but non-dilated left ventricle. This condition should be confirmed after the role out of other diagnosis accomplished with LV hypertrophy such as aortic valve stenosis, systemic hypertension, athlete's heart, and isolated basal septum hypertrophy in older adults [1, 2]. The clinical diagnosis of HCM has conventionally been made with 2D echocardiography. However, cardiovascular magnetic resonance (CMR) imaging has emerged with an expanded role in the diagnosis of HCM patients by virtue of its high-resolution tomographic imaging capability. CMR also allows for the quantification of late gadolinium enhancement (LGE), a marker for myocardial fibrosis [3, 4]. Imaging findings show an absolute increase in left ventricular wall thickness of 15 mm or more (to 21–22 mm on average), which can also be associated with mild right ventricular hypertrophy [2]. In some cases, apical hypertrophy in echocardiography is associated with giant T-wave inversion on electrocardiogram. Borderline LV wall thicknesses (13–15 mm in males and 11–12 mm in females) can create diagnostic ambiguity, particularly in the differential diagnosis of physiologic athlete's heart [1].

Hypertrophic cardiomyopathy is perhaps unique among cardiovascular diseases, with presentation at any age from infancy to old age. Many patients with hypertrophic cardiomyopathy achieve normal life expectancy with little or no disability and without the need for major therapeutic interventions. In some cases, symptoms of heart failure may develop at any age, with functional limitation predominantly resulting from exertional dyspnea and fatigue; orthopnea or paroxysmal nocturnal dyspnea occasionally occurs in advanced stages [1].

The complications attributable to HCM may progress in individual patients including: (1) sudden death (usually occurs in asymptomatic or mildly symptomatic patients); (2) progressive heart failure (with reduced or preserved systolic function); (3) repetitive, persistent, permanent atrial fibrillation (with risk for progressive heart failure symptoms and embolic stroke occurs in 20% of patients) [1]. Deep myocardial bridges over coronary arteries in patients with HCM have been reported in association with sudden cardiac death occurring during strenuous exercise, possibly caused by dynamic mechanical obstruction [5].

The surgical septal myectomy has been considered for disabled patients with severe drug-refractory symptoms (i.e., NYHA functional class III or IV due to significant obstruction to LV outflow more than 50 mm Hg or recurrent syncope) [6].

The primary objective of surgical myectomy is reduction in heart failure symptoms and improvement in the quality of life, by virtue of relieving the outflow obstruction (and SAM) and associated mitral regurgitation, resulting in the normalization of the LV pressures [5].

References

1. Maron BJ, Maron MS. Hypertrophic cardiomyopathy. Lancet. 2013;381:242.
2. Elliott PM, Anastasakis A, Borger MA, et al. ESC guidelines on diagnosis and management of hypertrophic cardiomyopathy: the task force for the diagnosis and Management of Hypertrophic Cardiomyopathy of the European Society of Cardiology (ESC). Eur Heart J. 2014;35:2733.
3. Maron MS, Maron BJ. Clinical impact of contemporary cardiovascular magnetic resonance imaging in hypertrophic cardiomyopathy. Circulation. 2015;132:292.
4. Chan RH, Maron BJ, Olivotto I, et al. Prognostic value of quantitative contrast-enhanced cardiovascular magnetic resonance for the evaluation of sudden death risk in patients with hypertrophic cardiomyopathy. Circulation. 2014;130:484.
5. Zipes DP, Libby P, Bonow RO, Mann DL, Tomaselli GF. Braunwald's heart disease E-book: a textbook of cardiovascular medicine. Philadelphia, PA: Elsevier; 2018.
6. Maleki M, Alizadehasl A, Haghjoo M. Practical cardiology. Philadelphia, PA: Elsevier; 2017.

Chapter 31
Coronary Artery Aneurysm

Mohammad Javad Alemzadeh-Ansari

Abstract A 33-year-old man presented in our emergency department with diagnosis of inferior ST-segment elevation myocardial infarction. The past medical history was positive for smoking. He was a bodybuilder and regularly consumed anabolic steroids and human growth hormone (hGH) for the past two years. The angiogram of right coronary artery (RCA) showed totally thrombotic cut off at mid part. After RCA wiring, the angiogram revealed ectasia in proximal part, a large coronary aneurysm in mid part with huge thrombus burden in mid to distal part segment.

History and Clinical Presentation

A 33-year-old man presented in our emergency department with acute chest pain from 6 months ago. The past medical history was positive for smoking. He was a bodybuilder and regularly consumed anabolic steroids and human growth hormone (hGH) for the past 2 years.

Para-Clinic Assessment

The first electrocardiogram showed ST-segment elevation in inferior leads and ST-segment depression with T-wave inversion in lateral leads.

M. J. Alemzadeh-Ansari (✉)
Cardiovascular Intervention Research Center, Cardio-Oncology Research Center, Rajaie Cardiovascular Medical and Research Center, Iran University of Medical Sciences, Tehran, Iran

M. Maleki, A. Alizadehasl (eds.), *Case-Based Clinical Cardiology*,
https://doi.org/10.1007/978-1-4471-7496-7_31

Managements

The patient immediately underwent coronary angiography with a diagnosis of inferior ST-segment elevation myocardial infarction. The angiogram of the left coronary system was unremarkable, but the right coronary artery (RCA) injection showed a totally thrombotic cut off at mid part (Figs. 31.1 and 31.2). After RCA wiring, the angiogram revealed ectasia in the proximal part, a large coronary aneurysm in mid part with a huge thrombus burden in mid to distal part segment (Fig. 31.2). After several manual thrombectomies, acceptable TIMI flow was achieved. Although in the final injection there is some thrombus in the coronary aneurysm at the mid part of RCA and also some in the ostio-proximal part of the posterior descending artery (PDA) (Fig. 31.3). Then, the patient was treated with an infusion of Glycoprotein IIb/IIIa inhibitor and heparin. Five days later the patient was discharged with dual antiplatelet and high dose statin.

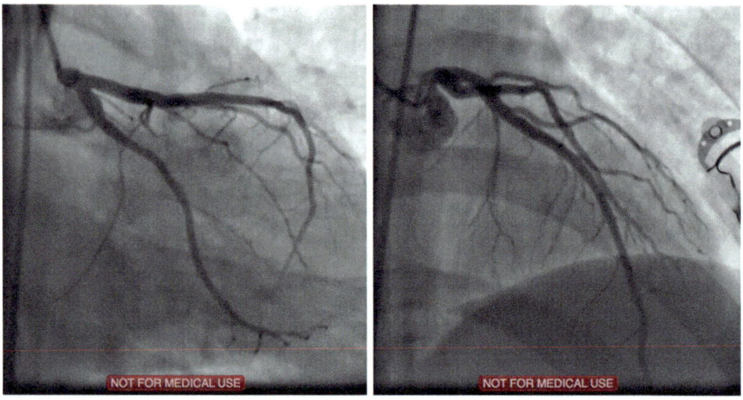

Fig. 31.1 The angiogram of left coronary system showed patient coronary arteries in RAO caudal (left figure) and AP cranial (right figure) view

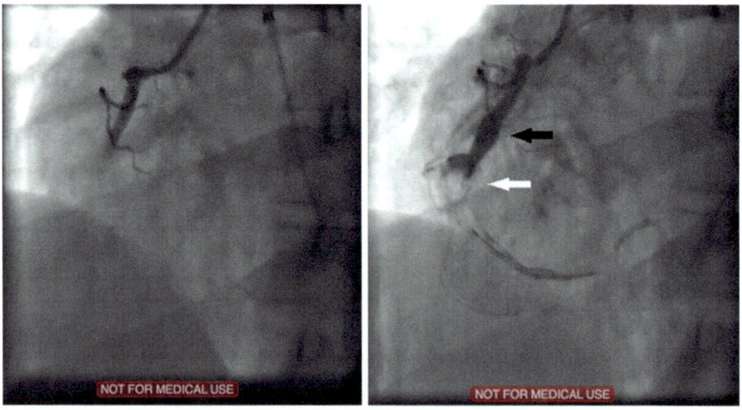

Fig. 31.2 The angiogram of RCA revealed totally thrombotic cut off at mid part (left figure). After wiring, the angiogram showed ectasia in proximal part (black arrow), a large coronary aneurysm (white arrow) in mid part with huge thrombus burden in mid to distal part segment (right figure)

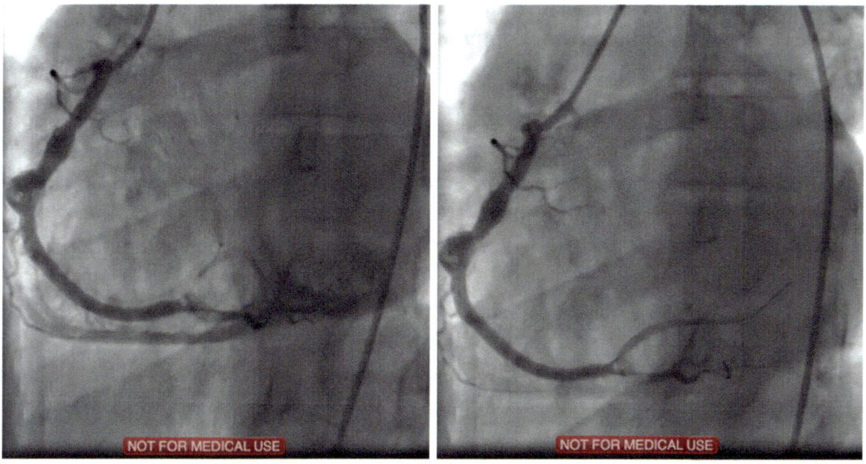

Fig. 31.3 After several manual thrombectomy, acceptable TIMI flow was achieved. The final injection showed some thrombus in the coronary aneurysm at the mid part of RCA and also some in the ostio-proximal part of posterior descending artery (PDA)

Conclusion

Aneurysmal dilation of coronary arteries is ranged from 0.3% to 5% among patients undergoing coronary angiography. Irrespective of the presence of concomitant atherosclerotic coronary artery disease, the presence of coronary aneurysm or ectasia has been associated with poor long-term outcomes. Clinical presentations range from incidental findings on cardiac imaging to acute coronary syndrome. There are criteria that distinguish between two phenotype types of coronary aneurysm and ectasia [1]. By these criteria, a focal dilation of coronary segments of at least 1.5 times the adjacent normal segment is described as a coronary aneurysm; whereas the term coronary ectasia is used to define similar, but more diffuse lesions where the length of the dilated segment is more than 50% of the diameter [1, 2].

Coronary aneurysms are most commonly found in the RCA (68%), followed by the proximal left anterior descending (60%) and left circumflex (50%). Aneurysms in the left main stem are exceedingly rare and occur in only 0.1% of the population [3]. Interestedly, the prevalence of coronary aneurysms is more in the men and also, in proximal than to distal segments of the coronary bed [4].

The most common cause of coronary aneurysms in adults is atherosclerosis, whereas Kawasaki disease is responsible for the majority of cases in children. Other etiologies such as inflammatory disorders, infectious, connective tissue disorders, drugs (cocaine and amphetamines), trauma, and iatrogenic are a less common cause of aneurysm formation [3]. Coronary aneurysms secondary to atherosclerosis or vasculitis usually affect more than one artery, whereas congenital and iatrogenic CAAs are typically confined to a single vessel [1].

Most coronary aneurysms are clinically silent and are only detected incidentally during coronary angiography or computed tomography. However, in some cases the clinical symptoms and presentation can develop due to one of the following reasons:

1. The presence of concomitant stenotic atherosclerotic disease can result in both effort angina or acute coronary syndrome.
2. Local thrombosis in the lumen of large aneurysms may lead to distal embolization and myocardial infarction.
3. Massive enlargement of some coronary aneurysms can result in compression of adjacent structures.
4. Stress-induced myocardial ischemia due to microvascular dysfunction has been documented even in the absence of significant coronary stenosis.
5. Myocardial ischemia due to the turbulence of flow and energy loss as blood passes through the coronary aneurysm in absent of significant coronary stenosis, especially in giant aneurysms.
6. Other complications such as sudden cardiac death, fistula formation, rupture, hemopericardium, tamponade are very rare [1, 3].

The most common imaging modality to assess ectatic or aneurysmal coronary arteries is coronary angiography. However, delayed antegrade contrast filling, segmental back flow, and contrast stasis in the dilated coronary segment often hamper optimal imaging during angiography [1, 4]. So, a forceful and prolonged contrast injection may be necessary to avoid misinterpreting slow aneurysmal filling as in situ thrombosis, especially in giant aneurysms. In some cases, intravascular ultrasound (IVUS) can be extremely helpful for better distinguishing of vessel wall structures (between true aneurysm, pseudoaneurysm) and also, selecting proper stent size if percutaneous coronary intervention is planned. Although, optical coherence tomography (OCT) in assessing coronary aneurysms is limited by the small scan diameter of the infrared light [1, 5]. Computed tomography is superior to invasive angiography for evaluation of coronary aneurysm size and degree of thrombus and calcification, particularly in those with giant aneurysm [6].

Our case was bodybuilder and used anabolic steroids and hGH, additional to smoking. Anabolic-androgenic steroids, including testosterone and its numerous derivatives that have been modified to improve anabolism, are usually used to boost protein synthesis, muscle growth, and erythropoiesis. The anabolic-androgenic steroids by a decrease in high-density lipoprotein, an increase in low-density lipoprotein, and an increase in homocysteine levels in the blood lead to increase the risk of Atherosclerosis development and cerebrovascular disease. Also, by direct effect on the coagulation/fibrinolysis system, can lead to an increased risk of thrombus formation. Other effects of anabolic-androgenic steroids on the cardiovascular system include hypertension, coronary spasm, myocardial apoptosis, cardiac hypertrophy, dilated cardiomyopathy, arrhythmia, and sudden cardiac arrest [7]. Additionally, hGH abuse contributes to increased heart rate and cardiac output, consequently leading to concentric ventricular hypertrophy and diastolic dysfunction. In some cases, hGH abuse may even promote ischemia/necrosis and heart failure associated with impairment of the systolic function [8].

References

1. Kawsara A, Gil IJN, Alqahtani F, Moreland J, Rihal CS, Alkhouli MJJCI. Management of coronary artery aneurysms. JACC. 2018;11(13):1211–23.
2. Abou Sherif S, Ozden Tok O, Taşköylü Ö, Goktekin O, Kilic ID. Coronary artery aneurysms: a review of the epidemiology, pathophysiology, diagnosis, and treatment. Front Cardiovasc Med. 2017;4:24.
3. Sheikh AS, Hailan A, Kinnaird T, Choudhury A, Smith D. Coronary artery aneurysm: evaluation, prognosis, and proposed treatment strategies. Heart Views. 2019;20(3):101–8.
4. Manginas A, Cokkinos DV. Coronary artery ectasias: imaging, functional assessment and clinical implications. Eur Heart J. 2006;27:1026–31.
5. Fathelbab H, Camacho Freire SJ, Leon JJ, et al. Detection of spontaneous coronary artery spasm with optical coherence tomography in a patient with acute coronary syndrome. Cardiovasc Revasc Med. 2017;18:7–9.
6. Murthy PA, Mohammed TL, Read K, Gilkeson RC, White CS. MDCT of coronary artery aneurysms. AJR Am J Roentgenol. 2005;184(Suppl):S19–20.
7. Liu J-D, Wu Y-QJC. Anabolic-androgenic steroids and cardiovascular risk. Chin Med J. 2019;132(18):2229–36.
8. Holt RI, Sönksen PH. Growth hormone, IGF-I and insulin and their abuse in sport. Br J Pharmacol. 2008;154(3):542–56.

Chapter 32
Conus Artery Injection: May Be Helpful?

Mohammad Javad Alemzadeh-Ansari

Abstract A 66-year-old man presented in our hospital with complain of exertional chest pain NYHA function class III from 8 months ago. The single-photon emission computed tomography (SPECT) scan revealed severe stress-induced ischemia in anterior and moderate ischemia in inferior and lateral territories. The angiogram of left coronary system showed that the left anterior descending artery (LAD) is totally cut off at mid part (after first large diagonal branch). The mid to distal part of LAD was not visualized at left coronary injection. In injection of right coronary artery (RCA), which was non-dominant, the LAD was not visualized. After withdrawal of catheter and selective conus artery injection, the mid to distal part of well-developed LAD was visualized by some collateral's branches.

History and Clinical Presentation

A 66-year-old man presented in our hospital with complain of exertional chest pain NYHA function class III from 8 months ago. The past medical history was positive for hypertension, dyslipidemia, and smoking.

Para-Clinic Assessment

The electrocardiogram showed non-specific ST-T change in pericardial leads; and the echocardiogram revealed preserved left ventricular systolic ejection fraction (LVEF: 55%), without significant valvular heart disease. Then,

---

M. J. Alemzadeh-Ansari (✉)
Cardiovascular Intervention Research Center, Cardio-Oncology Research Center, Rajaie Cardiovascular Medical and Research Center, Iran University of Medical Sciences, Tehran, Iran

M. Maleki, A. Alizadehasl (eds.), *Case-Based Clinical Cardiology*,
https://doi.org/10.1007/978-1-4471-7496-7_32

single-photon emission computed tomography (SPECT) scan was done and showed severe stress-induced ischemia in anterior and moderate ischemia in inferior and lateral territories.

Managements

By regarding the SPECT scan findings, the patient underwent coronary angiography. The angiogram of the left coronary system showed that the left anterior descending artery (LAD) is totally cut off at mid part (after first large diagonal branch), suggestive for chronic total occlusion (CTO). The mid to distal flow of LAD was not visualized in left coronary injection (Fig. 32.1). Other findings in left coronary injection revealed that first large diagonal had significant ostio-proximal lesion with good distal runoff; also, significant lesion was seen at proximal part of dominant left circumflex (LCx), significant lesion at proximal part of first large obtuse marginal (OM), and moderate lesion at proximal part of left posterior descending artery (PDA) (Fig. 32.1). The angiogram of right coronary artery (RCA) showed that this artery is nondominant artery and provides no collateral flow to the occluded LAD (Fig. 32.1). In this stage, we did not find the distal of LAD for decision about proper treatment strategy. So, by counterclockwise rotation and minimal withdrawal of right diagnostic Judkins (JR4) catheter and selective conus artery injection, good collaterals flow to a well-developed LAD with a well-preserved lumen distal to the occlusion (mid to distal parts with good runoff) was visualized (Fig. 32.2). Finally, by attention to angiogram findings, the patient referred to surgeon for coronary artery bypass grafting.

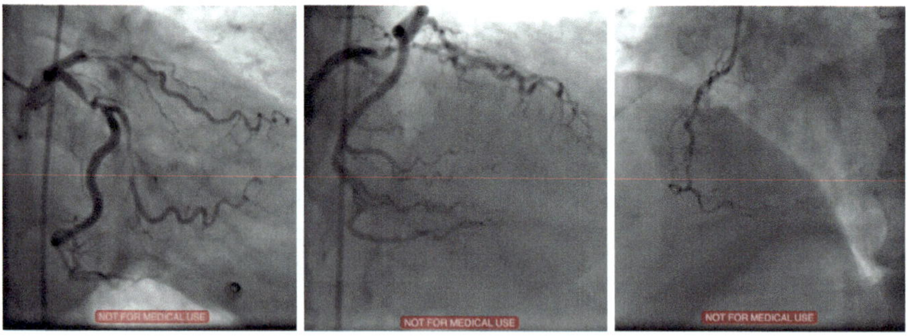

Fig. 32.1 The left anterior descending artery (LAD) is totally cut off at mid part (after first large diagonal branch). Also, significant ostio-proximal lesion at large first diagonal, significant lesions at proximal part of dominant left circumflex (LCx) and large first obtuse marginal (OM), and moderate lesion at proximal part of left posterior descending artery (PDA) was seen (left and middle figure). The right coronary artery (RCA) is nondominant artery (right figure). The mid to distal part of LAD was not visualized at left and right injection

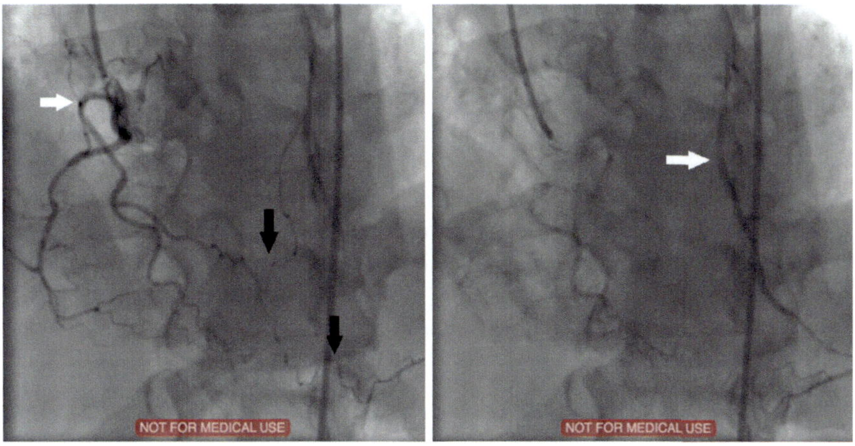

Fig. 32.2 After counterclockwise rotation and minimal withdrawal of JR4 catheter and selective conus artery (white arrow) injection the mid to distal part of well-developed LAD was visualized by some collateral's branches (black arrows) (left figure). Although this part of LAD (white arrow) was visualized fully with some delays (right figure)

Conclusion

The conus artery, first branch of the RCA, courses in anterior aspect of the heart and supplies the right ventricular outflow tract. This branch terminates near the anterior interventricular groove, which also contains the LAD. The conus artery can act as a major collateral source in patients with LAD or RCA occlusions. In about 50% of patients undergoing coronary angiography, the conus artery had a separate ostium near the RCA ostium [1]. Interestedly, in about 20% of patients undergoing coronary angiography and RCA injection, the conus artery was not adequately visualized due to injection of contrast distal to its origin or had a separate ostium [2]. In patients with CTO of the LAD or RCA, the conus artery often serves as a principal source of collateral circulation [2]. In patients with isolated conus artery, nonselective angiography or counterclockwise rotation and minimal withdrawal of JR catheter (same our case) could be helpful for better visualization of this artery. In other cases, multislice computed tomography may be an appropriate alternative diagnostic tool for detecting the isolated conus artery and also evaluation of collateral branches and occluded coronary bed [3].

In some patients undergoing percutaneous coronary intervention (PCI), especially in those with CTO of RCA or LAD, can be used from conus branch as an important collateral pathway for evaluation of the length and course of a totally occluded segment, that is very crucial. It is important that the acquisition must be prolonged to visualize the distal segments filled by collaterals. Also, in some CTO cases of RCA, can be used from conus branch for additional support; by the anchoring wire alone or, more commonly, by inflating the anchoring balloon at low pressure in this branch [4].

On the other hand, injection of contrast media directly into the conus branch may lead to ventricular fibrillation, especially in case of rapid intracoronary contrast medium injection on the condition of super-selective or deep engagement of right catheter [5]. Because in majority of cases, the lumen of the conus artery is small and its close proximity to the RCA ostium, inadvertent engagement of the conus artery by catheter is not uncommon. For the solution of this problem, re-position of the catheter with counterclockwise rotation and gentle withdrawal or re-engaging with a short tip catheter to prevent conus intubation may be helpful, especially when pressure damping has happened on selective engagement of the RCA. Also, for better evaluation of the anatomical location of the conus branch and severity of RCA ostium, a nonselective shot can be taken. If problem sustains and recurrent superselection of the conus branch has occurred, the other choices include using the other catheters such as Williams/3DRC catheters, catheter with a more down-sloping tip should be selected (e.g., JR4.5/JR5 or AR1/AR mod), 5 F JR catheter, or a guide catheter with side-holes [6].

References

1. Başkurt M, Ozkan A, Okçün B, Uzunhasan I, Ersanli M, Gürmen T. The conus artery injection in LAD occlusion. Anadolu Kardiyol Derg. 2008;8(6):E38–9.
2. Levin DC, Beckmann CF, Garnic JD, Carey P, Bettmann MAJC. Frequency and clinical significance of failure to visualize the conus artery during coronary arteriography. Circulation. 1981;63(4):833–7.
3. Andreini D, Mushtaq S, Pontone G, Cortinovis S, Annoni A, Formenti A, Agostoni P, Bartorelli AL, Fiorentini C, Ballerini G, Pepi M. Additional clinical role of 64-slice multidetector computed tomography in the evaluation of coronary artery variants and anomalies. Int J Cardiol. 2010;145(2):388–90.
4. Hirokami M, Saito S, Muto H. Anchoring technique to improve guiding catheter support in coronary angioplasty of chronic total occlusions. Catheter Cardiovasc Interv. 2006;67(3):366–71.
5. Chen J, Gao L, Yao M, Chen J. Ventricular arrhythmia onset during diagnostic coronary angiography with a 5F or 4F universal catheter. Rev Esp Cardiol. 2008;61:1092–5.
6. Lindsay A, Chitkara K, Di Mario C. Complications of percutaneous coronary intervention: the survival handbook: springer; 2016.

Chapter 33
Spontaneous Coronary Artery Dissection

Mohammad Javad Alemzadeh-Ansari

Abstract A 55-year-old woman presented in our hospital with complain of acute chest pain from one week ago. The past medical history was positive for only hypertension. The patient with diagnosis of non-ST segment elevation myocardial infarction (NSTEMI) underwent coronary angiography. The angiogram revealed long significant narrowing in mid part of left anterior descending artery (LAD) artery, which this segment was bordered by normal proximal and distal segments. The patient with diagnosis of spontaneous coronary artery dissection (SCAD type 2A) underwent conservative management.

History and Clinical Presentation

A 55-year-old woman presented in our hospital with complain of acute chest pain from 1 week ago. The past medical history was positive for only hypertension.

Para-Clinic Assessment

The electrocardiogram revealed T-wave inversion in pericardial leads. The echocardiogram showed normal left ventricle size with mid systolic left ventricle dysfunction (LVEF: 45%), hypokinesia in the anterior territory; without significant valvular heart disease. Also, in laboratory data, a rise in serum troponin level was seen.

M. J. Alemzadeh-Ansari (✉)
Cardiovascular Intervention Research Center, Cardio-Oncology Research Center, Rajaie Cardiovascular Medical and Research Center, Iran University of Medical Sciences, Tehran, Iran

M. Maleki, A. Alizadehasl (eds.), *Case-Based Clinical Cardiology*,
https://doi.org/10.1007/978-1-4471-7496-7_33

Managements

The patient with diagnosis of non-ST segment elevation myocardial infarction (NSTEMI) underwent coronary angiography. The angiogram revealed long significant narrowing in the mid part of left anterior descending artery (LAD) artery, which this segment was bordered by normal proximal and distal segments. This significant stenotic segment was smooth and tortuous (Fig. 33.1); other coronary segments were normal (Fig. 33.2). The patient with diagnosis of spontaneous coronary artery dissection (SCAD type 2A) underwent medical treatment with aspirin, metoprolol, atorvastatin, and losartan. Also, because of myocardial infarction, clopidogrel was started. The computed tomography angiography for screening the extra-coronary arteriopathy, especially in the carotid, renal, and iliac arteries was done and revealed no significant pathology in these arteries. After 2 days the patient was asymptomatic and after 7 days was discharged. In follow-up, 6 months later, the patient was asymptomatic.

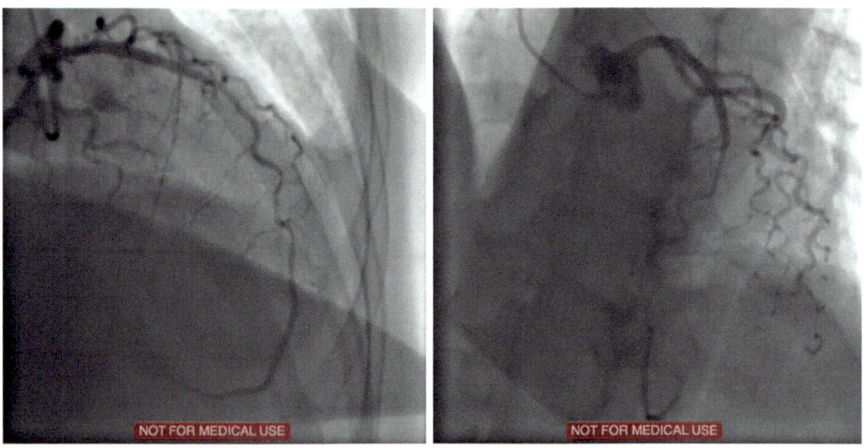

Fig. 33.1 The angiogram in RAO cranial view (left figure) and LAO cranial (right view) revealed long significant narrowing in mid part of left anterior descending artery (LAD) artery, which was bordered this segment by normal proximal and distal segments (SCAD type 2A). This significant stenotic segment was smooth and tortuous

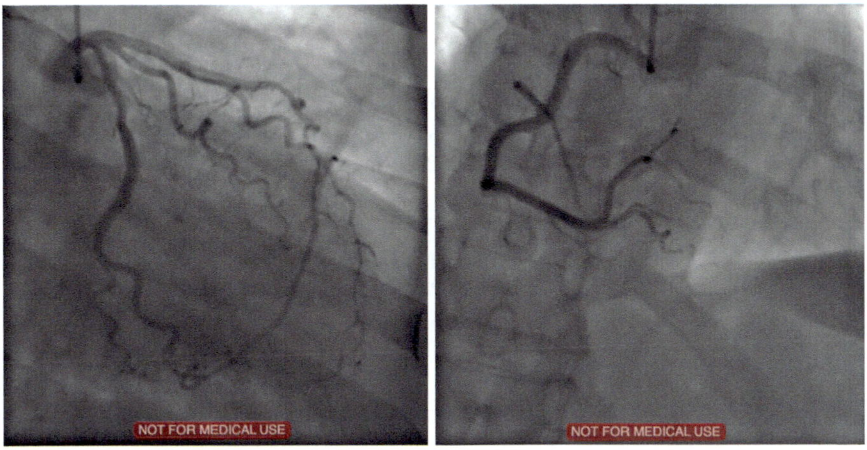

Fig. 33.2 The angiogram revealed that other coronary segments were patent without significant lesion

Conclusion

Epidemiology

The SCAD, a rare cause of acute coronary syndrome (ACS) or sudden cardiac death, is defined as an epicardial coronary artery dissection that is not associated with atherosclerosis or trauma and not iatrogenic. SCAD most commonly occurs in patients with few or no traditional cardiovascular risk factors. The true prevalence of SCAD remains uncertain, primarily because it is an underdiagnosed condition, but it is considered as a 1% to 4% of overall ACS cases. Although SCAD can occur in both men and women, it has occurred more in woman and it counts about 35% of MIs among women ≤50 years of age. The average age of women with SCAD ranges from 45 to 53 years. Interestedly, SCAD is the most common cause of pregnancy-associated MI (43%). The majority of patients with SCAD are white, but this condition has been reported in all major racial and ethnic groups. Although any coronary artery can be involved by SACD, the LAD artery is the most commonly involved (Table 33.1) [1]. The mid to distal segments of coronary arteries are more affected by SCAD, and only less than 10% of cases involved the proximal segment of coronary arteries [2].

Table 33.1 The coronary distribution of SCAD [1]

	Prevalence (%)
LAD and branches (septal and diagonal)	45–61
LCx and OM	15–45
RCA and branches (acute marginal, PDA, and PLB)	10–39
Left main	Up to 4
Multivessel	9–23

LAD left anterior descending; *LCx* left circumflex; *OM* obtuse marginal; *PDA* posterior descending artery; *PLB* posterolateral branch; *SCAD* spontaneous coronary artery dissection

Pathogenesis and Etiology

SCAD results from sudden disruption of the coronary artery wall and intramural hematoma (IMH) development in the outer third of the media or between the media and the adventitia in the absence of traumatic or iatrogenic causes, resulting in a false lumen. Expansion of false lumen through blood or clot accumulation leads to distal propagation of the dissection and to compression of the true lumen, causing myocardial ischemia [3]. There are two theories about SCAD development in coronary artery: (1) primary event is intimal tearing which allows blood from the true lumen to enter and generate a false lumen, (2) primary event is a spontaneous hemorrhage (IMH) arising from the vasa vasorum within the vessel wall. Although some believed that increasing pressure in the false lumen can cause reverse intimal rupture into the true lumen [1].

SCAD-Associated Conditions

The prevalence of traditional cardiovascular risk factors is low in patients with SCAD. On the other hand, other factors such as arteriopathies, genetic factors, hormonal influences, inherited or acquired arteriopathies, or systemic inflammatory diseases, often compounded by environmental precipitants or stressors have more effect on SCAD development. The most common associated condition associated with SCAD is multifocal fibromuscular dysplasia (FMD) in extracoronary arteries [1]. Thus, the screening for extracoronary arteriopathy by angiography, computed tomography angiography, or magnetic resonance angiography in these patients is recommended [1].

FMD, a nonatherosclerotic, noninflammatory vascular disease, most commonly affects the renal and internal carotid arteries but has been described in almost every arterial bed in the body. It can manifest as arterial stenosis, aneurysm, tortuosity, or dissection [4]. FMD according to the American Heart Association classification was defined in two types: (1) multifocal, most common type, is defined as the presence of sequential focal narrowing separated by focal dilations such as depicted in a classic string of beads pattern and (2) unifocal, less than 10% of cases, defined as single concentric or tubular narrowing [5].

The peripartum is another important condition associated with SCAD. The most common cause of MIs during pregnancy or in the 6-week postpartum period is SCAD [6, 7]. Although SCAD could be observed as early as 5 weeks of gestation and up to several months to a year or more postpartum, particularly in women who are still lactating, but the majority of pregnancy-associated SCAD events occur in the third trimester or early postpartum period. Also, the left main or LAD artery has been described as the most common coronary arteries which is affected. The most common hypothesis about pregnancy-associated SCAD is the hemodynamical and hormonal alternations during this period; resulting in an increase in spontaneous dissections in the arterial wall [1].

Clinical Presentation

There are wide ranges of clinical presentations ranges from unstable angina, acute MI, ventricular arrhythmias to sudden cardiac death. In rare instances, it can be asymptomatic and discovered incidentally on coronary angiography. Whenever a young patient, especially woman, without conventional major coronary risk factors or a woman in the postpartum period presents with an ACS or sudden cardiac death, the possibility of a SCAD should be suspected and an urgent coronary angiography should be performed [3].

Management

The conventional coronary angiography in ACS patients is the first-line diagnostic imaging method; although the major limitation of this method in patient with SCAD is that angiography is 2-dimensional lumenography and could not illustrate the structure of arterial wall and also, IMH. The SCAD based on angiographic appearance of stenotic segment and also severity and length of lesion divided into three types [1]:

- Type 1, Classic appearance of multiple radiolucent lumens or arterial wall contrast staining.
- Type 2, Presence of diffuse stenosis (usually >20 mm) divided into two variants: variant 2A, diffuse arterial narrowing bordered by normal segments proximal and distal to the IMH, and variant 2B, diffuse narrowing that extends to the distal tip of the artery.
- Type 3, Focal or tubular stenosis, usually <20 mm in length, that mimics atherosclerosis.

In some cases, intracoronary imaging including intravascular ultrasonography (IVUS) or optical coherence tomography (OCT) is required to confirm the presence of IMH. In patients with SCAD suspicious, catheter engagement in the coronary ostium and contrast injection should be done with great caution, because deep catheter engagement, noncoaxial positioning of the catheter tip, catheter dampening, and forceful contrast injection may lead to development or extension of the coronary dissection [8].

The conservative management is a preferred strategy for patients with SCAD and ACS, in contrast to the common atherosclerotic ACS. This decision is according on the natural history of spontaneous healing in SCAD, high rates of failure and/or complications during revascularization, and also poor clinical outcomes in those who underwent revascularization. Dual antiplatelet, beta-blockers, statins, ACE inhibitors, angiotensin, and mineralocorticoid receptor antagonists should be administrated according to ACS guidelines [9]. Interestedly, a large study showed that only the beta-blocker can reduce the risk of recurrent SCAD, whereas uncontrolled hypertension can increase this risk in long-term follow-up [10].

The conservative management may not be appropriate in high-risk patients with ongoing ischemia, left main artery dissection, or hemodynamic instability. The major complication during percutaneous coronary intervention in these patients include the entrance of coronary guidewires into false lumen and occlude the true lumen, extending dissection of the intima or propagating IMH upstream and downstream from the vessel following balloon dilation or stent placement, and long-term stent thrombosis resulting stent strut malapposition following resolving the IMH [11, 12].

References

1. Hayes SN, Kim ES, Saw J, Adlam D, Arslanian-Engoren C, Economy KE, et al. Spontaneous coronary artery dissection: current state of the science: a scientific statement from the American Heart Association. Circulation. 2018;137(19):e523–e57.
2. Saw J, Aymong E, Sedlak T, Buller CE, Starovoytov A, Ricci D, et al. Spontaneous coronary artery dissection: association with predisposing arteriopathies and precipitating stressors and cardiovascular outcomes. Circ Cardiovasc Interv. 2014;7:645–55.
3. Vrints CJ. Spontaneous coronary artery dissection. Heart. 2010;96(10):801–8.
4. Slovut DP, Olin JW. Fibromuscular dysplasia. N Engl J Med. 2004;350:1862–71.
5. Olin JW, Gornik HL, Bacharach JM, Biller J, Fine LJ, Gray BH, et al. Fibromuscular dysplasia: state of the science and critical unanswered questions: a scientific statement from the American Heart Association. Circulation. 2014;129:1048–78.
6. Elkayam U, Jalnapurkar S, Barakkat MN, Khatri N, Kealey AJ, Mehra A, Roth A. Pregnancy-associated acute myocardial infarction: a review of contemporary experience in 150 cases between 2006 and 2011. Circulation. 2014;129:1695–702.
7. Faden MS, Bottega N, Benjamin A, Brown RN. A nationwide evaluation of spontaneous coronary artery dissection in pregnancy and the puerperium. Heart. 2016;102:1974–9.
8. Prakash R, Starovoytov A, Heydari M, Mancini GB, Saw J. Catheter-induced iatrogenic coronary artery dissection in patients with spontaneous coronary artery dissection. JACC Cardiovasc Interv. 2016;9:1851–3.

9. Amsterdam EA, Wenger NK, Brindis RG, Casey DE, Ganiats TG, Holmes DR, et al. AHA/ACC guideline for the management of patients with non-ST-elevation acute coronary syndromes: executive summary: a report of the American College of Cardiology/American Heart Association task force on practice guidelines. Circulation. 2014;130:2354–94.
10. Saw J, Humphries K, Aymong E, et al. Spontaneous coronary artery dissection: clinical outcomes and risk of recurrence. J Am Coll Cardiol. 2017;70:1148–58.
11. Lempereur M, Fung A, Saw J. Stent mal-apposition with resorption of intramural hematoma with spontaneous coronary artery dissection. Cardiovasc Diagn Ther. 2015;5:323–9.
12. Alfonso F, Bastante T, García-Guimaraes M, Pozo E, Cuesta J, Rivero F, Benedicto A, Antuña P, Alvarado T, Gulati R, Saw J. Spontaneous coronary artery dissection: new insights into diagnosis and treatment. Coron Artery Dis. 2016;27:696–706.

Chapter 34
Catheter-Induced Severe Right Coronary Artery Dissection During Coronary Angiography: A Successful Aortocoronary Stenting

Bahram Mohebbi

Abstract A 42-year-old female patient complained with chest pain since three months ago. The physical examination was unremarkable. Patient was candidate for selective coronary angiography. Catheter induced dissection of right coronary artery (RCA) was occurred. Immediate stenting at the origin of the dissection, aortocoronary stenting, followed by stenting from proximal to distal part of RCA was performed to repair dissected RCA. After the procedure, patient was transferred to coronary care unit (CCU) and computed tomography (CT) angiography of aorta was performed and did not show any propagation of dissecting flap into the aorta. Post PCI course was uneventful and patient was discharged after a week. It is concluded that immediate coronary artery stenting at the origin of coronary artery can be a vital and emergent life-saving plan in catheter-induced coronary dissection.

History and Clinical Presentation

A 42-year-old female patient complained with chest pain since 3 months ago. The physical examination was unremarkable. Electrocardiography (ECG) showed normal sinus rhythm without any abnormality.

Electronic Supplementary Material The online version of this chapter (https://doi.org/10.1007/978-1-4471-7496-7_34) contains supplementary material, which is available to authorized users.

B. Mohebbi (✉)
Cardiovascular Intervention Research Center, Cardio-Oncology Research Center, Rajaie Cardiovascular Medical and Research Center, Iran University of Medical Sciences, Tehran, Iran

M. Maleki, A. Alizadehasl (eds.), *Case-Based Clinical Cardiology*,
https://doi.org/10.1007/978-1-4471-7496-7_34

Para-Clinic Assessment

Exercise test was positive. Selective Coronary angiography showed no significant lesion in the left coronary arteries (Fig. 34.1) (Video 34.1). Right coronary artery (RCA) injection revealed midpart 50% stenosis associated with dissection from ostium to the distal part which has been resulted during catheter manipulation in RCA angiography (Fig. 34.2) (Video 34.2). The patient developed chest pain associated with electrocardiographic evidence of ST-segment elevation in inferior leads. RCA was a dominant artery with a spiral dissection located between ostium and just before the proximal portion of the posterior descending and posterolateral artery bifurcation. Aortic root injection showed no retrograde propagation of dissecting flap into the aorta.

Managements

The decision was made to perform a PCI to the RCA lesion. Immediate stenting at the source of the dissection, aortoostial stenting, followed by stenting from proximal to distal part were performed successfully to repair the moderate stenotic and dissected RCA (Fig. 34.3) (Video 34.3). After the procedure, the patient was transferred to coronary care unit (CCU) and computed tomography (CT) angiography of ascending aorta was performed and did not show any propagation of dissecting flap into the aorta. There was no evidence in favor of PCI related myocardial infarction

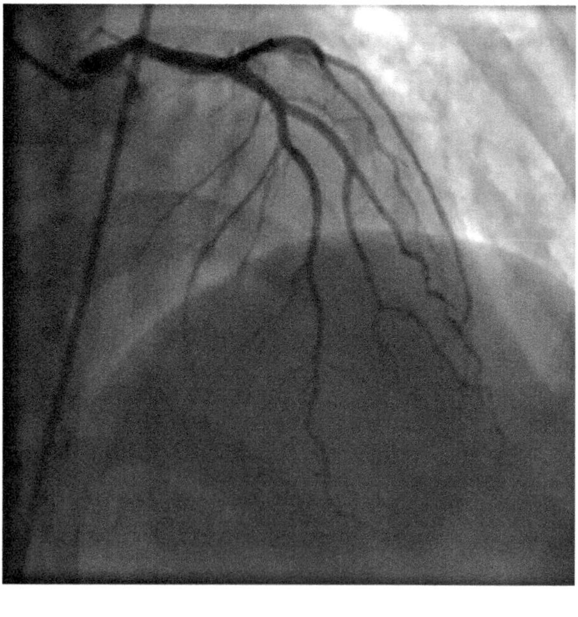

Fig. 34.1 Left coronary arteries angiography. There is no stenosis in left coronary artery system

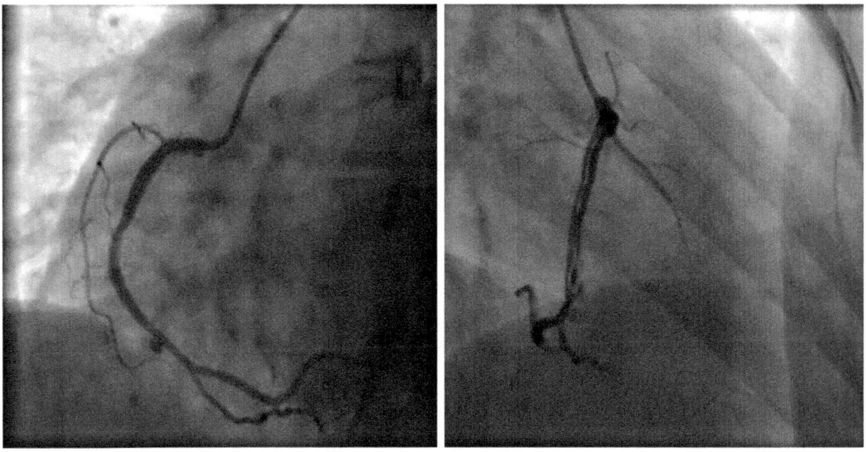

Fig. 34.2 Right coronary artery angiography. (**a**) Dominant RCA with midpart 50% stenosis. (**b**) dissection flap from ostium to distal part

Fig. 34.3 Stented right coronary artery. Final result of right coronary artery stenting

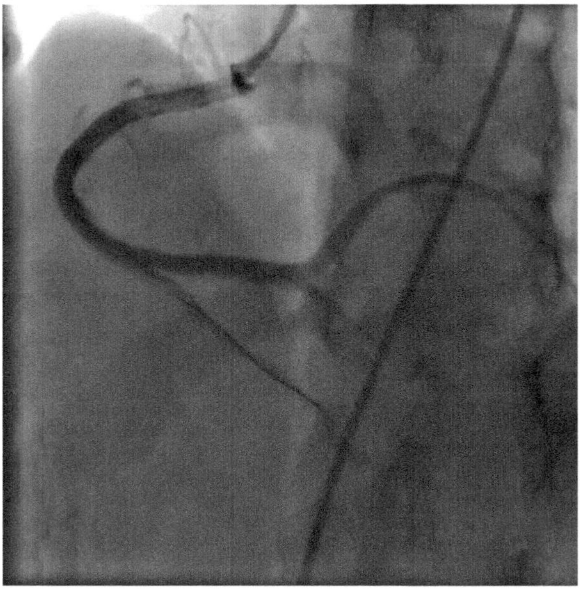

based on serial measurement of Troponin-T (cTn) level which was within normal limit [1]. Post-PCI course was uneventful and the patient was discharged after a week.

Catheter-induced coronary artery dissection is a rare but serious complication of diagnostic coronary angiography and percutaneous coronary intervention (PCI) [2]. Propagation of a coronary dissection resulting from mechanical trauma due to a catheter, wire, inflated balloon, or other device. Even this dissection can progress retrogradely to the ascending aorta [3]. Although treatment of coronary artery dissection may require surgical repair, coronary artery stenting is the mainstay treatment of dissection, even stenting at the origin of the dissection area may be sufficient in aortocoronary dissection [4].

Contrast injections may cause catheter-induced dissection to progress which was assumed by Perez-Castellano et al. [4] Also, ide branches rising from the epicardial vessels may be involved during propagation of coronary dissection. The shearing forces of blood flow during both systole and diastole could also probably explain the propagation of the dissection.

Conclusion

It is concluded that immediate coronary artery stenting at the aortocoronary dissection can be a vital and emergent life-saving plan in catheter-induced dissection. CT angiography can be safely conducted to more evaluation for residual aortic extension of the dissection and follow-up.

References

1. Maleki M, Alizadehasl A, Haghjoo M. Chapter 19 - ST-segment elevation myocardial infarction. In: Practical cardiology. Philadelphia, PA: Elsevier; 2017. p. 311–28.
2. Gur M, Yilmaz R, Demirbag R, Kunt AS. Large atherosclerotic plaque related severe right coronary artery dissection during coronary angiography. Int J Cardiovasc Imaging. 2006;22(3-4):321–5. https://doi.org/10.1007/s10554-005-9036-9.
3. Shah P, Dzavik V. Percutaneous treatment of dissection of the ascending aorta occurring as a complication during coronary angioplasty of a saphenous vein bypass graft. J Interv Cardiol. 2005;18:45–8.
4. Perez-Castellano N, Garcia-Fernandez MA, Garcia EJ, Delcan JL. Dissection of the aortic sinus of Valsalva complicating coronary catheterization: cause, mechanism, evolution, and management. Cathet Cardiovasc Diagn. 1998;43:273–9.
5. Carr JJ, Jacobs DR Jr, Terry JG, et al. Association of coronary artery calcium in adults aged 32 to 46 years with incident coronary heart disease and death. JAMA Cardiol. 2017;2:391–9.

Chapter 35
A Rare Case of Adult Type ALCAPA Syndrome

Bahram Mohebbi

Abstract A 43-year-old male patient complained with atypical chest pain and dyspnea on exertion since six months ago. In heart physical examination, S1, S2, and III/VI systolic murmur in left sternal border was detected. In transthoracic echocardiography, mild LV enlargement with severe systolic dysfunction, EF=30% was reported. Patient was candidate for selective coronary angiography. Based on coronary angiography, Anomalous origin of the left coronary artery from the pulmonary artery (ALCAPA) syndrome was confirmed and referred to cardiac surgeon to manage his condition.

History and Clinical Presentation

This case report described a 43-year-old male patient presented with atypical chest pain and dyspnea on exertion with slight limitation of physical activity, (New York Heart Association [NYHA] class II) since 6 months ago. The patient's vital signs were blood pressure 120/70 mmHg, pulse 80 beats/min with a regular rhythm. He did not report any cardiovascular risk factor. In heart physical examination, S1, S2, and III/VI systolic murmur in the left sternal border was detected.

Electronic Supplementary Material The online version of this chapter (https://doi.org/10.1007/978-1-4471-7496-7_35) contains supplementary material, which is available to authorized users.

B. Mohebbi (✉)
Cardiovascular Intervention Research Center, Cardio-Oncology Research Center, Rajaie Cardiovascular Medical and Research Center, Iran University of Medical Sciences, Tehran, Iran

M. Maleki, A. Alizadehasl (eds.), *Case-Based Clinical Cardiology*,
https://doi.org/10.1007/978-1-4471-7496-7_35

Para-Clinic Assessment

In transthoracic echocardiography, mild LV enlargement with severe systolic dysfunction, EF = 30% was reported. The patient underwent coronary angiography. Access was made through the right radial artery and due to the inability to engage the left coronary system, nonselective aortic root injection revealed only right coronary artery (RCA) origination from aorta which filled the left coronary system retrogradely (Video 35.1).

In selective RCA angiography, RCA was dominant and huge which retrogradely filled the left coronary system and drained to the pulmonary artery(PA) (Fig. 35.1) (Video 35.2). Actually, the left coronary system was originated from PA with retrogradely filled via RCA with good distal runoff.

Management

Because of enhancing survival rate due to performing surgery among pediatric ALCAPA patients, in this case, assessing the risk/benefit for surgery; finally, surgical correction was considered to the patient which was performed successfully.

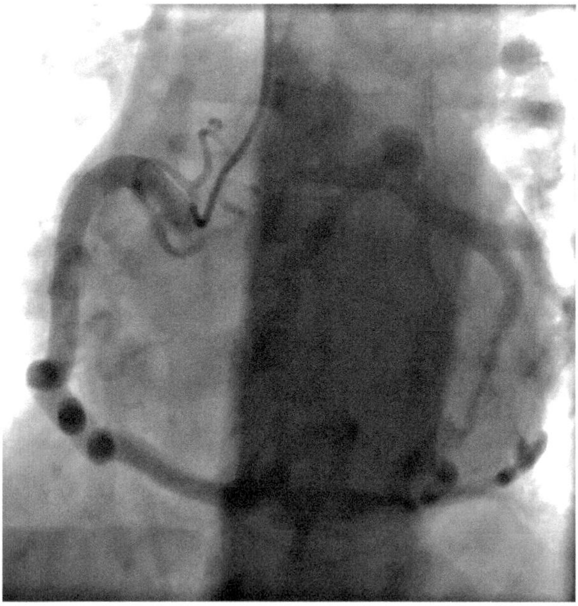

Fig. 35.1 Selective RCA angiography. RCA was dominant and huge which retrogradely filled left coronary system and drained to PA

Conclusion

Coronary artery anomalies consist of several variants with diverse cardiovascular manifestations. In order to categorize each anomaly, distinguishing any condition of anatomic pattern and clinical significance to understand the prognosis is crucial. ALCAPA syndrome is an uncommon diagnosis. Generally, it is very rare for ALCAPA syndrome to be diagnosed in adulthood, because if they did not receive on-time treatment in childhood, this malformation can lead to death [1]. Due to low pulmonary artery pressure, flow in the left coronary artery reverses and drains to the pulmonary artery instead of supplying the myocardium completely. So there is a steal phenomenon due to this left-to-right shunting [2]. The final decision in patients with ALCAPA syndrome is surgery. There are some surgical techniques as left main (LM) coronary artery reimplantation, Takeuchi procedure, left coronary artery ligation, and left coronary artery ligation with concomitant coronary artery bypass grafting [3].

References

1. Saedi S, Parsaee M, Farrashi M, Noohi F, Mohebbi B. The role of echocardiography in anomalous origin of coronary artery from pulmonary artery (ALCAPA): simple tool for a complex diagnosis. Echocardiography. 2019;36:177–81. https://doi.org/10.1111/echo.14236.
2. Elena P, Elsie TN, Naeem M, Carole D. ALCAPA syndrome: not just a pediatric disease. Radiographics. 2009;29:553–65.
3. Yew KL, Kang Z, Anum A. Late presentation of ALCAPA syndrome in an elderly Asian lady. Med J Malaysia. 2016;71(4):217–9.

Chapter 36
Takotsubo Syndrome

Bahram Mohebbi and Feridoun Noohi

Abstract A 64-year-old postmenopausal female patient complained with chest pain, dyspnea and palpitation referred to our center. Physical examination was unremarkable. She noted hypothyroidism in past medical history. In transthoracic echocardiography, normal LV size with severe systolic dysfunction, EF=25% with mild inferior hypokinesia and mild inferoseptal severe hypokinesia, apex and all related segments were akinetic with preserved tissue and moderate diastolic dysfunction were reported. Patient was candidate for selective coronary angiography. Based on coronary angiography and left ventriculography, Takotsubo syndrome was confirmed and appropriate medications was considered.

History and Clinical Presentation

This case report described a 64-year-old postmenopausal female patient complained with chest pain, dyspnea, and palpitation referred to our center. In heart physical examination, the patient's vital signs were blood pressure 105/70 mmHg, pulse 80 beats/min with regular rhythm. She noted hypothyroidism in past medical history. ECG revealed T-wave inversion in precordial leads and also there was mildly elevated troponin level.

Electronic Supplementary Material The online version of this chapter (https://doi.org/10.1007/978-1-4471-7496-7_36) contains supplementary material, which is available to authorized users.

B. Mohebbi (✉)
Cardiovascular Intervention Research Center, Cardio-Oncology Research Center, Rajaie Cardiovascular Medical and Research Center, Iran University of Medical Sciences, Tehran, Iran

F. Noohi
Interventional Cardiologist; Rajaie Cardiovascular Medical Center, Iran University of Medical Sciences, Tehran, Iran

M. Maleki, A. Alizadehasl (eds.), *Case-Based Clinical Cardiology*,
https://doi.org/10.1007/978-1-4471-7496-7_36

Para-Clinic Assessment

Transthoracic echocardiography showed normal LV size with severely decreased ejection fraction (EF = 25%), mid inferior hypokinesia, and mid inferoseptal severe hypokinesia, apex, and all related segments were akinetic with preserved tissue, and moderate diastolic dysfunction.

The patient underwent coronary angiography via right femoral access. There was only nonsignificant narrowing in the midpart of the left anterior descending (LAD) artery and the remaining coronary arteries were within the normal limit (Figs. 36.1 and 36.2). Left ventricle (LV) injection showed normal LV size with sever hypokinesia in all apical segments with good motion in the basal segments of LV (Apical ballooning) and severe LV dysfunction, LVEF = 20% (Fig. 36.3 and Video 36.1).

Management

In this case, medical treatment for LV dysfunction, including Beta-blockers, Diuretics, and Angiotensin II Receptor Blockers (ARB) inhibitors, was considered and the patient was referred to heart failure clinic for ambulate follow-up.

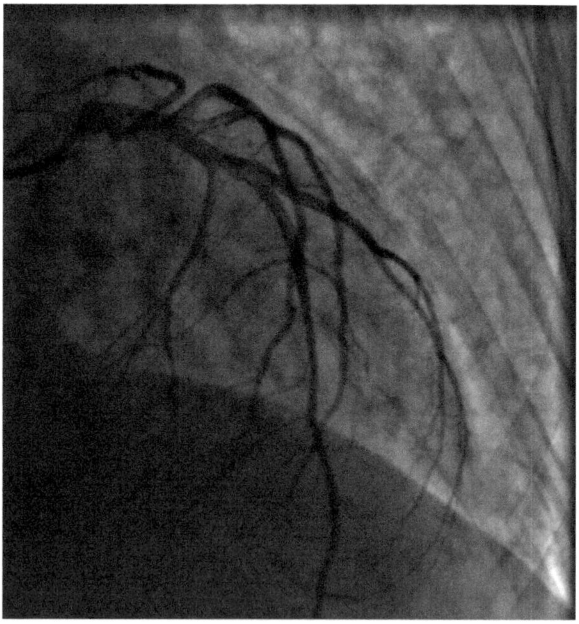

Fig. 36.1 Left coronary arteries angiography. There is nonsignificant narrowing in midpart of (LAD) artery

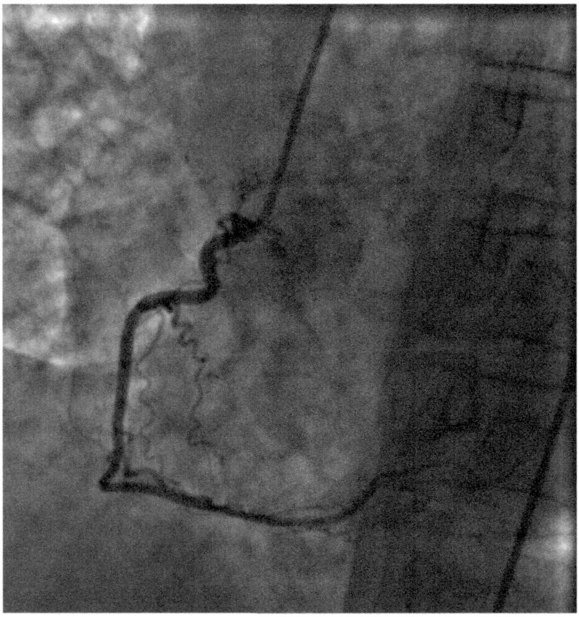

Fig. 36.2 Right coronary artery (RCA) angiography. Dominant and within normal limit

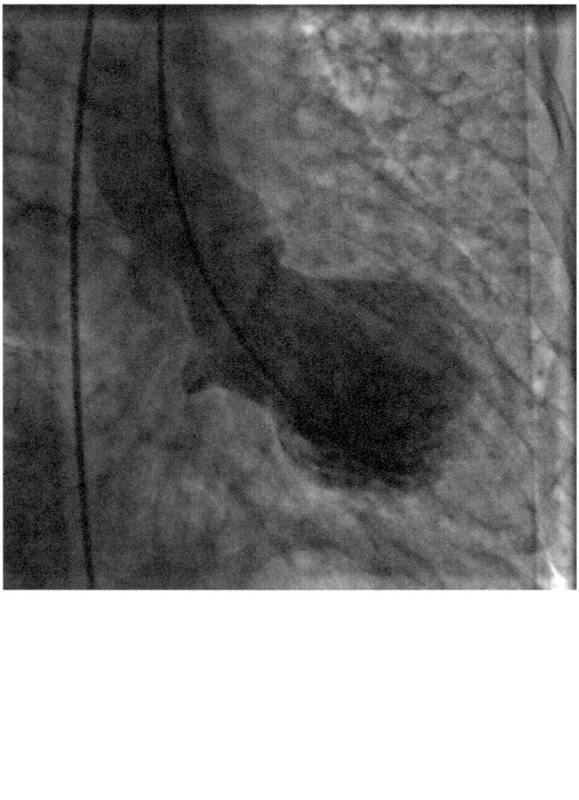

Fig. 36.3 Left ventriculography in right anterior oblique (RAO) projection. Normal LV size with apical ballooning morphology

Conclusion

Takotsubo syndrome described as a transient left ventricular systolic dysfunction, which frequently mimics a myocardial infarction activated by physical stress or emotional conditions [1]. Also, it is known as stress cardiomyopathy, apical ballooning syndrome, and broken heart syndrome. Takotsubo syndrome is an uncommon cardiomyopathy [2]. About 90% of Takotsubo cardiomyopathy cases happen in postmenopausal women aged between 58 and 75 years old [1]. Takotsubo syndrome presents with clinical features of acute myocardial infarction and LV dysfunction but there are normal coronary arteries in coronary angiography. The postulated mechanism seems to be catecholamine excess which may result in catecholamine intoxication, coronary spasm, and dysfunction of microvasculature causing myocardial damage [3]. As there are no evidence-based guidelines on Takotsubo management, patients are managed based on standard heart failure medications (Angiotensin-converting enzyme [ACE]/Angiotensin II Receptor Blockers [ARB] inhibitors, Beta-blockers, and Diuretics) [4]. It is concluded that facing patients (especially in postmenopausal female) with chest pain, ECG changes, and raising troponin level, besides to acute coronary syndrome (ACS), Takotsubo syndrome should be considered.

References

1. Barbaryan A, Bailuc SL, Patel K, Raqeem MW, Thakur A, Mirrakhimov AE. An emotional stress as a trigger for reverse Takotsubo cardiomyopathy: a case report and literature review. Am J Case Rep. 2016;17:137–42.
2. Ahmadjee A, Herzallah K, Saleh Y, Abela GS. Takotsubo cardiomyopathy presenting with different morphological patterns in the same patient: a case report and review of the literature. Cardiovasc Pathol. 2020;47:107204. https://doi.org/10.1016/j.carpath.2020.107204.
3. Pelliccia F, Kaski JC, Crea F, Camici PG. Pathophysiology of Takotsubo syndrome. Circulation. 2017;135(24):2426–41. https://doi.org/10.1161/CIRCULATIONAHA.116.027121.
4. Hollenberg SM, Warner Stevenson L, Ahmad T, Amin VJ, Bozkurt B, Butler J, Davis LL, et al. ACC expert consensus decision pathway on risk assessment, management, and clinical trajectory of patients hospitalized with heart failure: a report of the American College of Cardiology solution set oversight committee. J Am Coll Cardiol. 2019;74(15):1966–2011. https://doi.org/10.1016/j.jacc.2019.08.001.

Chapter 37
Hypertrophic Cardiomyopathy: A Case of Left Ventricle "Ballerina Foot" Morphology

Bahram Mohebbi and Feridoun Noohi

Abstract A 64-year-old male patient complained of dyspnea on exertion, New York Heart Association (NYHA) functional class II since six weeks ago. The physical examination revealed normal S1, S2 and II/VI systolic murmur in apex. Electrocardiography (ECG) revealed sinus rhythm with left bundle branch block (LBBB) QRS morphology. Transthoracic echocardiography showed normal LV size with LV EF=55%, asymmetric septal hypertrophy (anteroseptal wall thickness:1.8 cm), mild systolic anterior motion (SAM) of the anterior leaflet of mitral valve with mild mitral regurgitation (MR), no significant left ventricular outflow tract (LVOT) obstruction (LVOT peak gradient: 12mmHg). The echocardiographic findings were compatible with hypertrophic cardiomyopathy (HCM). Selective coronary angiography was performed, left and right coronary arteries were within normal limit, left ventriculography revealed normal LV size, EF= 55%, "Ballerina Foot" morphology without significant trans-left ventricular outflow tract (LVOT) gradient (peak gradient=10mmHg. It could be concluded that HCM should be considered in patients with dyspnea on exertion. Also, based on hereditary nature of disease, evaluating the family members of diagnosed patients is recommended.

History and Clinical Presentation

A 64-year-old male patient presented with dyspnea on exertion New York Heart Association (NYHA) functional class II since 6 weeks ago. Vital signs were blood pressure 120/80 mmHg, pulse 84 beats/min with a regular rhythm. Physical examination revealed normal S1, S2, and II/VI systolic murmur in apex. Electrocardiography (ECG) showed sinus rhythm with left bundle branch block (LBBB) QRS morphology.

B. Mohebbi (✉)
Cardiovascular Intervention Research Center, Cardio-Oncology Research Center, Rajaie Cardiovascular Medical and Research Center, Iran University of Medical Sciences, Tehran, Iran

F. Noohi
Interventional Cardiologist; Rajaie Cardiovascular Medical Center, Iran University of Medical Sciences, Tehran, Iran

M. Maleki, A. Alizadehasl (eds.), *Case-Based Clinical Cardiology*,
https://doi.org/10.1007/978-1-4471-7496-7_37

Para-Clinic Assessment

Transthoracic echocardiography showed normal LV size with LV EF = 55%, mild LV diastolic dysfunction, asymmetric septal hypertrophy (anteroseptal wall thickness: 1.8 cm), mild systolic anterior motion (SAM) of the anterior leaflet of mitral valve with mild mitral regurgitation (MR), no significant left ventricular outflow tract (LVOT) obstruction (LVOT peak gradient: 12 mmHg). The echocardiographic findings were compatible with hypertrophic cardiomyopathy (HCM). Selective coronary angiography and left heart catheterism were also performed. Left and right coronary arteries were within normal limit (Figs. 37.1 and 37.2); left ventricle (LV) injection revealed normal LV size, EF = 55%, "Ballerina Foot" morphology (LV anterior convexity with early robust contraction of the posteromedial portion of LV, resulting in the morphology similar to a ballet dancer's foot) without significant trans-left ventricular outflow tract (LVOT) gradient (peak gradient = 10 mmHg) (Fig. 37.3).

Managements

Since the patient was symptomatic without LVOT obstruction, beta-blocker was started for him and his symptom improved dramatically in follow-up.

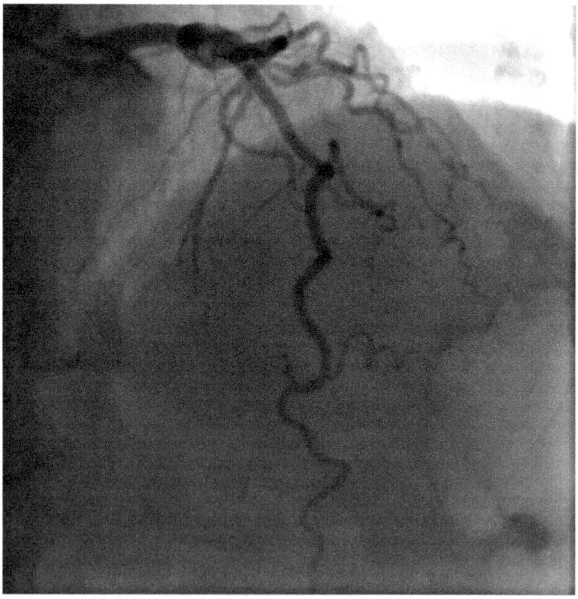

Fig. 37.1 Left coronary arteries angiography. There is no stenosis in left coronary artery system

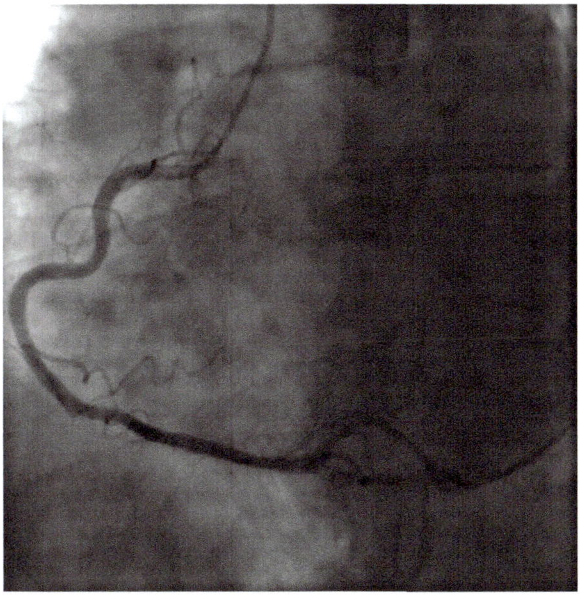

Fig. 37.2 Right coronary artery angiography. There is no stenosis in right coronary artery

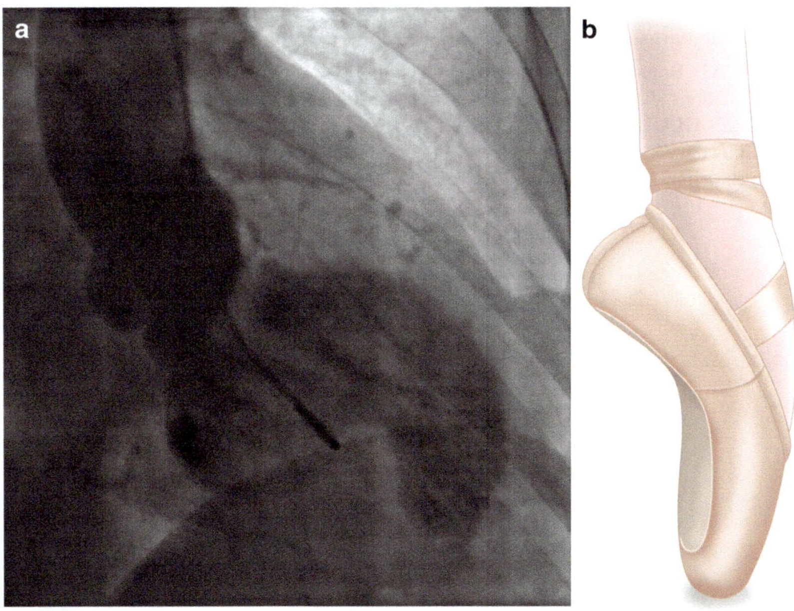

Fig. 37.3 Left ventriculography in right anterior oblique (RAO) projection. LV anterior convexity with early robust contraction of the posteromedial portion of LV, resulting in "Ballerina foot" morphology (**a**) similar to a ballet dancer's foot (**b**)

Conclusion

HCM as a genetic disorder described with left ventricular hypertrophy based on a non-dilated LV with preserved/increased ejection fraction [1]. Maximum disease-related mortality is related to sudden cardiac death, followed by heart failure and stroke-related embolism [2]. Clinical assessment of patients with HCM consists of a detailed personal and family history for HCM, sudden cardiac death, and heart failure, physical examination, 12-lead ECG, and complete echocardiographic assessment. Cardiac magnetic resonance (CMR) imaging sometimes considers as a complementary tool besides to echocardiography for the assessment of HCM. All patients should be counseled to the genetic nature of the disease. Because of being asymptomatic or minimally symptomatic of most patients with HCM, they do not feel the need to adherence medical treatment. Periodic re-evaluation in asymptomatic patients seems necessary [2]. Health care workers should encourage them to have a healthy lifestyle to reach a better quality of life. Patients with HCM may be optimistic to have a near-normal life expectancy using modern management strategies including family screening, risk stratification, thromboembolic prophylaxis, and implantation of cardioverter-defibrillators [2].

References

1. Marian AJ, Braunwald E. Hypertrophic cardiomyopathy: genetics, pathogenesis, clinical manifestations, diagnosis, and therapy. Circ Res. 2017;121(7):749–70. https://doi.org/10.1161/CIRCRESAHA.117.311059.
2. Sen-Chowdhry S, Jacoby D, Moon J, et al. Update on hypertrophic cardiomyopathy and a guide to the guidelines. Nat Rev Cardiol. 2016;13:651–75. https://doi.org/10.1038/nrcardio.2016.140.

Chapter 38
Device Closure of Multi-Fenestrated Atrial Septal Defect

Sedigheh Saedi

Abstract Atrial septal defects (ASD) are categorized into ostium primum, ostium secundum, sinus venosus, and coronary sinus types with the secundum type being the most prevalent form. ASD should be repaired once diagnosed to prevent progressive right ventricular enlargement and volume overload. With the advances in the field of structural heart disease interventions and advent of new occluder devices many secundum type ASDs are amenable to catheter closure. The major limitations of the percutaneous method are insufficient rims, multiple ASDs and highly aneurysmal atrial septum. However new devices have been developed for closure of the multi-fenestrated or "Cribriform" defects that help the patients benefit from a less invasive repair method. Here we present a patient with multiple defects successfully managed by catheter intervention.

History and Clinical Presentation

A 31-year-old female presented with recent onset palpitation and mild exertional dyspnea. Past medical history was negative and she had no history of drug use. Physical examination was normal except for wide fixed splitting of the second heart sound in cardiac auscultation.

Para-Clinic Assessment

Twelve lead ECG showed normal sinus rhythm with incomplete right bundle branch block and T wave inversion in V2–V3 precordial leads. Chest X-ray depicted evidence of right ventricular (RV) enlargement and pulmonary overflow.

S. Saedi (✉)
Rajaei Cardiovascular Medical and Research Center, Iran University of Medical Sciences, Tehran, Iran

M. Maleki, A. Alizadehasl (eds.), *Case-Based Clinical Cardiology*,
https://doi.org/10.1007/978-1-4471-7496-7_38

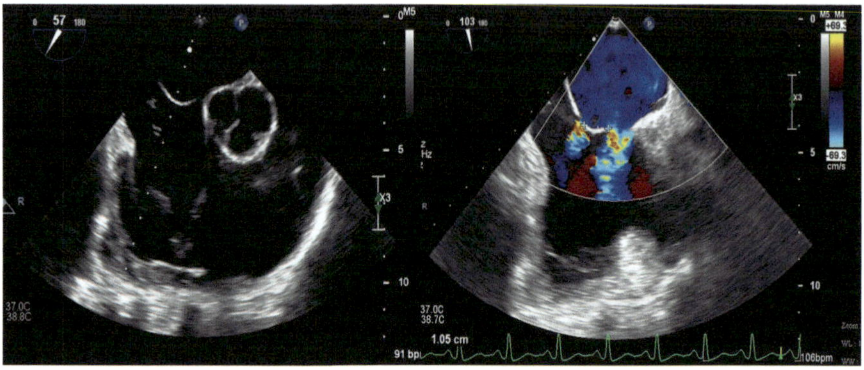

Fig. 38.1 Two-dimensional and color Doppler TEE views showing aneurysmal IAS with multiple defects in different echocardiographic planes

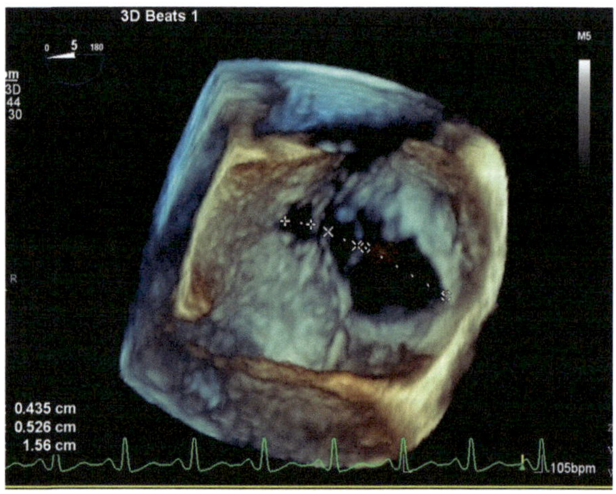

Fig. 38.2 Three-dimensional echocardiography image of multiple ASDs

Transthoracic and transesophageal (TEE) echocardiography was performed that showed moderate RV enlargement with normal RV systolic function, mildly increased pulmonary arterial pressure(40 mmHg), aneurysmal interatrial septum (IAS), and multiple secundum type ASDs (three defects measuring 16, 7, and 5 mm) with significant left to right shunt. IAS was redundant and aneurysmal (Figs. 38.1 and 38.2).

Management

Cardiac catheterization and hemodynamic assessment showed significant left to right shunt and a Qp/Qs: 2.9:1. Under TEE guidance a superstiff guidewire was passed through the most central defect and a dedicated Figulla® Flex II UNI 33 mm Occlutech device was deployed with good final results. Intra-procedural TEE showed that all the defects were covered by the device (Figs. 38.3 and 38.4).

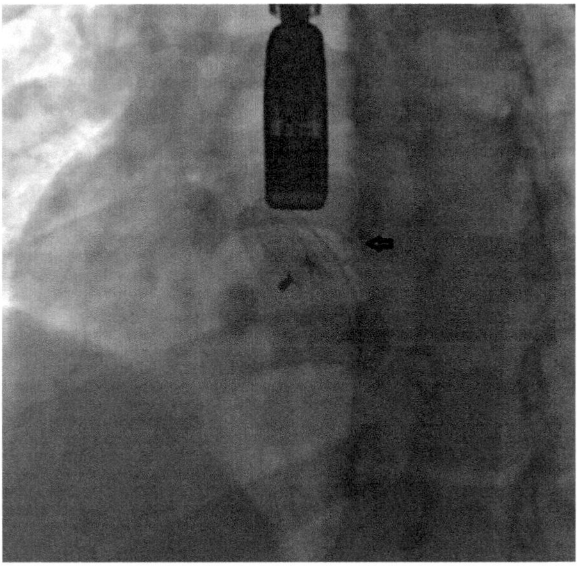

Fig. 38.3 Fluoroscopic image showing implanted occlude device

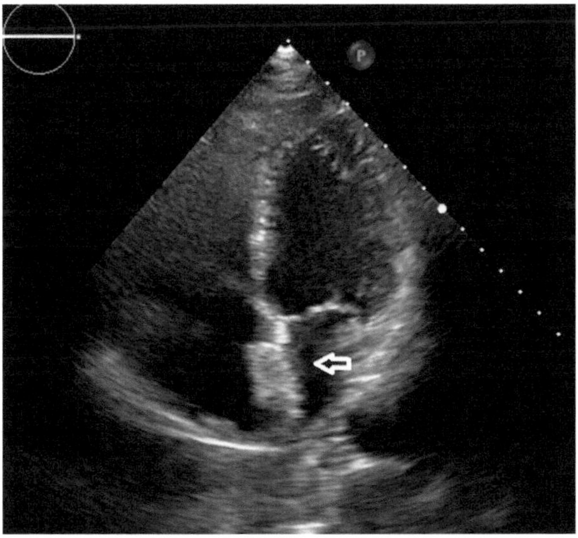

Fig. 38.4 Post-procedural echocardiography showing the occlude device on IAS (arrow)

Conclusion

Transcatheter device closure of multiple secundum ASDs that was once considered an indication for surgical repair is evolving. Various methods including covering all the defects by an oversized device, use of two separate devices, or dedicated devices for cribriform IAS has been carried on with satisfactory results. Three-dimensional (3D) echocardiography facilitates the definition of the IAS and defect anatomy as well as planning of the procedure and guiding the device deployment [1–3].

References

1. Khajali Z, Saedi S. Chapter 28 – Congenital heart disease. In: Practical cardiology. New York: Elsevier; 2017. p. 477–98. https://doi.org/10.1016/B978-0-323-51149-0.00028-6
2. Nasiri Brojeni M, Seilan P, Parsaee M, Saedi S. Postoperative outcome of the transcatheter closure of atrial septal defects using the AMPLATZER septal occluder. Iran Heart J. 2016;17(4):30–5.
3. Saedi S, Aliramezany M, Khajali Z, Sanati HR. Transcatheter closure of large atrial septal defects: a single-center experience. Res Cardiovasc Med. 2018;7(3):148.

Chapter 39
Partial Anomalous Pulmonary Venous Return with Scimitar Vein

Sedigheh Saedi and Tahereh Saedi

Abstract Partial anomalous pulmonary venous drainage/connection (PAPVC/D) results from the failure of the normal return of a single or multiple pulmonary veins to the left atrium. Instead the abnormal pulmonary veins (PVs) connect to the systemic veins (including superior vena cava, inferior vena cava (IVC) and coronary sinus) or directly to the right atrium. Connection of the right sided veins to the IVC is a rare congenital anomaly and is usually through a vein that appears as a curvilinear shadow on Chest x-ray resembling a "scimitar sword" and hence termed scimitar vein. If scimitar vein and PAPVC are associated with other anomalies including right pulmonary hypoplasia and lung sequestration, cardiac shift to the right and aortic collaterals to the right lung the term scimitar syndrome is used. Here we describe a young patient in whom all the right sided PVs drained to the IVC via a scimitar vein.

History and Clinical Presentation

A 17-year-old female with a history of occasional palpitation was referred to our clinic due to abnormal finding of right ventricular (RV) enlargement during transthoracic echocardiography in another center. On thorough questioning, she expressed mildly diminished exercise capacity. There was no relevant past medical history. In physical exam, a II/VI ejection type systolic murmur could be heard in the left sternal border.

S. Saedi (✉) · T. Saedi
Rajaei Cardiovascular Medical and Research Center, Iran University of Medical Sciences, Tehran, Iran

M. Maleki, A. Alizadehasl (eds.), *Case-Based Clinical Cardiology*,
https://doi.org/10.1007/978-1-4471-7496-7_39

Para-Clinic Assessment

ECG showed evidence of RV dilatation. Chest X-ray depicted a curvilinear silhouette in the right lung and around right heart border suggesting a scimitar sign (Fig. 39.1).

In transesophageal echocardiography there was severe RV enlargement and mild systolic dysfunction and a large secundum type ASD. All left-sided PVs drained to left atrium but right pulmonary veins flow was seen to enter IVC-right atrium junction.

Cardiac computed tomographic (CT) angiography confirmed the echocardiographic findings and showed all right-sided PVs draining to scimitar vein and then to suprahepatic portion of the IVC (Fig. 39.2).

Catheterization was performed to determine the precise pulmonary arterial pressure (PAP) as it could not be optimally measured by echocardiography and showed top normal systolic PAP of 30 mmHg (Fig. 39.3).

Management

Cardiac surgery was performed and the scimitar vein and the PVs were baffled to the left atrium through IVC, right atrium, and the ASD. The ASD was then repaired with satisfactory post-op results.

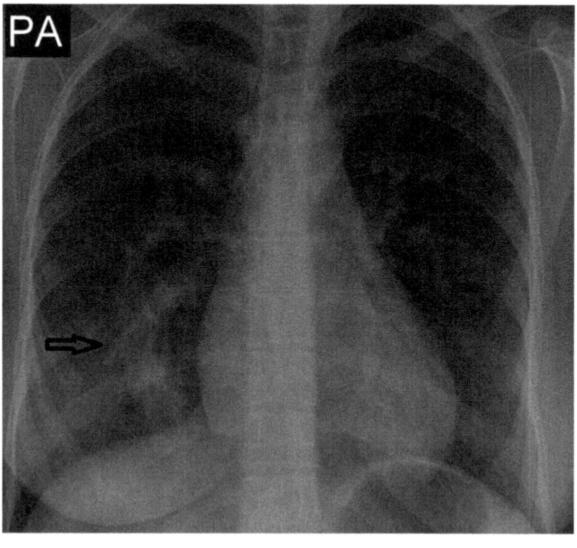

Fig. 39.1 Chest X-ray depicting the scimitar vein (arrow)

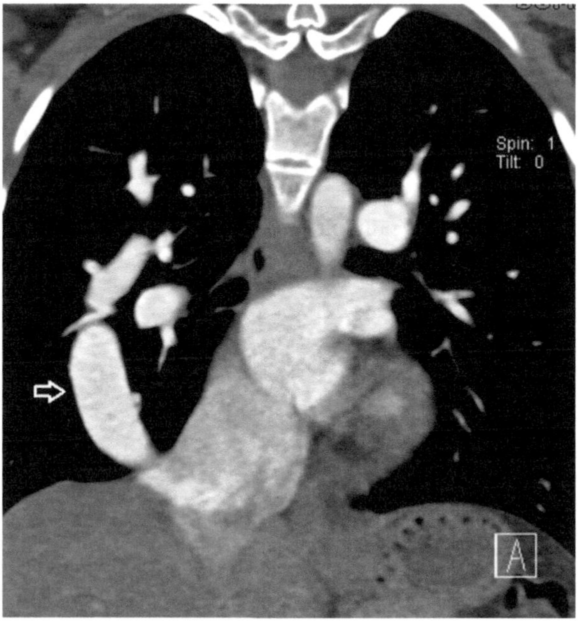

Fig. 39.2 Coronal projection image in computed tomographic pulmonary angiogram showing right-sided PVs connecting to scimitar vein (arrow) and then to the IVC

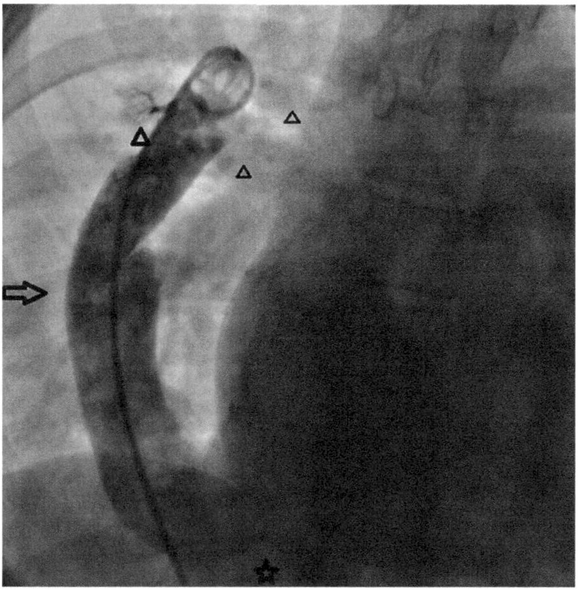

Fig. 39.3 Catheter angiogram image showing a pigtail catheter advanced from IVC (star) up to the scimitar vein (arrow) and connection to pulmonary veins (arrowheads)

Conclusion

Patients with PAPVC might be asymptomatic for many years. Hemodynamic effects of the PAPVC depends on the degree of left to right shunting and associated anomalies. An isolated PAPVC usually does not lead to a significant shunt but if there are multiple PAPVCs or concomitant defects such as ASD with cardiac chamber enlargement and pulmonary overflow corrective surgery should be considered [1–5].

References

1. Khajali Z, Saedi S. Chapter 28 – Congenital heart disease. In: Practical cardiology. New York: Elsevier; 2017. p. 477–98. https://doi.org/10.1016/B978-0-323-51149-0.00028-6
2. Eidem BW, Cetta F, O'Leary PW, editors. Echocardiography in pediatric and adult congenital heart disease. 2nd ed: Lippincott Williams & Wilkins; 2015.
3. Thangarajah A. A rare case of isolated partial anomalous pulmonary venous connection to the inferior vena cava. J Clin Diagn Res. 2015;9(3):TJ01.
4. Saedi S, Salehi A, Saedi T, Hashemi MJ. Association of left ventricular diverticula and sinus venosus atrial septal defect. Congenit Heart Dis. 2013;8(5):E145–8.
5. Parsaee M, Saedi S, Salehi N, Saedi T. Altered pulmonary venous flow pattern in young adults with atrial septal defect. Int J Cardiovasc Pract. 2016;1(2):41–4.

Chapter 40
Left Sided Partial Anomalous Pulmonary Venous Drainage with Vertical Vein

Sedigheh Saedi

Abstract Partial anomalous pulmonary venous drainage/connection (PAPVC/D) is abnormal connection of a single or multiple pulmonary veins to systemic veins including superior vena cava (SVC), inferior vena cava (IVC), coronary sinus or the right atrium. Right side PAPVCs that connect to SVC are frequently associated with SVC type sinus venosus atrial septal defect. Left sided PAPVCs and more commonly anomalous left upper pulmonary vein usually drains to the left innominate vein via a persistent fetal period structure called the vertical vein and thereby to SVC and the right atrium creating a left to right shunt. Here we present a middle age patient with isolated abnormal drainage of left pulmonary veins.

History and Clinical Presentation

A 41-year-old female presented with dyspnea on exertion and atypical chest discomfort since a year ago. She had no coronary artery disease risk factors and did not use any medication. There was no relevant familial history. Physical examination findings were unremarkable.

Para-Clinic Assessment

Twelve lead ECG showed normal sinus rhythm, normal QRS axis, and T wave inversion in V1–V3 precordial leads. Chest X-ray depicted evidence of right atrial and right ventricular (RV) enlargement. A prominent abnormal shadow could be seen on the left side of the aortic knob (Fig. 40.1). In transthoracic echocardiography, she had normal left ventricle size and function but moderate RV enlargement and mild systolic dysfunction. No intracardiac defect was detected. In the

S. Saedi (✉)
Rajaei Cardiovascular Medical and Research Center, Iran University of Medical Sciences, Tehran, Iran

M. Maleki, A. Alizadehasl (eds.), *Case-Based Clinical Cardiology*,
https://doi.org/10.1007/978-1-4471-7496-7_40

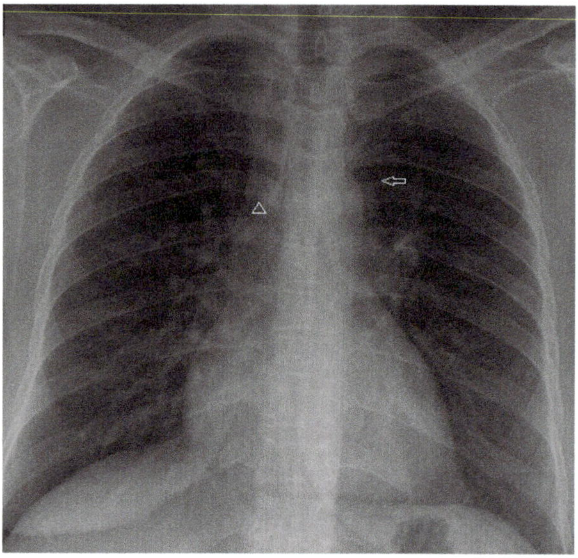

Fig. 40.1 Posteroanterior (PA) projection chest x-ray with abnormal silhouette beside aortic knob (arrow) in favor of a vertical vein. SVC shadow is also prominent that could result from overflow (arrowhead)

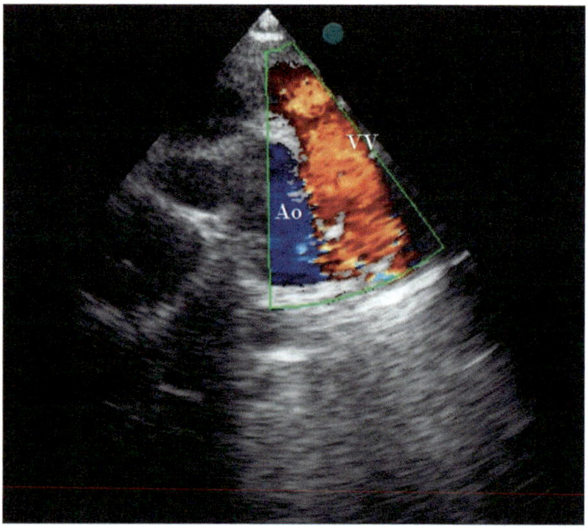

Fig. 40.2 Echocardiographic image from suprasternal window with color Doppler imaging showing vertical vein (VV) parallel to the aortic arch and proximal of descending thoracic aorta with a cephalad (red) flow toward the innominate vein. Ao: proximal part of descending thoracic aorta, *VV* vertical vein

suprasternal notch window, a vessel with cephalad flow was seen running parallel to the proximal part of descending thoracic aorta compatible with vertical vein and emptying to innominate vein (Fig. 40.2). In transesophageal echocardiography there was normal drainage of right PVs to the left atrium (LA) but left side PV drainage to LA was not seen and there was no atrial septal defect. With the diagnosis of left side PAPVC computed tomographic (CT) angiogram was performed and reported most left-sided PVs drained to the vertical vein except for a small left lower lobe PV that returned to the left atrium (Fig. 40.3). Cardiac catheterization was done for shunt evaluation and there was a Qp/Qs: 2:1. Pulmonary artery pressure and coronary arteries were normal (Fig. 40.4).

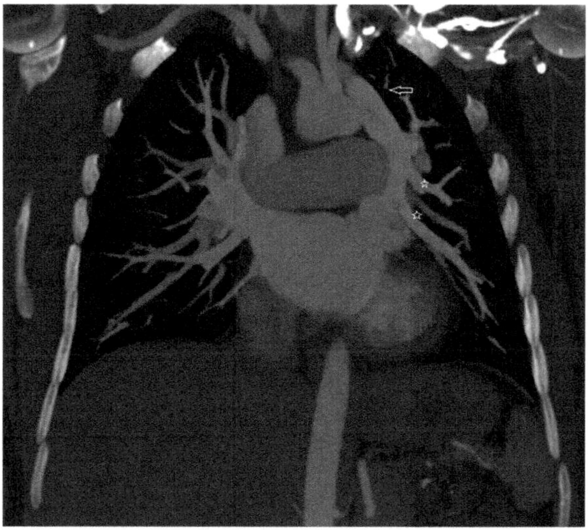

Fig. 40.3 Reconstructed CT angiogram image of vertical vein (arrow) draining most left PVs (stars)

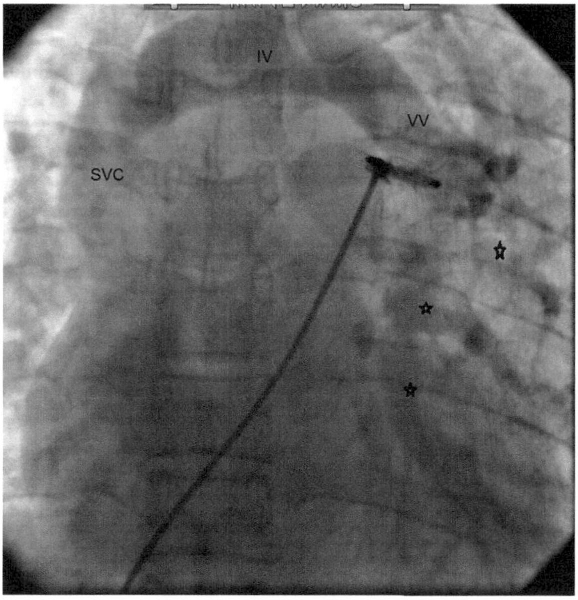

Fig. 40.4 Pulmonary angiogram in levophase showing the left PVs (star) draining to vertical vein (VV), innominate vein (IV) and thereby to SVC

Management

Due to significant left to right shunt corrective surgery was performed in which the vertical vein was transected and anastomosed to the left atrial appendage.

Conclusion

Management of PAPVCs is based on the level of overflow and left to right shunting. If the shunt leads to RV enlargement, significant pulmonary overflow (pulmonary blood flow more than1.5 times systemic blood flow), or pulmonary hypertension reparative surgery is indicated. Patients with isolated single PAPVC and no significant left to right shunt could be followed clinically and generally do not need further intervention [1–4].

References

1. Khajali Z, Saedi S, Khajali Z, Saedi S. Chapter 28 – Congenital heart disease. In: Practical cardiology. New York: Elsevier; 2017. p. 477–98. https://doi.org/10.1016/B978-0-323-51149-0.00028-6
2. Saedi S, Salehi A, Saedi T, Hashemi MJ. Association of left ventricular diverticula and sinus venosus atrial septal defect. Congenit Heart Dis. 2013;8(5):E145–8.
3. Brown DW, Geva T, Anomalies of pulmonary veins, In Moss and Adams' heart disease in infants, children, and adolescents: including the fetus and young adult. 9th ed. Wolters Kluwer Health Adis (ESP); 2016.
4. Saedi S, Saedi T. Catheter intervention for abnormal pulmonary venous drainage. The Egypt Heart J. 2018;70(2):125–7.

Chapter 41
Coronary Artery Abnormality and Atrial Septal Defect

Sedigheh Saedi

Abstract Congenital coronary artery (CA) anomalies might be isolated or in in association with other congenital heart defects and carry a risk of sudden cardiac death (SCD) in young individuals and athletes. There are various classifications for CA anomalies but clinically they are categorized based on anatomy or the potential to cause myocardial ischemia. Anatomic subtypes include coronary ostial anomaly/hypoplasia/atresia, anomalies of origin or course of the CA or absence/hypoplasia of the CA.

Secundum type atrial septal defect (ASD) is the most common form of atrial septal defects but concomitant coronary artery anomaly is rare. Here we report incidental finding of associated coronary abnormality in a young patient with ASD.

History and Clinical Presentation

A 25 year-old female presented with a prolonged history of occasional palpitation. She did not have chest pain, dyspnea, syncope, or family history of heart disease, and her past history was unremarkable. In physical examination, there was an ejection type systolic murmur in the left sternal border and fixed splitting of the second heart sound.

Para-Clinic Assessment

Twelve lead ECG showed normal sinus rhythm, the normal axis with incomplete right bundle branch block pattern. Chest X-ray showed evidence of pulmonary overflow and shunt vascularity.

S. Saedi (✉)
Rajaei Cardiovascular Medical and Research Center, Iran University of Medical Sciences, Tehran, Iran

M. Maleki, A. Alizadehasl (eds.), *Case-Based Clinical Cardiology*,
https://doi.org/10.1007/978-1-4471-7496-7_41

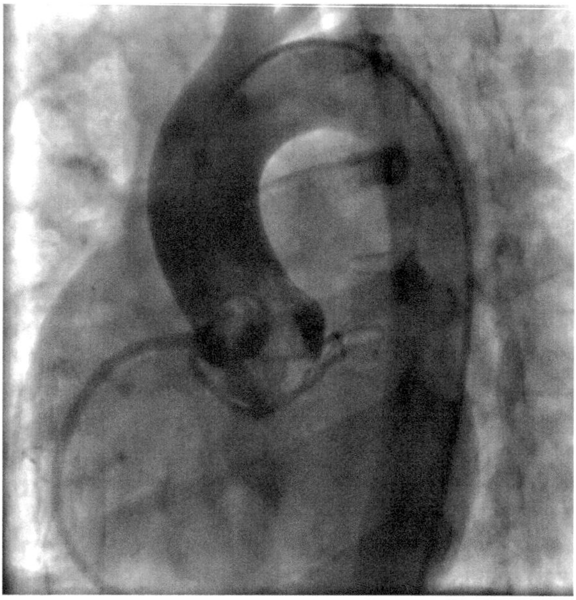

Fig. 41.1 Aortic root injection in LAO (Left anterior oblique) projection, No coronary artery originated from the left sinus

Transthoracic and transesophageal echocardiography (TEE) showed normal left ventricle size and function, moderate right ventricular (RV) enlargement with normal RV systolic function, normal pulmonary artery pressure and a moderate-sized (1.4 cm) secundum type ASD with sufficient rims for transcatheter device closure.

Hemodynamic study showed significant left to right shunt. During cardiac catheterization aortic root injection revealed that no coronary artery originated from the left aortic sinus and selective coronary angiography showed all the coronary arteries arising from the right coronary cusp (Figs. 41.1 and 41.2).

Management

As the left anterior descending artery (LAD) gave rise to septal perforator branches and regarding negative past history for syncope or chest pain and no family history of sudden cardiac death the coronary course was not expected to be of interarterial or malignant type. However coronary computed tomographic (CT) angiography was performed for better evaluation. CT reported anomalous origin of LAD and the left circumflex artery (LCx) from the right coronary cusp but with a retroaortic course (Fig. 41.3). As coronary artery anomaly was not of the malignant type and is not reported to be associated with a high risk of SCD or ischemia, successful ASD device closure was performed under TEE guidance (Fig. 41.4). There was no compressive effect on coronary arteries post-procedurally.

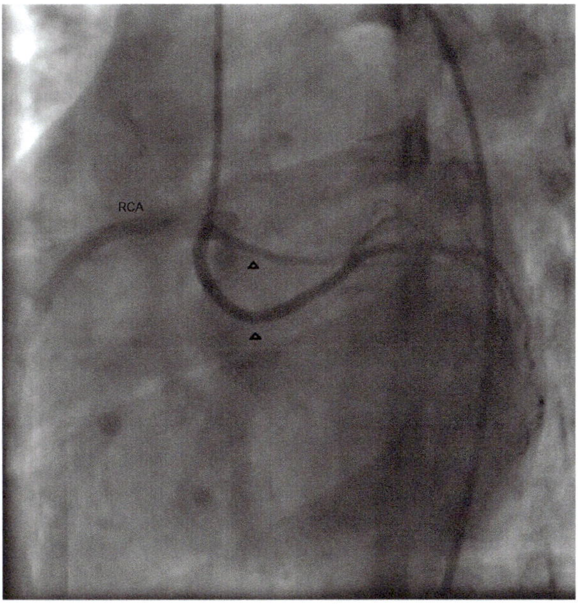

Fig. 41.2 Anomalous origin of left coronary artery from right coronary sinus, *RCA* Right coronary artery; arrowheads point to left coronary artery branches

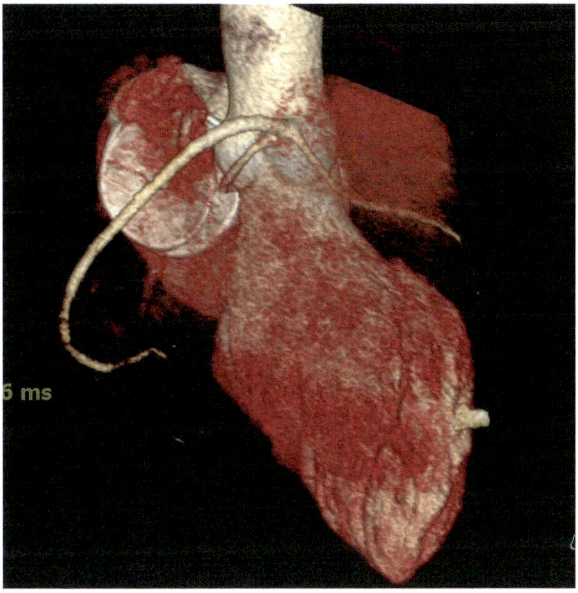

Fig. 41.3 3D reconstruction of coronary CT angiogram showing anomalous origin of all coronary arteries from the right aortic cusp

Conclusion

Left coronary arteries arising from the right aortic cusp may follow four different courses and are anatomically classified as retroaortic, interarterial, prepulmonic, or intramyocardial/transeptal course. The interarterial course is malignant and can result in myocardial ischemia and SCD. When this type of anomaly is diagnosed coronary artery bypass grafting (CABGs) is warranted [1–5].

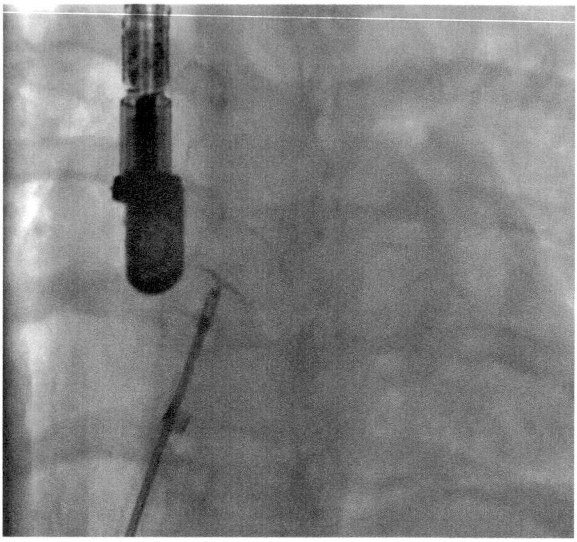

Fig. 41.4 ASD occluder device deployment under TEE guidance

References

1. Nasiri Brojeni M, Seilan P, Parsaee M, Saedi S. Postoperative outcome of the Transcatheter closure of atrial septal defects using the AMPLATZER septal occluder. Iran Heart J. 2016;17(4):30–5.
2. Braunwald's heart disease: a textbook of cardiovascular medicine. 11th ed. Philadelphia, PA: Elsevier; 2019.
3. Saedi S, Parsaee M, Farrashi M, Noohi F, Mohebbi B. The role of echocardiography in anomalous origin of coronary artery from pulmonary artery (ALCAPA): simple tool for a complex diagnosis. Echocardiography. 2019;36(1):177–81.
4. Saedi S, Pouraliakbar HR, Ghaderian H, Saedi T. Congenital atresia of left main coronary artery. Egypt Heart J. 2018;70(4):451–3.
5. Saedi S, Ghavidel AA, Panahifar N. Anomalous origin of the left coronary artery from the pulmonary artery-adult type with heart failure and ventricular arrhythmia presentation. Res Cardiovasc Med. 2019;8(3):84.

Chapter 42
Transcatheter Repair of Residual Postsurgical Ventricular Septal Defect

Sedigheh Saedi and Tahereh Saedi

Abstract Transcatheter closure of muscular and perimembranous ventricular septal defect (VSD) is becoming the technique of choice in patients with suitable anatomy and has superior patient comfort compared to surgery. However, there are subsets of patients with complex forms of congenital heart disease that have often undergone multiple reparative surgeries and yet suffer from clinically significant residual post-surgical VSDs. Transcatheter closure of a post-surgical VSD is much more challenging due to the variable and unusual form and location of the residual VSD or the previous repair patch and renders the device positioning and stability more unpredictable. Careful pre-procedural evaluation with use of multi-modality imaging could help choose the right candidates and decrease the complications. We report an adolescent with residual VSD and tricuspid regurgitation in whom successful device closure was achieved percutaneously.

History and Clinical Presentation

A 15-year-old male with a history of surgical VSD and pulmonary stenosis repair at age three came for follow-up visit after the transition to adult congenital heart disease care. In his previous pediatric post-op echocardiograms, small residual VSD was reported. Physical exam showed normal growth for age. In cardiac auscultation, there was a III/VI holosystolic murmur in the left sternal border.

S. Saedi (✉) · T. Saedi
Rajaei Cardiovascular Medical and Research Center, Iran University of Medical Sciences, Tehran, Iran

M. Maleki, A. Alizadehasl (eds.), *Case-Based Clinical Cardiology*,
https://doi.org/10.1007/978-1-4471-7496-7_42

Para-Clinic Assessment

In chest X-ray, the left ventricle was mildly enlarged with evidence of pulmonary overflow. Transthoracic (TTE) and transesophageal echocardiography (TEE) showed mild left ventricular (LV) enlargement and systolic dysfunction (estimated EF: 50%), mild aortic regurgitation (AI) and moderate tricuspid valve regurgitation (TR). There was no residual pulmonary stenosis and no regurgitation. A moderate size (about 8 mm) residual VSD at the previous repair site was visible with left to right shunt. The interventricular septum (IVS) around the VSD was aneurysmal and redundant. Distance of the VSD from aorta was 8 mm and from tricuspid valve 5 mm which is considered acceptable for device closure (Fig. 42.1).

Management

Cardiac catheterization was performed for hemodynamic study and device closure of the residual VSD. The calculated Qp/Qs was 2.3:1 implying significant left to right shunt. LV injection showed a residual VSD and aneurysmal IVS that measured larger than that reported by the echocardiography (Fig. 42.2). Wiring of the VSD was done from the LV side and the wire was snared in the superior vena cava to exit the femoral vein access. Then a long femoral sheath was inserted and passed the VSD to ascending aorta. Device closure was done with a 16 mm muscular VSD occluder under TEE guidance. TEE confirmed an acceptable device position with no compressive effect on adjacent structures so the device was released with no complications (Fig. 42.3). TTE prior to discharge showed the device in proper position with no residue and no change in TR or AI severity (Fig. 42.4). The patient was monitored for 48 h to detect possible arrhythmias and complete heart block and was then discharged home with aspirin and clopidogrel.

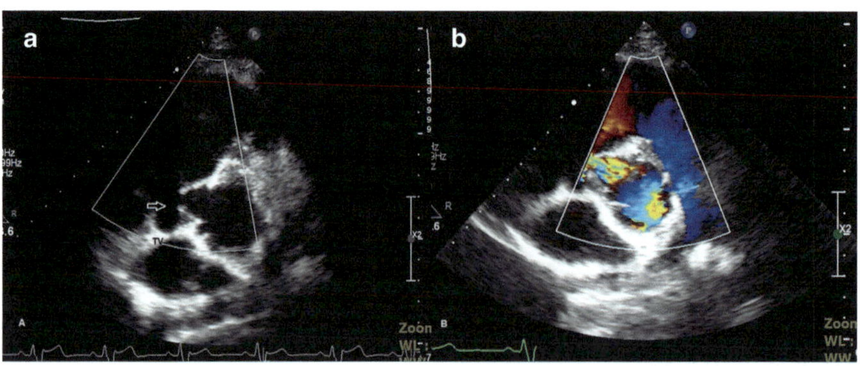

Fig. 42.1 Short-axis echocardiography view in 2D (**a**) and color Doppler (**b**) showing residual VSD (arrow) near tricuspid valve

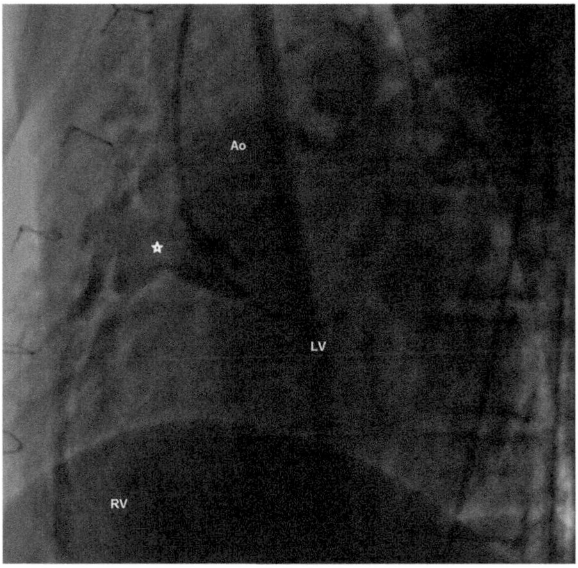

Fig. 42.2 Angiographic injection in LAO (left anterior oblique) caudal view showing residual VSD (star) and opacification of the right ventricle (RV) via VSD. *Ao* aorta, *LV* left ventricle

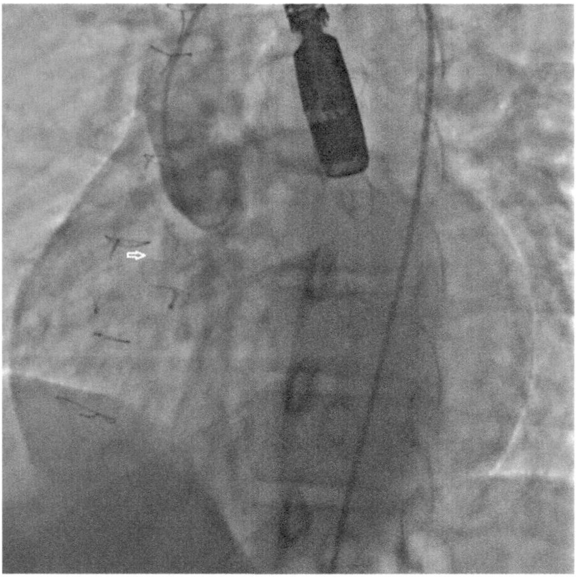

Fig. 42.3 Angiogram image showing occluder device obstructing the VSD flow (arrow)

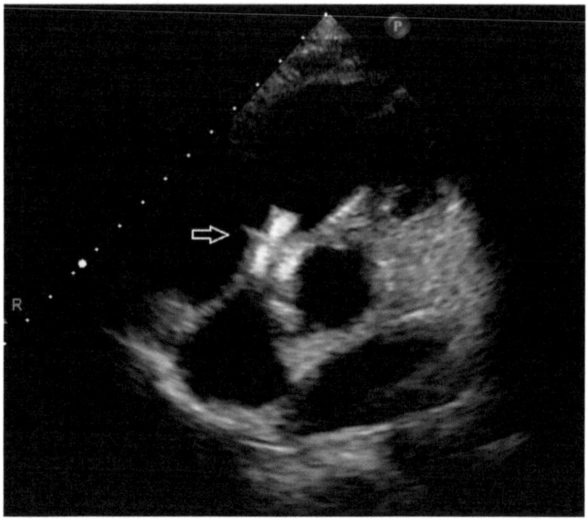

Fig. 42.4 Transthoracic echocardiography in short-axis view showing the proper position of the occluder device (arrow)

Conclusion

Before proceeding with VSD device closure presence of adequate distance and a safe margin from adjacent structures and most importantly aorta and tricuspid valve should be evaluated, otherwise, device-related complications including device embolization, tricuspid or aortic regurgitation, and heart rhythm abnormalities may occur.

Post-operation residual VSDs are often hemodynamically remarkable but hard to repair surgically. Device closure is a safe and effective method for residual postsurgical VSD closure in meticulously selected patients [1–4].

References

1. Khajali Z, Saedi S. Chapter 28 – Congenital heart disease. In Practical Cardiology (pp. 477–498). Elsevier 2017. https://doi.org/10.1016/B978-0-323-51149-0.00028-6
2. Carminati M, Butera G, Chessa M, De Giovanni J, Fisher G, Gewillig M, Peuster M, Piechaud JF, Santoro G, Sievert H, Spadoni I. Transcatheter closure of congenital ventricular septal defects: results of the European Registry. Eur Heart J. 2007;28(19):2361–8.
3. Saedi S, Saedi T. Directly ventricular septal defect closure without using arteriovenous wire loop: our adult case series using transarterial retrograde approach. Anatol J Cardiol. 2017;17(6):469.
4. Saedi S, Parsaee M. Intramural ventricular septal defect. Int J Cardiovasc Pract. 2017;2(3):70–2.

Chapter 43
Percutaneous Device Closure of Ruptured Sinus of Valsalva Aneurysm

Sedigheh Saedi

Abstract Aneurysm of the aortic sinus of Valsalva is a rare anomaly and could be congenital or acquired. The aneurysms could rupture, most commonly to the right side heart chambers and lead to severe left-to-right shunt. If left untreated ruptured sinus of Valsalva (ROSV) causes cardiac chamber dilation, failure and pulmonary hypertension. Surgical correction is the standard procedure but catheter intervention can alternatively be performed.

History and Clinical Presentation

A 52-year-old female with a history of hypertension presented with atypical chest discomfort. In a physical examination a loud continuous machinery cardiac murmur was heard with the maximal intensity in the left sternal border.

Para-Clinic Assessment

Transthoracic (TTE) and later transesophageal echocardiography (TEE) showed mild left ventricular (LV) enlargement and systolic dysfunction (estimated EF: 50%), ruptured right aortic sinus to right atrium (RA) with high-velocity continuous flow, windsock was seen at the site of rupture (Fig. 43.1).

Computed tomographic (CT) angiography showed a rupture size of about 6 mm and a good distance from the right coronary artery (RCA) but close proximity to tricuspid valve (Fig. 43.2).

S. Saedi (✉)
Rajaei Cardiovascular Medical and Research Center, Iran University of Medical Sciences, Tehran, Iran

M. Maleki, A. Alizadehasl (eds.), *Case-Based Clinical Cardiology*,
https://doi.org/10.1007/978-1-4471-7496-7_43

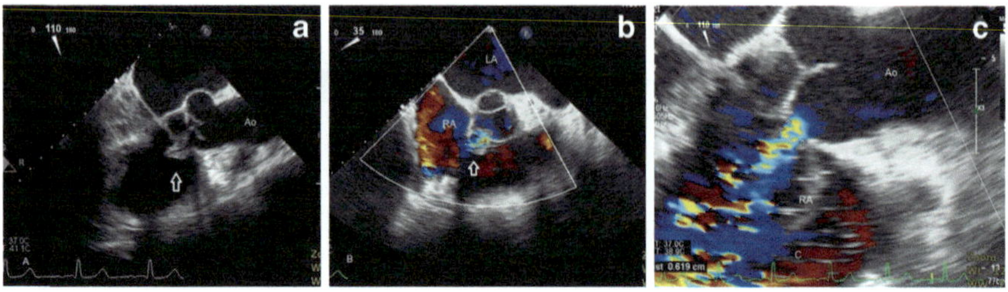

Fig. 43.1 TEE 2D and color Doppler images of RSOV, (**a**) windsock appearance of the ruptured RCC (arrow), (**b**, **c**) color flow from ruptured cusp to RA, *Ao* aorta, *RA* right atrium, *LA* left atrium

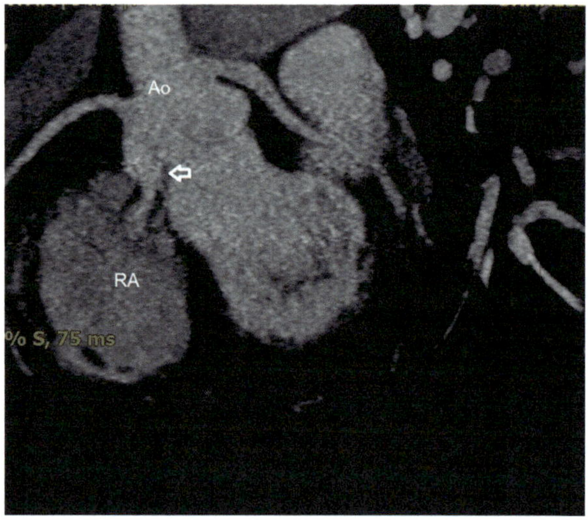

Fig. 43.2 CT angiography mage of rupture of the aortic cusp to RA

Management

The patient was scheduled for device closure of ROSV. Under TEE guidance wiring of the rupture site from the aortic side and snaring was performed, device closure was attempted with a patent ductus arteriosus (PDA) occluder 10/8 mm, but the device failed to stabilize and there was significant residue so the device was retrieved. Successful closure was then achieved with a 12/10 mm PDA occluder (Fig. 43.3).

Intra and post-procedure echocardiography showed proper device position with no residue and no compressive effect on tricuspid valve or other adjacent structures (Fig. 43.4).

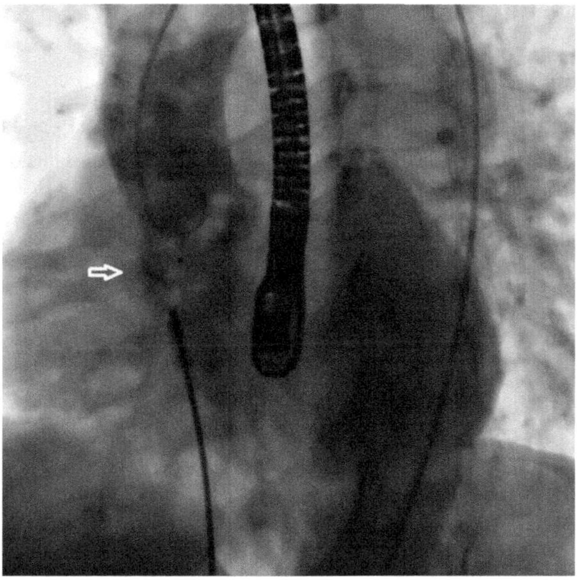

Fig. 43.3 Device closure of ROSV with a PDA occluder under TEE guidance

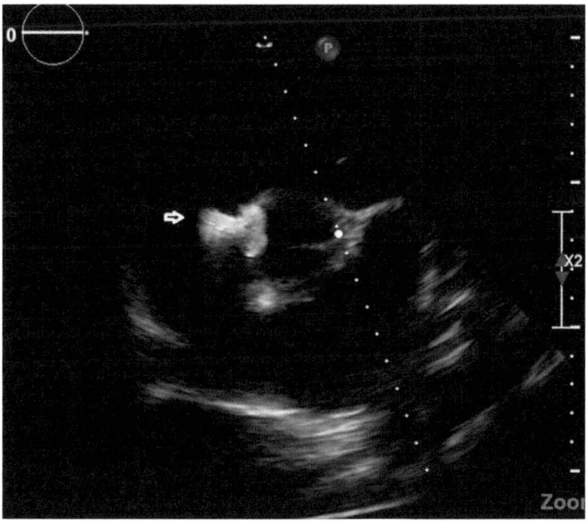

Fig. 43.4 Predischarge echocardiogram in short-axis view showing the device in the proper position (arrow)

Conclusion

With improvement in catheter intervention techniques, percutaneous device closure of ROSV has become an alternative to surgery and could be performed feasibly in expert centers. Randomized clinical trials comparing the percutaneous and surgical methods are needed to evaluate the long-term outcomes [1–3].

References

1. Weinreich M, Yu PJ, Trost B. Sinus of valsalva aneurysms: review of the literature and an update on management. Clin Cardiol. 2015;38(3):185–9.
2. Khajali Z, Maleki M, Amin A, Saedi S, Arabian M, Moosazadeh M, Naderi N, Mozzafari K, Khalaj H, Aliramezani M. Prevalence of cardiac dysfunction among adult patients with congenital heart disease: a single-center investigation. Iran Heart J. 2019;20(3):12–9.
3. Kuriakose EM, Bhatla P, McElhinney DB. Comparison of reported outcomes with percutaneous versus surgical closure of ruptured sinus of Valsalva aneurysm. Am J Cardiol. 2015;115(3):392–8.

Chapter 44
Cor Triatriatum Sinistrum

Sedigheh Saedi

Abstract Cor triatriatum sinisterum (triatrial heart) is a congenital heart defect where the left atrium is divided to two chambers by a membrane due to failure of normal absorption of common pulmonary vein to left atrium (LA). Embryologically pulmonary intra-parenchymal veins connect to left atrium via a common pulmonary vein. If the orifice of the common pulmonary vein to left atrium is stenotic a membrane like structure forms in LA and divides it in to two compartments: One receiving the pulmonary veins and the other with LA appendage and mitral valve. Stenosis severity is variable and could result in increased pulmonary venous and pulmonary capillary wedge pressures with ensuing pulmonary arterial hypertension and right sided heart failure. Here we present a young adult presenting with this rare congenital anomaly.

History and Clinical Presentation

A 16 years old female presented with palpitation since a year ago. She had been diagnosed with congenital heart disease and proposed surgery at childhood but had refused and had no follow-up since. Physical examination revealed III/VI systolic murmur in left sternal border, loud P2, and fine bibasilar rales in lung auscultation. There was no peripheral edema, ascites, or cyanosis.

Para-Clinic Assessment

ECG showed normal sinus rhythm and left atrial abnormality. Chest X-ray showed evidence of pulmonary congestion with prominent pulmonary arteries and LA enlargement (Fig. 44.1). Lab data were unremarkable.

S. Saedi (✉)
Rajaei Cardiovascular Medical and Research Center, Iran University of Medical Sciences, Tehran, Iran

M. Maleki, A. Alizadehasl (eds.), *Case-Based Clinical Cardiology*,
https://doi.org/10.1007/978-1-4471-7496-7_44

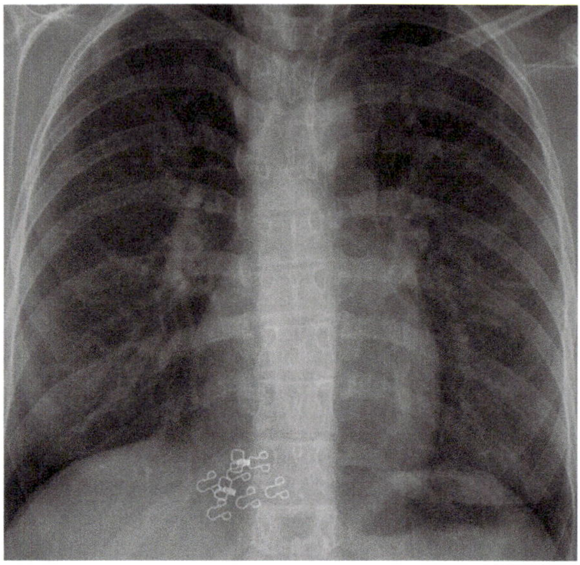

Fig. 44.1 Chest X-ray depicting pulmonary congestion and LA enlargement

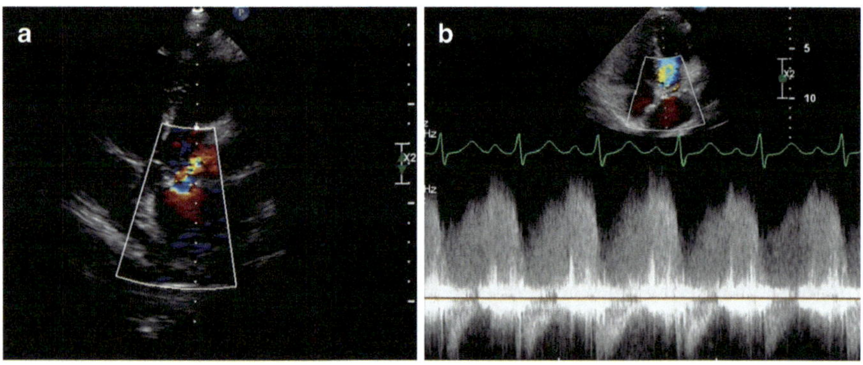

Fig. 44.2 Color (**a**) and Doppler flow (**b**) study of the cor triatriatum

Echocardiography showed normal left ventricle but moderate left atrial(LA) enlargement, there was a thick membrane in LA resulting in division of LA into two chambers with a small orifice connecting the chambers, posterosuperior chamber received all pulmonary veins and anteroinferior chamber emptied into mitral valve. LA appendage was connected to the latter chamber, compatible with cor triatriatum with severe obstruction (mean gradient: 26 mmHg). There was characteristic continuous systolic and diastolic flow through mitral inflow in Doppler study (Fig. 44.2). The estimated systolic pulmonary arterial pressure was about 50 mmHg (Fig. 44.3a, b). Cardiac CT was performed to better evaluate the drainage of pulmonary veins and possible associated anomalies and confirmed the presence of a dividing membrane in LA (Fig. 44.4).

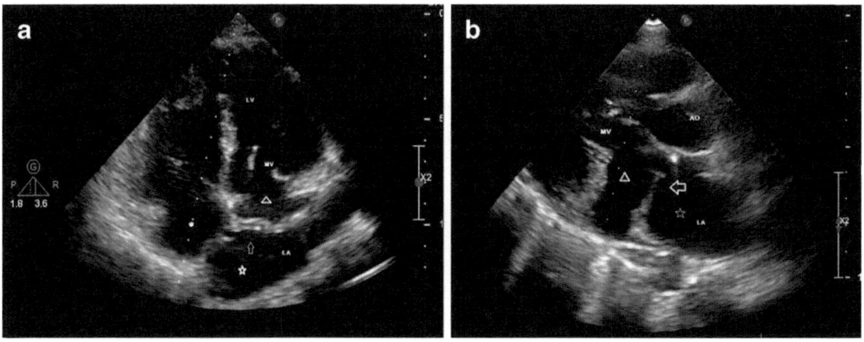

Fig. 44.3 (**a**) Echocardiographic four-chamber and (**b**) parasternal long-axis views of the obstructive membrane in the left atrium (arrow) dividing the LA to posterosuperior (asterisk) and antero-inferior chambers(arrowhead). *LA* left atrium, *LV* left ventricle, *MV* mitral valve

Fig. 44.4 Axial CT image of intra-left atrium membrane (arrow). *LA* left atrium, *LAA* left atrial appendage

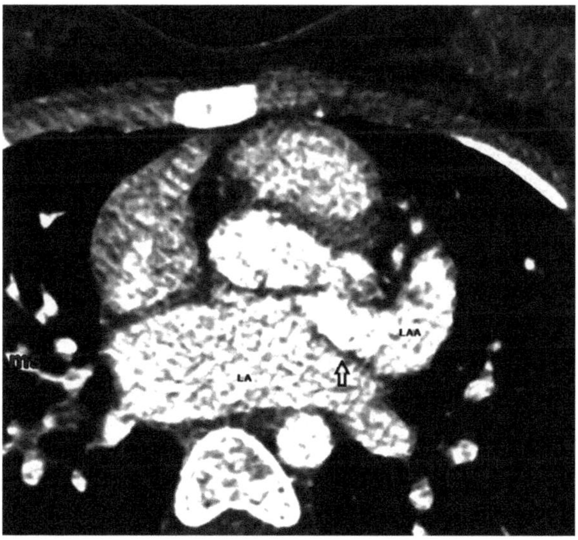

Management

Due to significant obstruction and pulmonary hypertension surgery was planned to respect the obstructive membrane and mitral valve repair.

Conclusion

Congenital obstruction in the path of pulmonary vein emptying results in increased pulmonary venous pressure, pulmonary hypertension, and heart failure if left untreated. Symptoms vary based on the degree of obstruction. Diagnosis is usually established by echocardiography. The obstructing membrane is detected superior to LA appendage which distinguishes this anomaly from supramitral ring. Cardiac catheterization is occasionally necessary for hemodynamic evaluation and determination of the degree of pulmonary hypertension. Treatment involves surgical resection of the stenotic membrane and repair of associated anomalies [1–3].

References

1. Khajali Z, Saedi S. Chapter 28 – Congenital heart disease. In: Practical cardiology. New York: Elsevier; 2017. p. 477–98. https://doi.org/10.1016/B978-0-323-51149-0.00028-6
2. Saedi S, Aliramezany M, Khajali Z, Sanati HR. Transcatheter closure of large atrial septal defects: a single-center experience. Res Cardiovasc Med. 2018;7(3):148.
3. Brown DW, Geva T, Anomalies of pulmonary veins, In Moss and Adams' heart disease in infants, children, and adolescents: including the fetus and young adult. 9th ed. Wolters Kluwer Health Adis (ESP); 2016.

Chapter 45
Coarctoplasty in Gothic Type Aortic Arch

Sedigheh Saedi and Tahereh Saedi

Abstract Aortic coarctation is a congenital narrowing and stenosis in the aorta that is most frequently located near the ligamentum arteriosum and the left subclavian artery. Coarctation in adults is now usually treated with catheter intervention with good follow-up results. However there are coarctation types that are anatomically challenging for catheter intervention. Here we present a patient with an angulated aortic arch who underwent successful coarctoplasty and stenting.

History and Clinical Presentation

A 18-year-old female was referred to our clinic with dyspnea on exertion and resistant hypertension that was not controlled despite the use of multiple antihypertensive medications including calcium-channel blockers, beta-blockers, diuretics, and angiotensin converting enzyme inhibitors (ACE inh). Physical examination showed diminished and delayed bi-femoral pulses compared to radial artery pulse. Systolic blood pressure was 160 mmHg in the upper extremity and 100 mmHg in the lower extremity.

Para-Clinic Assessment

Twelve lead ECG showed normal sinus rhythm, left axis deviation, and left ventricular hypertrophy (LVH). Chest X-ray had evidence of rib notching in the inferior aspect of posterior ribs (Fig. 45.1). In transthoracic echocardiography, she had normal left ventricle size and function with severe LVH. Aortic valve was bicuspid with fusion of left and non-coronary cusps but no stenosis and mild regurgitation. Pulsed Doppler in abdominal aorta from sub-xyphoid window showed abnormal and

S. Saedi (✉) · T. Saedi
Rajaei Cardiovascular Medical and Research Center, Iran University of Medical Sciences, Tehran, Iran

M. Maleki, A. Alizadehasl (eds.), *Case-Based Clinical Cardiology*,
https://doi.org/10.1007/978-1-4471-7496-7_45

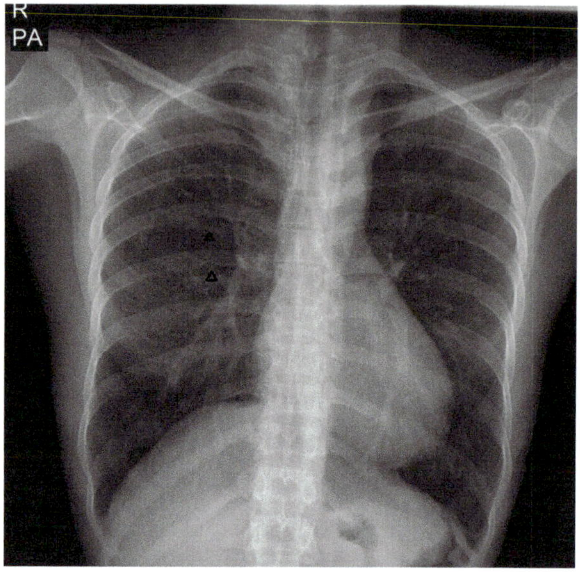

Fig. 45.1 Chest X-ray showing rib notching in the inferior borders of the posterior ribs (arrowhead)

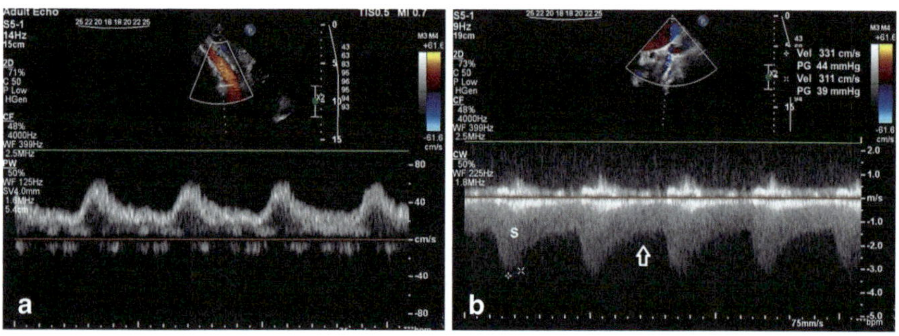

Fig. 45.2 (**a**) Abdominal aorta pulsed Doppler flow pattern showing slow and delayed upstroke. (**b**) Continuous-wave Doppler from suprasternal notch showing increased gradients across coarctation site (S)

delayed upstroke. In the suprasternal notch, an angulated aorta was evident with turbulency and increased gradients at proximal of descending aorta after subclavian artery(Fig. 45.2). With the diagnosis of coarctation of aorta and aortic arch anomaly a computed tomographic (CT) angiogram was performed and showed a high arch aorta with angulated geometry and discrete post-ductal coarctation (Fig. 45.3).

Management

Interventional coarctoplasty and stenting was planned. Catheterization showed 70 mmHg gradient across the coarctation site. Despite the use of several guidewires and different maneuvers in various projections, the guidewire could not be passed to the ascending aorta. Eventually, a hydrophilic wire was used and after multiple

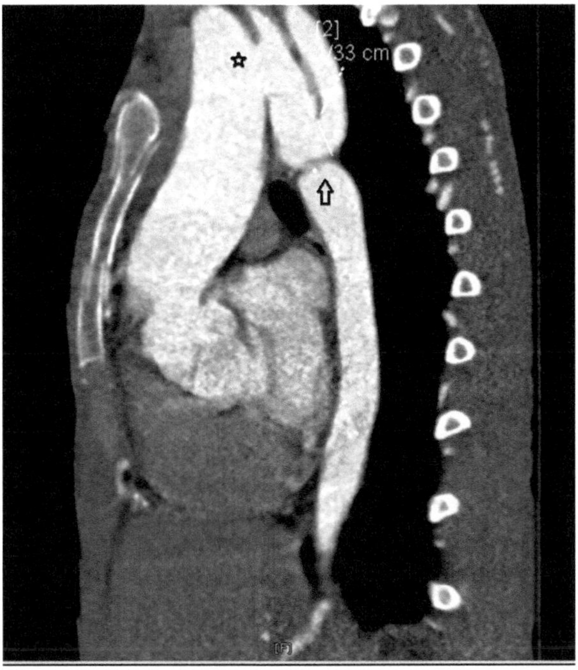

Fig. 45.3 Computed tomographic angiogram showing high position and angulated aortic arch (star) and discrete coarctation after subclavian artery (arrow)

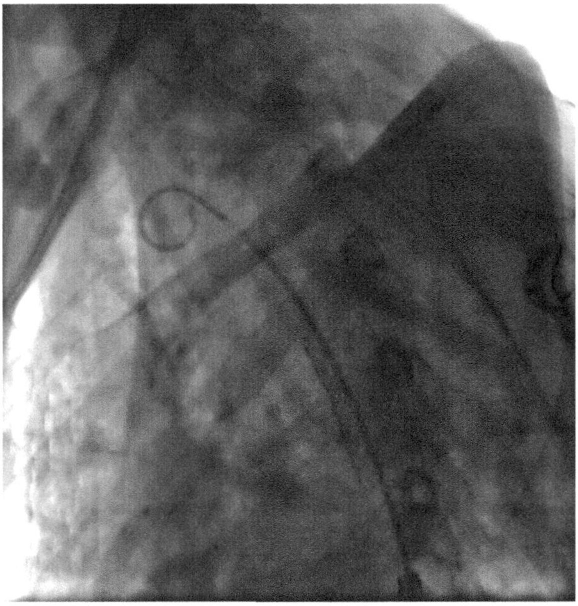

Fig. 45.4 Post-procedure angiogram with fully dilated stent in the proper position

attempts, the wire and a multipurpose catheter were passed to the ascending aorta and the wire was exchanged for a super stiff guidewire. Coarctoplasty was done with a BeGraft (Bently Aortic Stent Graft) 16 × 48 mm with zero residual gradients at coarctation site (Fig. 45.4). In 6 months follow-up visit the patient's blood pressure was normalized in ambulatory blood pressure monitoring with no need for drug therapy.

Conclusion

Angular, Gothic, or high aortic arch is a rare type of aortic arch geometry in which there is a sharp angle between the ascending and the proximal part of descending thoracic aorta. This abnormal form may also develop following surgical repair of complex congenital heart disease and has been described after surgery for coarctation repair and arterial switch procedure in the transposition of great arteries. Gothic arch has been reported to cause exercise-induced hypertension in patients after reparative surgery. Interventional procedures although the first choice for coarctation repair could be more challenging in patients with this type of anomaly [1–5].

References

1. Khajali Z, Saedi S. Chapter 28 – Congenital heart disease. In: Practical cardiology. New York: Elsevier; 2017. p. 477–98. https://doi.org/10.1016/B978-0-323-51149-0.00028-6
2. Ou P, Celermajer DS, Raisky O, Jolivet O, Buyens F, Herment A, Sidi D, Bonnet D, Mousseaux E. Angular (Gothic) aortic arch leads to enhanced systolic wave reflection, central aortic stiffness, and increased left ventricular mass late after aortic coarctation repair: evaluation with magnetic resonance flow mapping. J Thorac Cardiovasc Surg. 2008;135(1):62–8.
3. Bassiri HA, Abdi S, Shafe O, Sarpooshi J. Early and midterm results following interventional coarctoplasty: evaluation of variables that can affect the results. Korean Circ J. 2017;47(1):97–106.
4. Saedi S, Aliramezany M, Moosavi J, Saedi T. Successful thoracic endovascular aortic repair for post-coarctoplasty aneurysm. Egypt Heart J. 2020;72(1):1–5.
5. Rezaee A, Ebrahimi L, Saedi S. Diagnosis of aortic coarctation using renal doppler sonography, a case report. Case Rep Clin Med. 2015;4(05):189.

Chapter 46
Severe Subpulmonary Right Ventricular Outflow Obstruction in an Adult Patient

Sedigheh Saedi

Abstract Double chambered right ventricle (RV) is a form of sub pulmonary right ventricular outflow obstruction resulting from presence of abnormal, hypertrophied and aberrant muscle bundles in the RV cavity dividing it to proximal high pressure and distal low pressure chambers. This congenital anomaly is frequently associated with a small perimembranous ventricular septal defect. Here we present a young female with a severe RV intracavitary obstruction successfully treated by surgery.

History and Clinical Presentation

A 28-year-female presented with dizziness, progressive dyspnea, and a decline in functional capacity. She had not been evaluated for cardiac problems before but mentioned an abnormal heart murmur detected recently by his family physician during a visit for the common cold. In physical examination, there was a harsh pan-systolic murmur best heard at the left sternal border. There was a prominent jugular venous pulse, no ascites, and no pedal edema.

Para-Clinic Assessment

Twelve lead ECG showed normal sinus rhythm, right axis deviation, and RV hypertrophy. In echocardiography, there was moderate RV enlargement and systolic dysfunction. An aberrant hypertrophied muscle band was seen in the RV outflow tract resulting in severe stenosis and turbulent flow in favor of double-chambered RV (DCRV). There was a small perimembranous VSD. Precise RV pressure could not be estimated due to the VSD jet flow overlap (Fig. 46.1).

S. Saedi (✉)
Rajaei Cardiovascular Medical and Research Center, Iran University of Medical Sciences, Tehran, Iran

M. Maleki, A. Alizadehasl (eds.), *Case-Based Clinical Cardiology*,
https://doi.org/10.1007/978-1-4471-7496-7_46

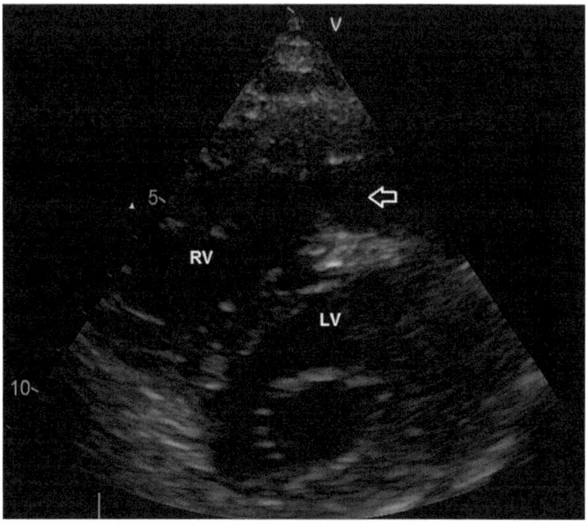

Fig. 46.1 Transthoracic echocardiography in parasternal short-axis view showing aberrant muscle band in RVOT (arrow). *RV* right ventricle, *LV* left ventricle

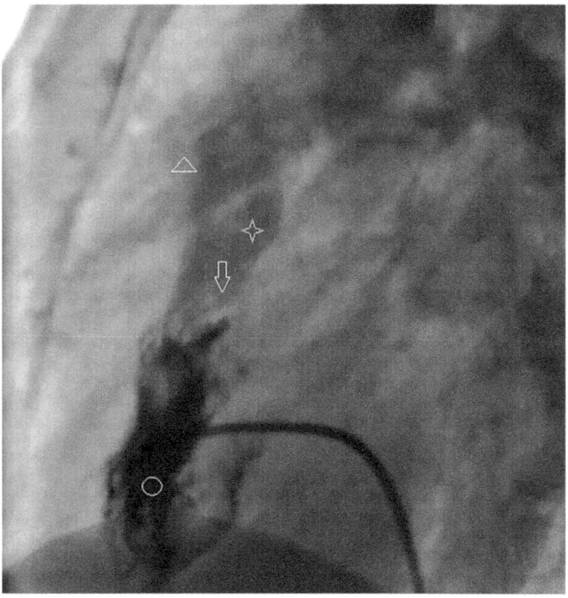

Fig. 46.2 Angiogram image in lateral projection depicting double-chambered RV, Star: proximal high-pressure chamber, circle: distal subpulmonic low-pressure chamber, arrow: aberrant muscle band, arrowhead: pulmonary valve

Cardiac catheterization was performed for hemodynamic evaluation and there was 120 mmHg gradient between proximal and distal parts of the RV.RV pressure in the proximal chamber was supersystemic and pulmonary artery pressure was normal . Proximal chamber was highly trabeculated and separated from the distal, smooth, low-pressure chamber with a hypertrophied muscle bundle. There was a small perimembranous VSD with nonsignificant left to right shunt (Fig. 46.2).

Management

The patient underwent reparative surgery during which the abnormal muscle bundle was resected and VSD closed. She had symptomatic relief early after surgery and RV showed degrees of functional improvement in 6 months follow-up echocardiography.

Conclusion

Abnormal muscle bands can cause varying severities of obstruction in RV. If RV pressure is more than 60% of the left ventricle pressure surgery is warranted. DCRV is usually corrected in childhood and rarely seen in adults. Unrepaired DCRV tends to worsen overtime and patients might present with dyspnea, angina pectoris, exertional syncope, and eventually RV failure at older ages [1–3].

References

1. Khajali Z, Saedi S. Chapter 28 – Congenital heart disease. In: Practical cardiology. New York: Elsevier; 2017. p. 477–98. https://doi.org/10.1016/B978-0-323-51149-0.00028-6
2. Prieto LR, Latson LA. Pulmonary stenosis. In Moss and Adams' heart disease in infants, children, and adolescents: including the fetus and young adult. 9th ed. Wolters Kluwer Health Adis (ESP); 2016.
3. Saedi S, Oraii S, Hajsheikholeslami F. A cross sectional study on prevalence and etiology of syncope in Tehran. Acta Med Iran. 2013;51(10):715–9.

Chapter 47
Very Severe Pulmonary Valve Stenosis in a Middle-Aged Male Treated Percutaneously

Sedigheh Saedi

Abstract Pulmonary valve stenosis is a most often a congenital anomaly and acquired forms are very rare. Patients with mild or moderate stenosis could be asymptomatic. In severe stenosis patients might present with exertional dyspnea, fatigue or even syncope due to low right sided cardiac output and eventually right sided heart failure. Most patients with severe degrees of stenosis will have had a form of intervention in childhood or early adolescence. We present a middle aged man with very severe stenosis and no prior intervention managed successfully with balloon valvuloplasty.

History and Clinical Presentation

A 43 year-old male was referred to our clinic with progressive shortness of breath that exacerbated following a recent upper respiratory tract infection. He had been diagnosed with chronic obstructive pulmonary disease (COPD) previously but never had a cardiac evaluation. Physical examination revealed cyanosis and finger clubbing. There was a IV/VI harsh systolic murmur best heard in the left second intercostal space and a trill, right ventricular lift, and elevated jugular venous pulse (JVP). Systemic oxygen saturation at room air was 60% with no significant change after administration of 100% supplementary oxygen.

S. Saedi (✉)
Rajaei Cardiovascular Medical and Research Center, Iran University of Medical Sciences, Tehran, Iran

M. Maleki, A. Alizadehasl (eds.), *Case-Based Clinical Cardiology*,
https://doi.org/10.1007/978-1-4471-7496-7_47

Para-Clinic Assessment

ECG showed normal sinus rhythm, evidence of right atrial (RA) enlargement, right axis deviation and right ventricular hypertrophy (RVH). Chest X-ray depicted reduced pulmonary vascularity with post-stenotic dilation of the main pulmonary artery trunk and RA and right ventricle (RV) enlargement (Fig. 47.1).

Echocardiography reported normal left ventricular (LV) size and mild systolic dysfunction. There was severe RV enlargement with severe RVH and severe systolic dysfunction. Pulmonary valve (PV) leaflets were thickened with severe stenosis (PG = 160 mmHg, MG = 100 mmHg) and mild pulmonary regurgitation. Cardiac catheterization showed thick and dome (PV) with post-stenotic dilation (Fig. 47.2). There was about 190 mmHg gradient across the valve and normal pulmonary artery pressure while LV pressure was about 140 mmHg and RV pressure much higher than the systemic pressure.

Management

Successful percutaneous balloon pulmonary valvuloplasty was performed with a 24 × 40 mm balloon-in-balloon catheter (BIB) with good final results (Fig. 47.3). RV pressure post-intervention was about 90mHg.The patient was started on selective beta-blockers. In 12 months clinical follow-up valvular gradient was significantly decreased and the patient was asymptomatic. O_2 saturation at room air was about 93%.

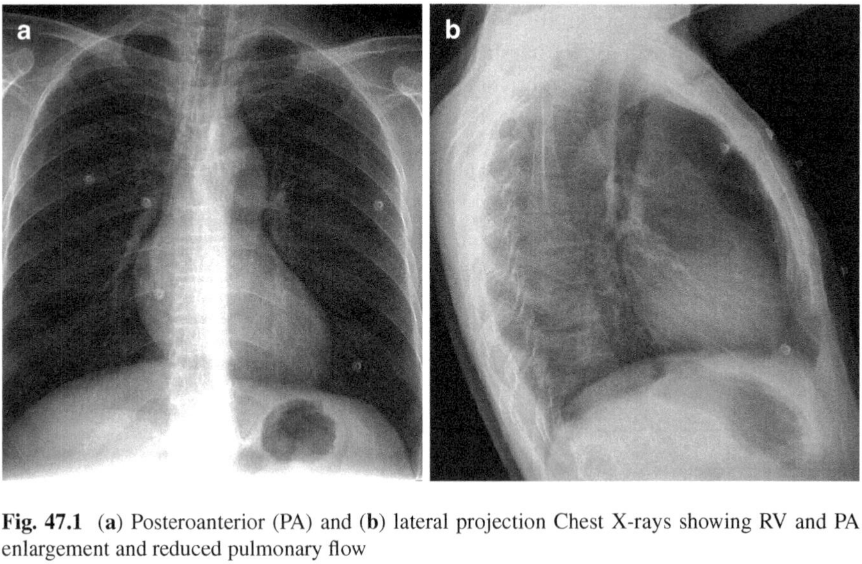

Fig. 47.1 (**a**) Posteroanterior (PA) and (**b**) lateral projection Chest X-rays showing RV and PA enlargement and reduced pulmonary flow

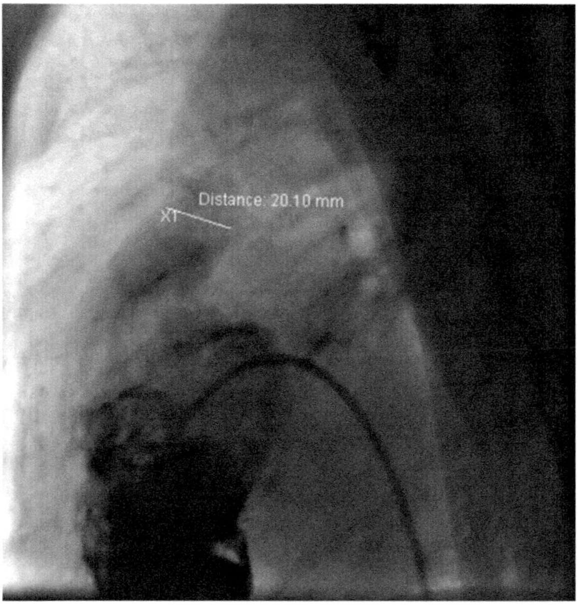

Fig. 47.2 Lateral view of thickened PV in catheterization. X1: measured RV outflow diameter just beneath the pulmonic valve

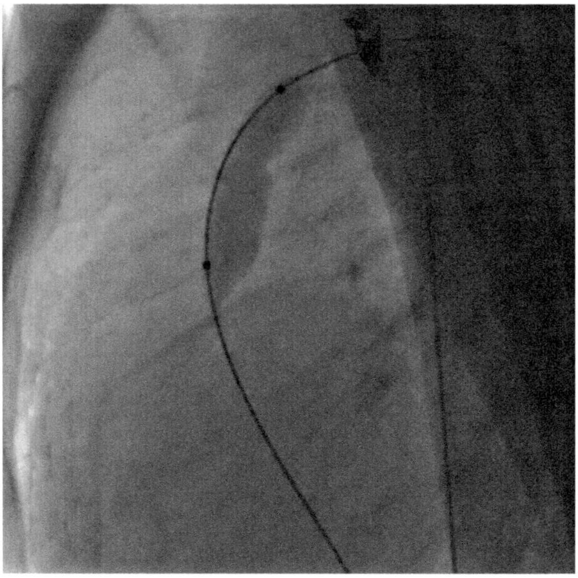

Fig. 47.3 Balloon valvuloplasty of PV

Conclusion

Pulmonic valve stenosis has three forms: Dome and thick pulmonary valve with post-stenotic dilation, dysplastic pulmonary valve, and bicuspid or unicuspid pulmonary valve which is more common in tetralogy of Fallot. The doming type is usually amenable to catheter intervention and percutaneous valvuloplasty can successfully be performed at any age with low complication rates. In the other forms, often pulmonary valve replacement with a biologic or mechanical valve is required. If left untreated right ventricular failure would ensue [1–5].

References

1. Khajali Z, Saedi S. Chapter 28 – Congenital heart disease. In Practical Cardiology (pp. 477–498). Elsevier 2017. https://doi.org/10.1016/B978-0-323-51149-0.00028-6
2. Eidem BW, Cetta F, O'Leary PW, editors. Echocardiography in pediatric and adult congenital heart disease. 2nd ed: Lippincott Williams & Wilkins; 2015.
3. Webb GD, Smallhorn JF, Therrien J, Redington AN. Congenital heart disease in the adult and pediatric patient. Braunwald's heart disease: a textbook of cardiovascular medicine. 11th ed. Philadelphia, PA: Elsevier; 2019.
4. Saedi S, Oraii S, Hajsheikholeslami F. A cross sectional study on prevalence and etiology of syncope in Tehran. Acta Med Iran. 2013;51(10):715–9.
5. Seilani P, Nasiri-Brojeni M, Saedi S, Maleki M, Saedi T. Midterm longevity of bioprosthetic pulmonary valves in congenital heart disease patients. Iran Heart J. 2017;18(3):21–7.

Chapter 48
Percutaneous Pulmonary Valve in Valve Implantation

Sedigheh Saedi

Abstract Tetralogy of Fallot (TOF) is the most common cyanotic congenital heart disease and consists of right ventricular outflow tract (RVOT) obstruction, right ventricular(RV) hypertrophy, outlet ventricular septal defect(VSD) and overriding of aorta. After reparative surgery and during follow-up to adulthood some of these patients have residual defects including pulmonary regurgitation often due to shaving of RVOT to relieve the stenosis or augmenting patches used at the time of initial surgery. These patients have to undergo pulmonary valve replacement with a mechanical or bioprosthetic valve. Limitations of the mechanical valves include the need for lifelong anticoagulation and the adherent risk of malfunction. Bioprosthetic valves on the other hand have limited durability especially in younger patients. With the advent of percutaneous pulmonary valve in valve procedures patients with degenerated previous biologic pulmonary valves and suitable anatomies could undergo transcatheter valve implantation and avert the high risk of redo surgeries.

History and Clinical Presentation

A 17-year-old female with history of the palliative shunt at infancy, TOF total repair at age four and redo surgery with biologic pulmonary valve(PV) replacement (Carpentier-Edwards 23 mm) due to severe pulmonary regurgitation(PI) at age nine presented to the clinic for routine follow-up. She mentioned mild dyspnea during exercise in the past months. In a physical examination a III/VI diastolic murmur was audible in the left second intercostal space. There was no cyanosis, ascites, or pedal edema.

S. Saedi (✉)
Rajaei Cardiovascular Medical and Research Center, Iran University of Medical Sciences, Tehran, Iran

M. Maleki, A. Alizadehasl (eds.), *Case-Based Clinical Cardiology*,
https://doi.org/10.1007/978-1-4471-7496-7_48

Para-Clinic Assessment

Twelve lead ECG showed normal sinus rhythm and right bundle branch block. Chest X-ray depicted right ventricular (RV) enlargement and bulging of RVOT (Fig. 48.1). In echocardiography, there was normal left ventricular (LV) size with mild systolic dysfunction, severe RV enlargement with moderate systolic dysfunction. Bioprosthetic PV had degenerative change and increased gradients (Peak pressure gradient: 50 mmHg) and severe regurgitation (Fig. 48.2).

Management

Redo surgery and transcatheter options were discussed with the patient and her family. They chose the percutaneous method as the patient did not wish to undergo another surgery . Cardiac catheterization was performed and a Edwards SAPIEN XT 23 mm valve was successfully implanted inside the previous bioprosthesis (Figs. 48.3 and 48.4).

In post-procedure echocardiography the new stented bioprosthetic PV had good leaflets motion, good alignment, and hemodynamic study (Peak pressure gradient: 19 mmHg) and no paravalvular or transvalvular leakage. The patient was discharged home one day after the procedure with aspirin and clopidogrel.

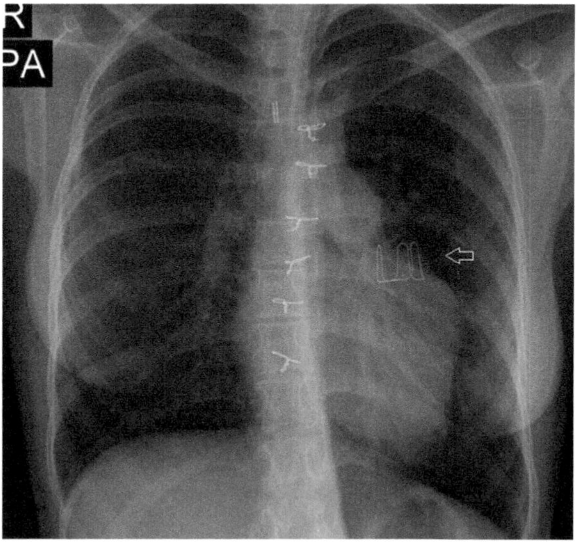

Fig. 48.1 Chest X-ray showing post sternotomy status and the biologic pulmonary valve (arrow)

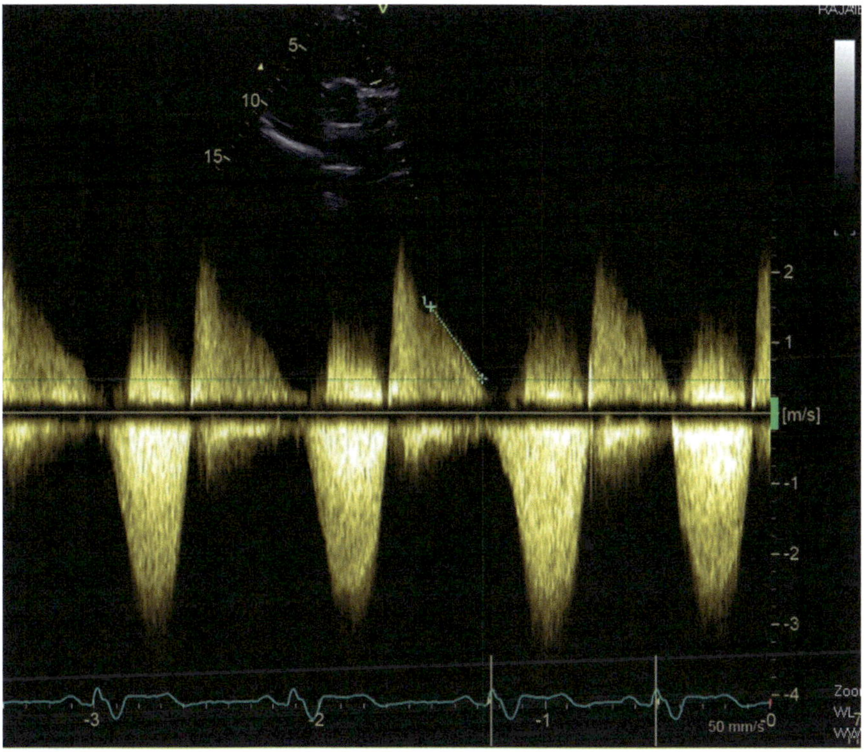

Fig. 48.2 Continuous wave Doppler of biologic pulmonary valve with severe regurgitation and pressure half time below 100 ms and significant increased gradients

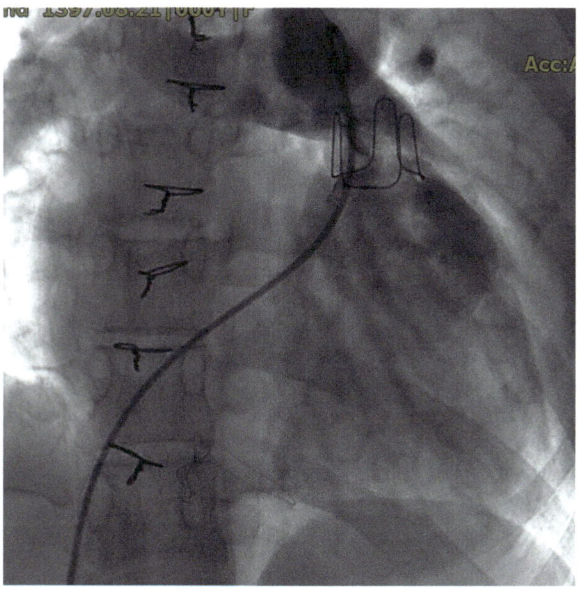

Fig. 48.3 Fluoroscopic image of first biologic PV and injection in pulmonary artery with a pigtail catheter. There are significant regurgitation and RV enlargement

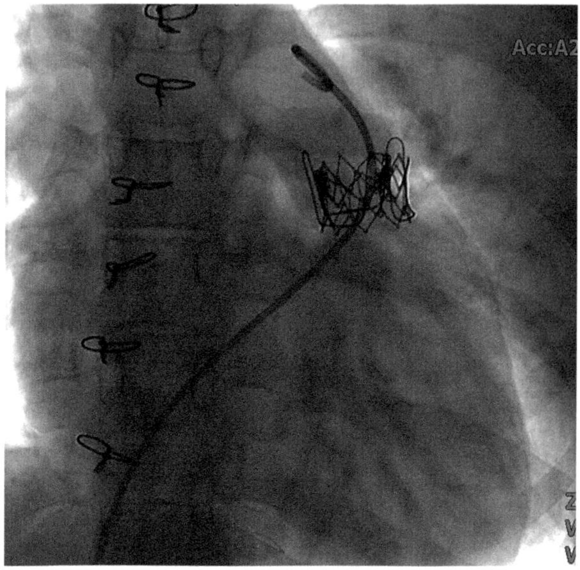

Fig. 48.4 Successful implantation of the second biologic prosthesis inside the degenerated valve

Conclusion

Percutaneous valve in valve implantation (PVVI) is an evolving technique for patients with degenerated bioprosthesis and has shown promising results. PVVI unlike percutaneous valve implantation (PVI) in the native valves can apply to a greater subset of patients as there is already a frame with known size in the valve were as PVI cannot be performed in many patients due to variations in the anatomy, coronary anomalies or aneurysmal RVOTs. In appropriately selected patients, transcatheter valve implantation helps to improve patient symptoms and exercise tolerance as well as cardiac hemodynamics [1–3].

References

1. Khajali Z, Saedi S. Chapter 28–Congenital heart disease. In: Practical Cardiology (pp. 477–498). Elsevier; 2017. https://doi.org/10.1016/B978-0-323-51149-0.00028-6
2. Seilani P, Nasiri-Brojeni M, Saedi S, Maleki M, Saedi T. Midterm longevity of bioprosthetic pulmonary valves in congenital heart disease patients. Iran Heart J. 2017;18(3):21–7.
3. Ansari MM, Cardoso R, Garcia D, Sandhu S, Horlick E, Brinster D, Martucci G, Piazza N. Percutaneous pulmonary valve implantation: present status and evolving future. Journal of the American College of Cardiology. 2015 Nov 17;66(20):2246–55.

Chapter 49
Quadricuspid Aortic Valve

Sedigheh Saedi

Abstract Normal aortic valve has three leaflets. Quadricuspid aortic valve(QAV) is a rare congenital anomaly of aortic valve in which there are four cusps. These patients should be diagnosed and clinically monitored as they are prone to developing aortic regurgitation in their life. Other structural anomalies and aortic dilation are also common in these patients. Advances in cardiac imaging have resulted in more and earlier detection of QAV.

History and Clinical Presentation

A 58-year-old asymptomatic female was referred to our clinic with incidental finding of severe aortic regurgitation in transthoracic echocardiography. She had a history of hypertension and was on antihypertensive medications. In physical exam loud III/IV diastolic murmur in the left sternal border was audible. Other clinical findings were within normal limits.

Para-Clinic Assessment

Twelve lead ECG showed normal sinus rhythm and normal axis. In chest X-ray, the left ventricle seemed enlarged. Transthoracic and transesophageal echocardiography was performed and showed moderate left ventricular (LV) enlargement and systolic dysfunction (estimated EF: 40%), AV was thickened and had four almost equal cusps with a central regurgitant orifice, severe regurgitation and holodiastolic flow reversal in proximal of descending aorta. There was no valvular stenosis or aortic root dilation (Figs. 49.1 and 49.2).

S. Saedi (✉)
Rajaei Cardiovascular Medical and Research Center, Iran University of Medical Sciences, Tehran, Iran

M. Maleki, A. Alizadehasl (eds.), *Case-Based Clinical Cardiology*,
https://doi.org/10.1007/978-1-4471-7496-7_49

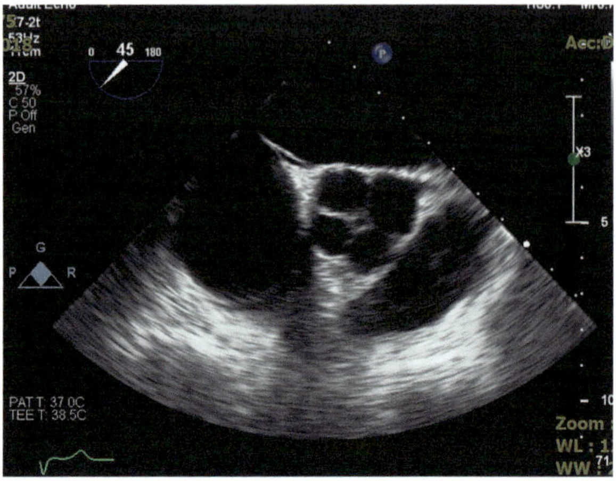

Fig. 49.1 Transesophageal echocardiography short-axis view of the aortic valve showing four almost equal aortic cusps and a small central orifice of aortic regurgitation

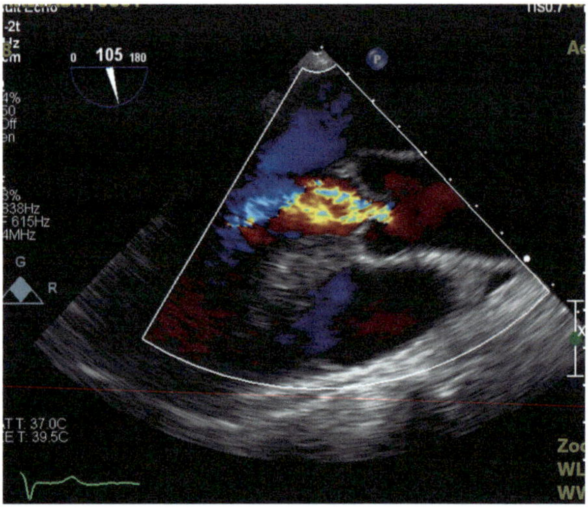

Fig. 49.2 Transesophageal echocardiography long-axis view of the aortic valve with severe regurgitation

In cardiac catheterization, the coronary arteries were patent and had a normal course. There was QAV with severe regurgitation and no stenosis (Fig. 49.3).

Management

Due to LV enlargement and dysfunction, the patient was scheduled for surgical aortic valve replacement.

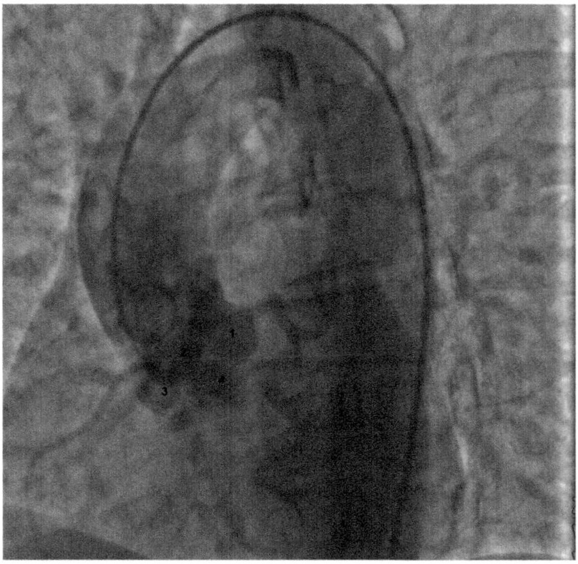

Fig. 49.3 Angiogram in LAO (left anterior oblique) caudal projection of aortic root injection with four separate cusps

Conclusion

Aortic regurgitation is the predominant sequel of QAV but stenosis could also occur. Most of these patients need aortic valve repair or replacement in the fifth to the sixth decade of life. The classification by Hurwitz and Roberts is widely used and categorizes the QAV to A to G subtypes based on the symmetry and size of the cusps. Infective endocarditis is more frequent in these patients particularly in those with asymmetric cusps due to flow turbulency. Coronary artery anomalies are also reported to be more prevalent in QAV. Surgical indications follow the guidelines for aortic regurgitation, stenosis, or associated anomalies. Successful transcatheter aortic valve implantation (TAVI) has been reported in these patients [1–4].

References

1. Yuan SM. Quadricuspid aortic valve: a comprehensive review. Braz J Cardiovasc Surg. 2016;31(6):454–60.
2. Ibrahim M, Wattanakit K, Barzallo M, Mungee S. Quadricuspid aortic valve stenosis: expanding our experience in transcatheter aortic valve implantation. J Invasive Cardiol. 2018;30(3):E27.
3. Tsang MY, Abudiab MM, Ammash NM, Naqvi TZ, Edwards WD, Nkomo VT, Pellikka PA. Quadricuspid aortic valve: characteristics, associated structural cardiovascular abnormalities, and clinical outcomes. Circulation. 2016;133(3):312–9.
4. Hammermeister K, Sethi GK, Henderson WG, Grover FL, Oprian C, Rahimtoola SH. Outcomes 15 years after valve replacement with a mechanical versus a bioprosthetic valve: final report of the Veterans Affairs randomized trial. J Am Coll Cardiol. 2000;36:1152–8.

Chapter 50
Stenting of Stenotic Modified Blalock-Taussing Shunt in Adult with Pulmonary Atresia

Sedigheh Saedi

Abstract In patients with complex and cyanotic congenital heart disease it is not always possible to perform complete reparative surgery. These patients are candidates for palliative systemic to pulmonary shunts to increase pulmonary blood flow and oxygen saturation and to alleviate cyanosis, secondary erythrocytosis, hyperviscosity syndrome and hemostatic abnormalities . These shunts could be arterial with a surgically created connection (shunt) between aorta or its branches and the pulmonary artery (PA)or venous connecting superior vena cava(SVC) to PA(Glenn shunt) or both SVC and inferior vena cava to PA (Fontan procedure).However palliative shunts have their own pitfalls and could become thrombosed and obstructed leading to worsening patient condition. On the other hand repeat surgery for another shunt is extremely high risk in most of these patients. Here we present a young male with occluded palliative shunt successfully treated with catheter intervention.

History and Clinical Presentation

A 27-year-old male with a history of pulmonary atresia and cardiac dysfunction who had undergone right modified Blalock-Taussing (BT) shunt palliation (shunt between the right subclavian artery and right pulmonary artery branch) in childhood presented with increasing cyanosis, dyspnea and severely limited functional capacity. In the physical exam, there was severe cyanosis and finger clubbing. Oxygen saturation at room air was about 65%.

S. Saedi (✉)
Rajaei Cardiovascular Medical and Research Center, Iran University of Medical Sciences, Tehran, Iran

M. Maleki, A. Alizadehasl (eds.), *Case-Based Clinical Cardiology*,
https://doi.org/10.1007/978-1-4471-7496-7_50

Para-Clinic Assessment

In lab tests, the patient had significant erythrocytosis with a hemoglobin concentration of 23 mg/dl. In echocardiography, the morphologic right ventricle was moderately enlarged with moderate dysfunction and the left ventricle was relatively small and had moderate dysfunction. Aorta originated from the RV and the pulmonary valve and main pulmonary artery were atretic. There was a large subaortic ventricular septal defect (VSD).Previous right BT shunt was small and had diminished flow.

Computed tomography (CT) angiography showed narrowing and partial occlusion in the BT shunt. There were multiple aorto-pulmonary collaterals.

Management

The patient was scheduled for shunt angioplasty. Phlebotomy was performed before the procedure to lower the bleeding tendency. After wiring of the shunt, balloon predilation and then stenting with a 5 × 57 mm stent was done with good final results. Oxygen saturation increased from 65% to 85% post-procedure (Figs. 50.1, 50.2, and 50.3). The patient had acceptable function capacity in 6 months follow-up visit.

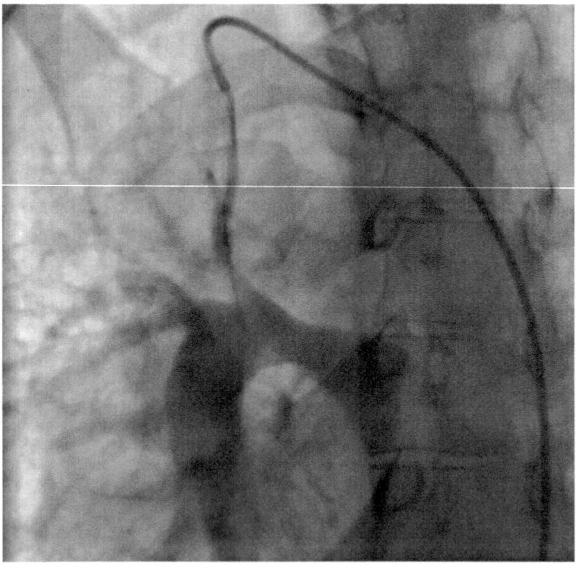

Fig. 50.1 Angiogram image of the modified BT shunt, Course of catheter is from the aorta to left subclavian artery and BT shunt with selective injection showing a narrowed and stenotic shunt

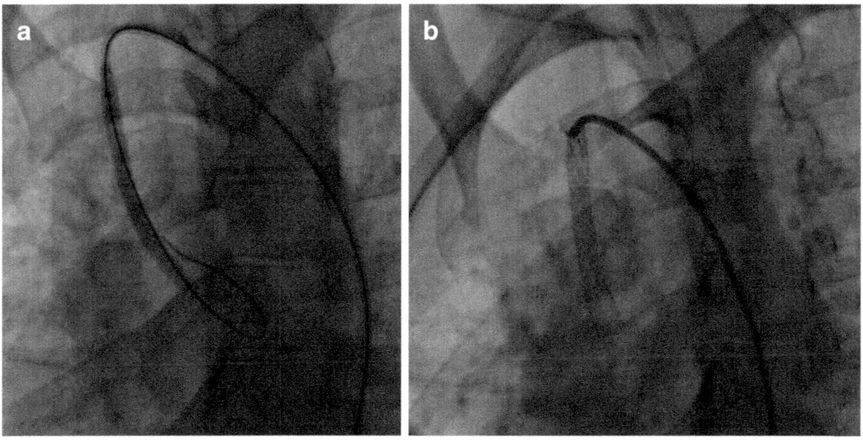

Fig. 50.2 Fluoroscopic image of balloon angioplasty (**a**) and stenting (**b**) of the right BT shunt

Fig. 50.3 Chest X-ray in follow-up showing the stented palliative shunt

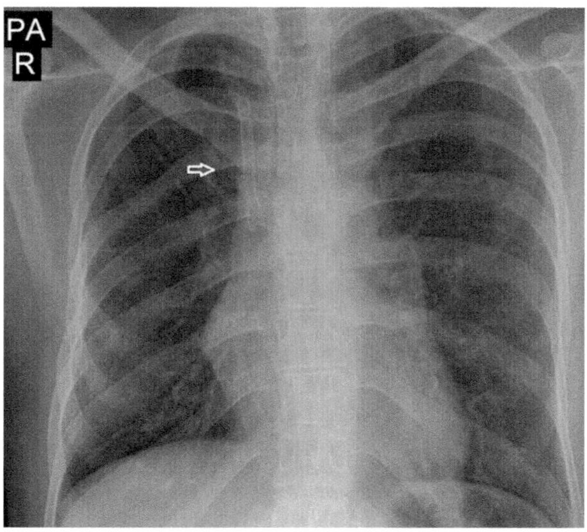

Conclusion

In adult patients with complex congenital heart disease, particularly pulmonary atresia surgery is challenging due to extensive aorto-pulmonary collateral formation and high bleeding risk. Catheter intervention and shunt angioplasty offers a chance for improvement in symptoms, functional capacity, and cardiovascular hemodynamics [1, 2].

References

1. Khajali Z, Saedi S. Chapter 28–Congenital heart disease. In: Practical Cardiology (pp. 477–498). Elsevier; 2017. https://doi.org/10.1016/B978-0-323-51149-0.00028-6
2. Webb GD, Smallhorn JF, Therrien J, Redington AN. Congenital heart disease in the adult and pediatric patient. Braunwald's Heart Disease: A Textbook of Cardiovascular Medicine. 11th ed. Philadelphia, PA: Elsevier; 2019.

Chapter 51
ASD Device Closure in Isolated Right Ventricular Hypoplasia

Zahra Khajali

Abstract The patient is a 23 years old lady whom came to us with cyanosis and history of abortion. In first echocardiography we found moderate size atrial septal defect with right to left shunt and small ventricular septal defect with normal size of right ventricle, that this size of RV was not in proportion of ASD size. After other workup and imaging modality we concluded this case had hypoplastic RV with ASD. After some months medical treatment for lowering of RA pressure, we closed ASD by occlutech device, and cyanosis eliminated completely. Patient had not any symptoms after closure and during one-year follow-up.

History and Clinical Presentation

A 23-year-old lady presented for evaluation of cyanosis and an elevated hemoglobin level which were noted as part of a complete blood count obtained after two miscarriages that had occurred at 6 and 8 weeks' gestational age. She denied dyspnea at rest or orthopnea, hemoptysis, and chest pain. She was admitted to our hospital in October 2018. The patient had not been diagnosed with a cardiac abnormality or heart murmur in childhood and had not undergone prior cardiac evaluation. However, her only symptom was mild dyspnea on exertion. The family history was remarkable for the death of her paternal uncle and her brother due to unidentified congenital heart diseases that there were not any medical documentaries about them.

Physical Examination

Blood Pressure: 110/70 mmHg, **Heart Rate**: 76 beats per minute, **Oxygen Saturation**: 83% in the air room.

Z. Khajali (✉)
Rajaei Cardiovascular Medical and Research Center, Iran University of Medical Sciences, Tehran, Iran

M. Maleki, A. Alizadehasl (eds.), *Case-Based Clinical Cardiology*,
https://doi.org/10.1007/978-1-4471-7496-7_51

General appearance: On examination, the patient was well developed. The nailbeds, lips, and mucous membranes were cyanotic, and digital clubbing was noted, there was not any respiratory distress at rest.

Lung/chest: No deformity of the chest wall, the lungs were clear.

Heart: Cardiac auscultation revealed a normal first heart sound, decreased pulmonary component of second heart sound, and a grade III/VI systolic murmur at the left sternal border, with no diastolic murmur or gallop. The rhythm was regular.

Abdomen: The abdomen was soft with normal sounds, and also the abdominal examination showed that the liver was on the right side with a normal span.

Extremities: There was no peripheral edema, but there was a digital clubbing. The pulses were regular and symmetric.

Laboratory Data

Hemoglobin	18 gr/dl
Hematocrit	50.5%
White Blood Count	5800 cells/mm3
Platelet	207,000 cells/mm3
Creatinine	0.7 mg/dl
Blood urea nitrogen	13 mg/dl
Cholesterol	115 mg/dl
Triglyceride	86 mg/dl
ALT (Alanine transaminase)	19 IU/L
AST (Aspartate transaminase)	15 IU/L
TSH (Thyroid stimulating hormone)	1.7 micro IU/ml

Electrocardiogram

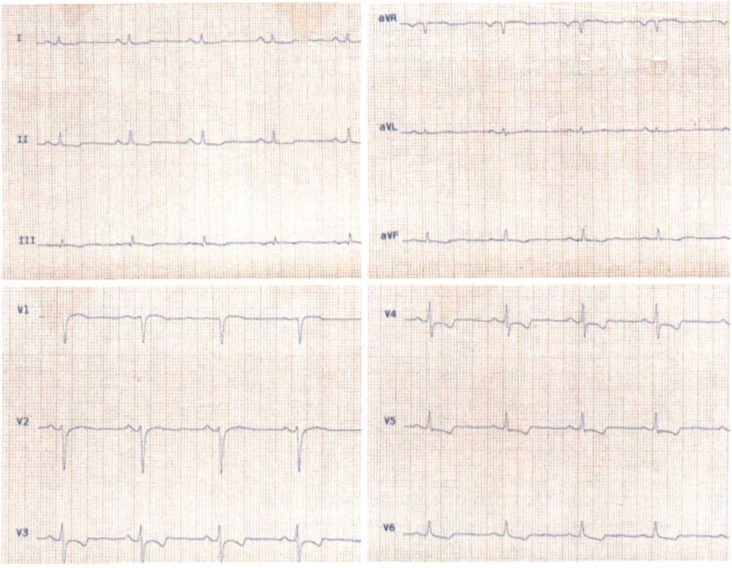

Twelve lead standard electrocardiogram
Normal sinus rhythm
Heart rate: 62 beats per minute, regular
Normal axis deviation
Normal PR interval
Peaked P in leads V1–V4 suggesting Right Atrium overload
Normal QRS duration
Mild ST-T changes in inferior leads and leads V1–V3 in favor of LV strain pattern

Chest X-Ray

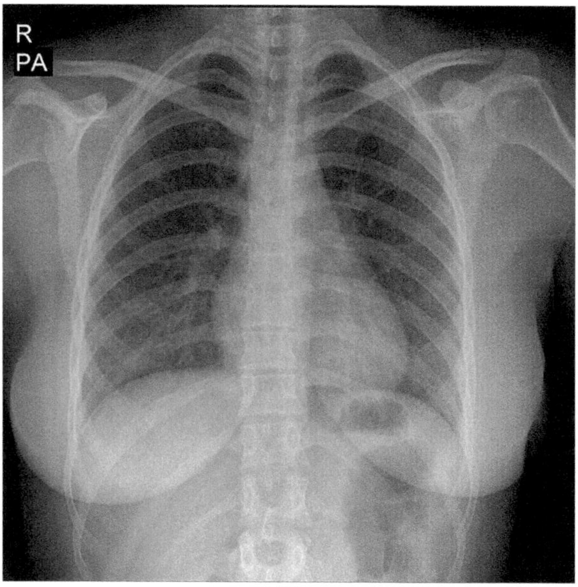

Posteroanterior projection, full inspiration

Levocardia (apex orientation to the left), situs solitus (The gastric bubble is seen in the left)

Left aortic arch
Normal cardiothoracic ratio
Normal pulmonary parenchyma and vascularity
Small aortic knob

Echocardiography

- Normal left ventricle size with mild systolic dysfunction (left ventricle ejection fraction = 45%)
- Small apical ventricular septal defect (2 mm)
- Small right ventricle size based on intracardiac shunt with mild to moderate systolic dysfunction, a significantly calcified bundle in right ventricle apex
- Normal mitral valve leaflets, no mitral stenosis, mild mitral regurgitation
- Normal tricuspid aortic Valve, no aortic stenosis, no aortic insufficiency
- Normal tricuspid valve leaflets, no tricuspid valve stenosis, mild tricuspid valve regurgitation (TRG = 22 mmHg)
- Normal pulmonary valve, no pulmonary stenosis, mild to moderate pulmonary insufficiency
- Moderate size secundum type atrial septal defect with the bidirectional shunt (size:16 mm), predominant flow from right to left (Figs. 51.1, 51.2, and 51.3)

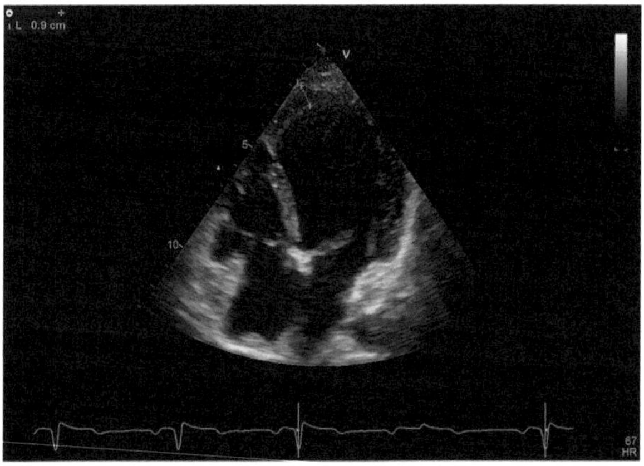

Fig. 51.1 Four-chamber view showed small right ventricle size

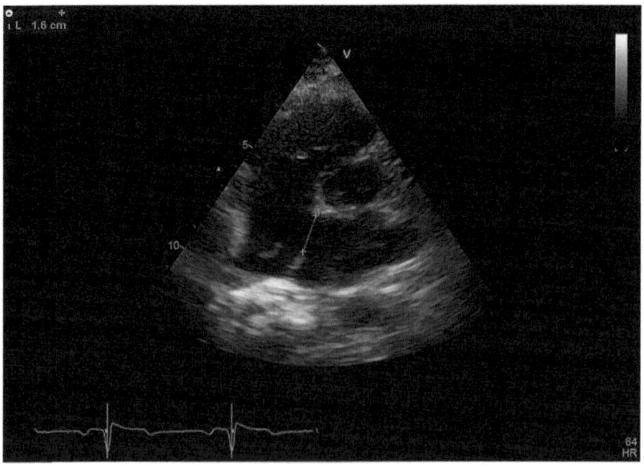

Fig. 51.2 Parasternal short-axis view showed moderate size secundum type ASD

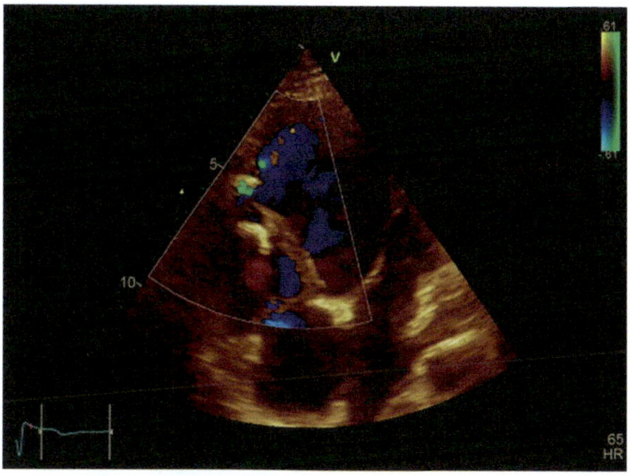

Fig. 51.3 Small VSD, significantly calcified bundle in right ventricle apex was seen

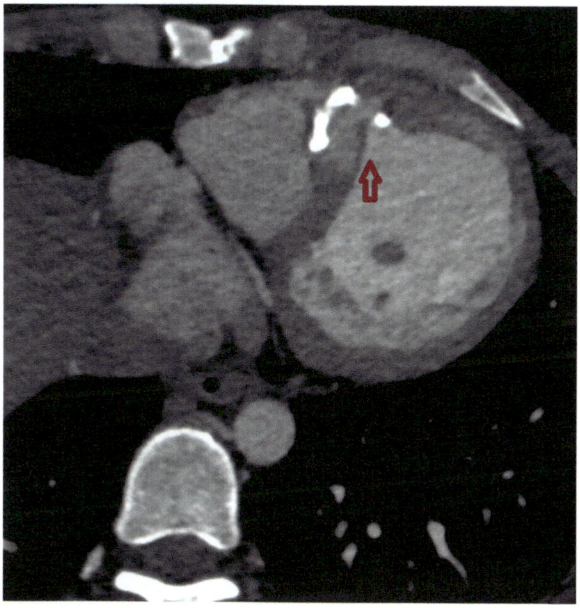

Fig. 51.4 Calcified moderator band and hypoplastic apical portion of RV was noted

Congenital and Coronary CT Angiography

Normal epicardial coronary arteries. Cardiomegaly and small ventricular septal defect and a secundum type atrial septal defect with mild RA enlargement are noted. Curvilinear calcification is visible in right ventricle (Figs. 51.4 and 51.5).

Cardiac MRI (Magnetic Resonance Imaging)

- Normal left ventricle size with preserved systolic function, left ventricle apical and lateral hyper trabeculation, left ventricular ejection fraction = 50%.

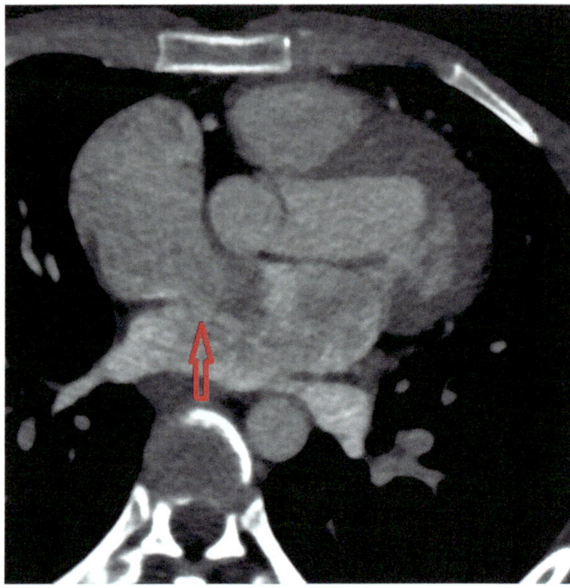

Fig. 51.5 Secundum type ASD

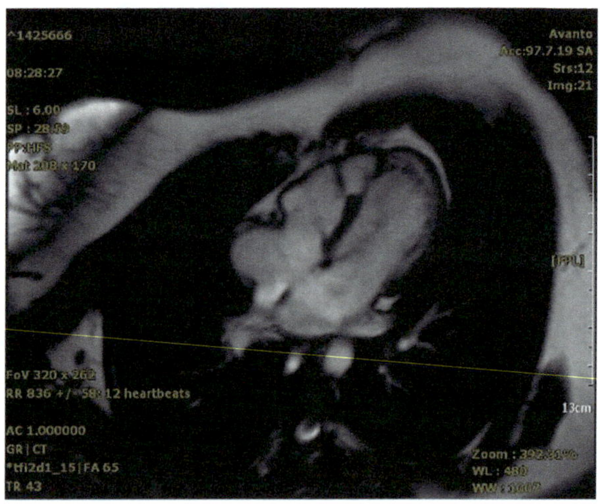

Fig. 51.6 Small right ventricle, calcified bundle in right ventricle apex, secundum type atrial septal defect, left ventricle apical hyper trabeculation was seen in axial view

- Small right ventricle size with right ventricle end diastolic volume index: 40 ml/ m^2 and right ventricle Ejection Fraction: 40%.
- The left atrium is normal in size, and the right atrium is enlarged.
- A secundum atrial septal defect measured 17 mm with the right to left shunt.
- Redundant interatrial septum is seen.
- The interventricular septum shows the small near closed apicoseptal muscular Ventricular Septal Defect with nonsignificant left to right shunt (Fig. 51.6).

Catheterization

- Hemodynamic and pressure study showed evidence of bidirectional shunt, elevated Right Atrium Pressure and Right Ventricular End Diastolic Pressure (RVEDP) that they were about 10 mmHg. Pulmonary arterial pressure was normal.
- Left ventricle injection showed normal left ventricular size and mild systolic dysfunction, hyper trabeculated left ventricle, and small apical ventricular septal defect.
- Right ventricle injection showed the normal size of inlet and outlet parts of the right ventricle with severe hypoplastic of apical part and moderate right ventricle systolic dysfunction.
- Right ventricle was hypoplastic so atrial septal defect was closed temporarily with sizing balloon for evaluation of the hemodynamic response of right ventricle to the closing of the atrial septal defect. Sizing balloon test performed and there was a significant increase in right atrium pressure and right ventricular end diastolic pressure, so the patient underwent diuretic therapy and after 6 months, again catheterization performed. After sizing balloon inflation there was no significant increase in right atrium pressure and right ventricular end diastolic pressure, and there was up to 25% rising in O_2 saturation (O_2 saturation increased from 83% to 94%). Atrial septal defect closure was done by occlutech device 21 mm successfully (Figs. 51.7, 51.8, 51.9, and 51.10).

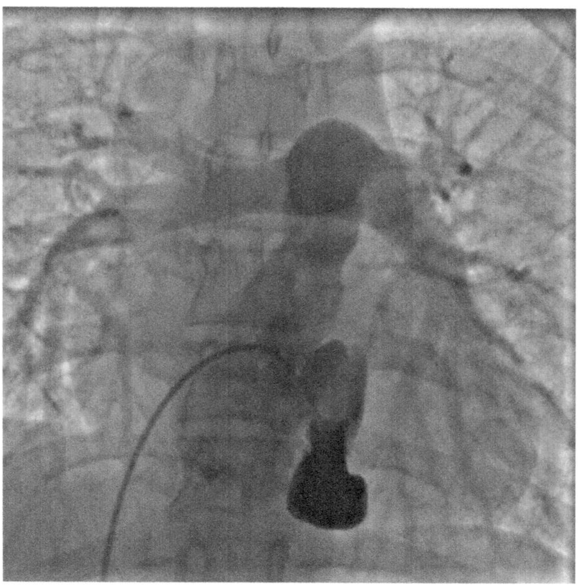

Fig. 51.7 RV angiogram showed hypoplastic apical part of RV with well-developed inlet and outlet part

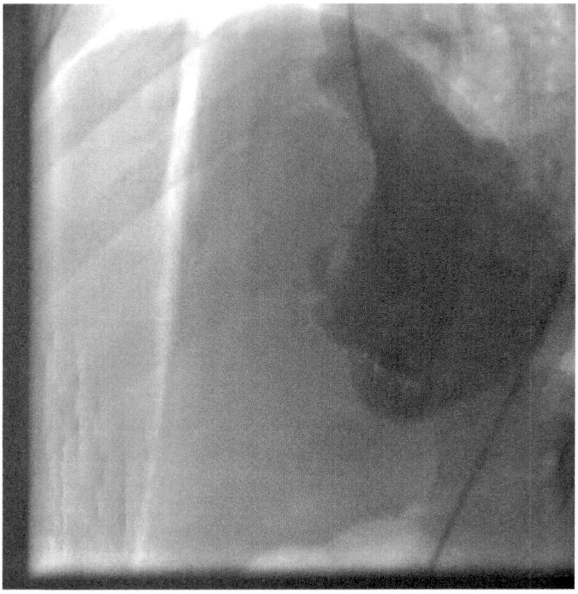

Fig. 51.8 Left ventricle injection showed apical hyper trabeculation, small VSD

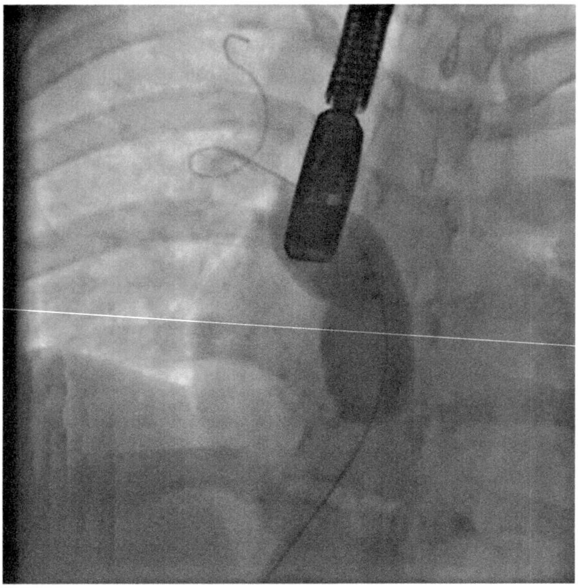

Fig. 51.9 Sizing balloon test

Echocardiography a Day After Device Closure

Echocardiography a day after device closure showed the proper position of the device and acceptable systolic and diastolic function of both ventricles (Fig. 51.11).

Discussion Isolated right ventricle hypoplasia is an anomaly that inlet and outlet parts of the right ventricle are normal but the apical portion of right ventricle is

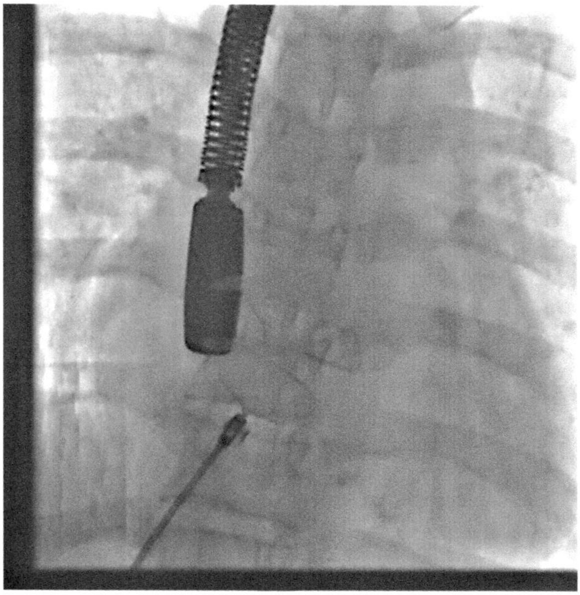

Fig. 51.10 Deployment of ASD device

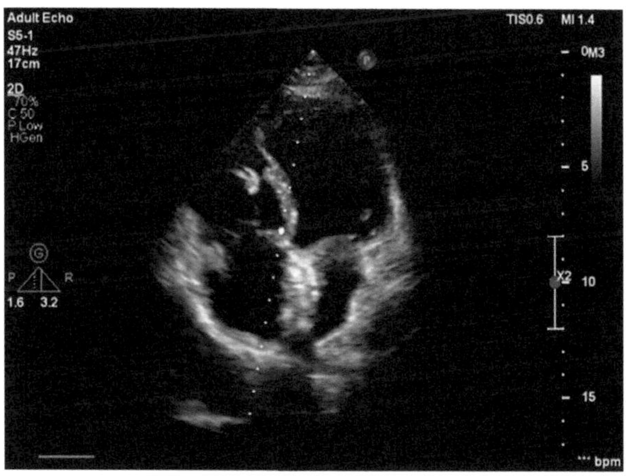

Fig. 51.11 Echocardiography after ASD device closure showed proper position of the device and no bulging to LA

absent or underdeveloped [1]. In more usual circumstances a small cavity of the right ventricle is associated with a malformed inlet or outlet portion of the chamber. This anomaly always is associated with patent foramen oval or atrial septal defect as an escape valve. For diagnosis and management of this anomaly multi modalities are practical [2]. In this particular patient, there was hypoplastic right ventricle with an atrial septal defect that the outlet and the inlet portions were normal size and the right ventricle was smaller than normal because of the absence of apical trabecular component. The poor compliant ventricle resulted in elevation of the diastolic pressure, raising in RA pressure and inducing right to left shunt. Because of small and low volume, underfilled right ventricle, output into pulmonary artery was reduced.

Clinical management in this anomaly depends on right ventricle size and hemodynamics. In some groups atrial septal defect surgical or device closure is reasonable and some of these patients cannot tolerate atrial septal defect closure alone and need to one and half repair [3] or even Fontan operation. An obvious benefit of closure would be the elimination of the right to left shunting, which in this patient was considerable, and improved oxygen saturation. Furthermore, the risk of paradoxical embolism will be aborted.

References

1. Lombardi M, Tagliente MR, Pirolo T, Massari E, Vairo U. Transient and anatomic isolated right-ventricular hypoplasia. J Cardiovasc Med (Hagerstown). 2016;17(Suppl 2):e257–e63.
2. Zhou D, Liao HQ, Ouyang MZ, Shang QL, Zhang M. Isolated right ventricular apical hypoplasia characterized by computed tomography and echocardiography. J Clin Ultrasound. 2018;46(1):82–4.
3. Hata H, Sumitomo N, Ayusawa M, Shiono M. Biventricular repair of pulmonary atresia with intact ventricular septum and severely hypoplastic right ventricle: a case report of a minimum intervention surgical approach. J Cardiothorac Surg. 2016;11(1):94.

Chapter 52
Complicated Case of Device Closure of Large Patent Ductus Arteriosus Associated with Significant Mitral Valve Regurgitation

Zahra Khajali

Abstract A 29-year-old lady referred to us for work-up of valvular heart disease. She had mild dyspnea, and did not aware of her problem. In physical examination we noticed continuous machinery murmur. In ECG had evidence of bi-ventricular hypertrophy especially LV volume overload. In echocardiography the patient had large PDA, moderate to severe MR due to MVP and severe PAH. In cardiac catheterization we resulted evidence of significant left to right shunt via PDA, and pulmonary artery vasoreactivity, so we decided to close PDA by device to improving PAP and also MR severity. We performed closure of defect by the largest available device (muscular VSD18mm). It seems that the procedure was successful but the day after procedure we found embolized device on RPA, patient transferred to operating room, the device was removed from RPA, the PDA and mitral valve was repaired and the patient transferred uneventfully from operating room to ICU.

History and Clinical Presentation

A 29 years old female referred to our clinic with valvular disease diagnosis. She came to our clinic with mild dyspnea. The patient did not receive any drug or management before.

Electronic Supplementary Material The online version of this chapter (https://doi.org/10.1007/978-1-4471-7496-7_52) contains supplementary material, which is available to authorized users.

Z. Khajali (✉)
Rajaei Cardiovascular Medical and Research Center, Iran University of Medical Sciences, Tehran, Iran

M. Maleki, A. Alizadehasl (eds.), *Case-Based Clinical Cardiology*,
https://doi.org/10.1007/978-1-4471-7496-7_52

Physical Examination

Blood Pressure: 120/80 mmHg, **Heart Rate**: 75 beats per minute, **Oxygen Saturation**: 94% in room air.

General appearance: On examination, the patient was well developed. The nailbeds, lips, and mucous membranes were normal.

Lung/chest: No deformity of the chest wall, the lungs sound was normal.

Heart: Cardiac auscultation revealed a normal first heart sound, increased pulmonary component of second heart sound, and a continuous murmur at the left sternal border and at the back in interscapular region. The rhythm was regular.

Abdomen: The abdominal examination had no remarkable abnormality.

Extremities: There was no peripheral edema. The pulses were regular and symmetric.

Electrocardiogram

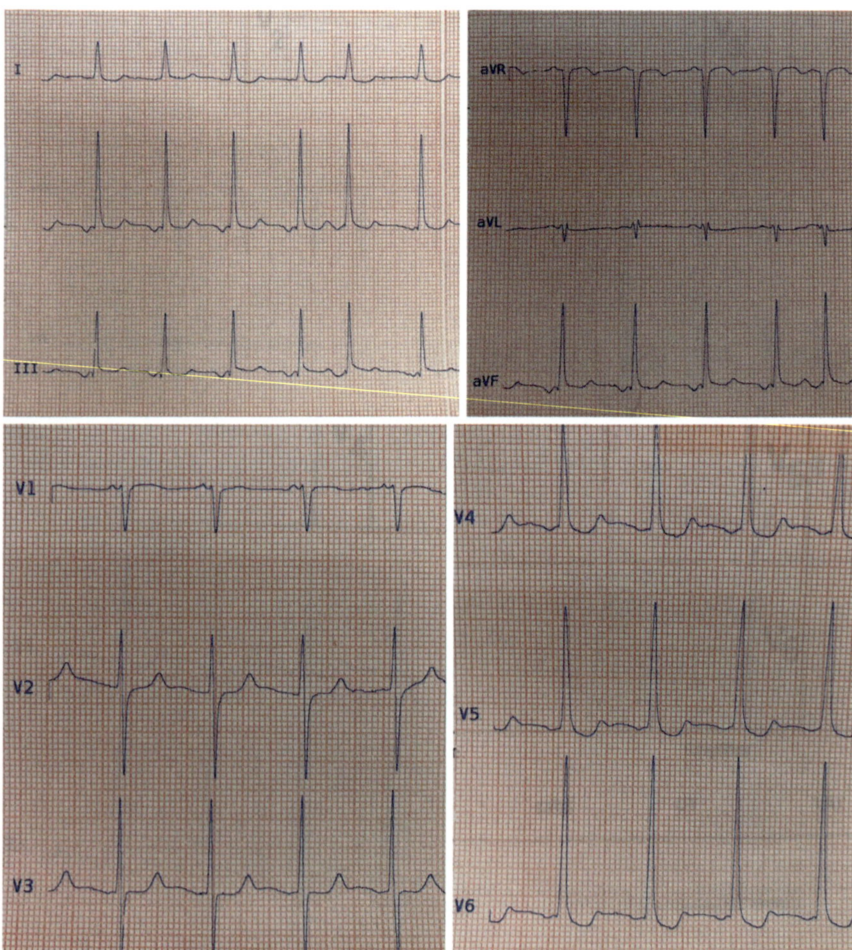

Twelve lead standard electrocardiogram

Low atrial rhythm, PAC

Heart Rate: 85 beats per minute

Normal axis deviation

Tall R in V5, V6, and inverted T in favor of LV volume overload and diphasic V3 and V4 in favor of BVH

Chest X-Ray

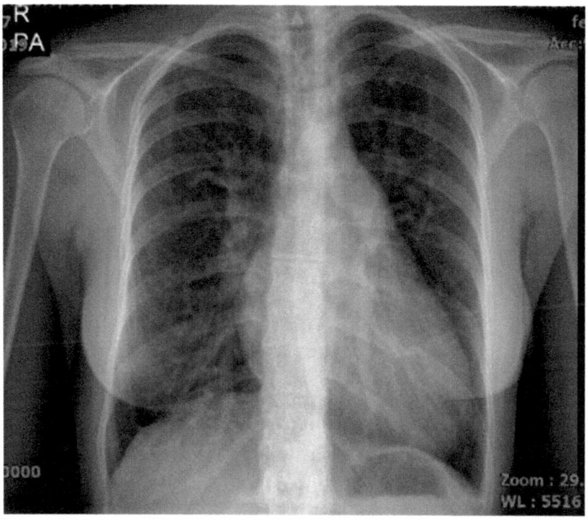

Posteroanterior projection, full inspiration

Levocardia (apex orientation to the left), situs solitus (The gastric bubble is seen in the left)

Left aortic arch

Increased cardiothoracic ratio(downward displacement of apex in favor of LV enlargement)

Increased pulmonary vascularity

Dilated PA border

Dilate aorta

All data in favor of shunt vascularity and PDA

Echocardiography

- Moderate left ventricle enlargement with mild systolic dysfunction (left ventricle ejection fraction = 45%)

- No ventricular septal defect
- Moderate enlargement of right ventricle with mild systolic dysfunction
- Prolaptic both mitral valve leaflets with no mitral stenosis, moderate to severe mitral regurgitation
- Normal tricuspid aortic valve, no aortic stenosis, no aortic insufficiency
- Normal tricuspid valve leaflets, no tricuspid valve stenosis, moderate tricuspid valve regurgitation (tricuspid regurgitation gradient = 75 mmHg, severe PAH)
- Normal pulmonary valve, no pulmonary stenosis, moderate pulmonary insufficiency
- Large size PDA with left to right shunt (size: 14 mm)
- No coarctation of aorta (Fig. 52.1)

Cardiac Catheterization and Procedure

- Hemodynamic and pressure study showed evidence of left to right shunt via PDA, elevated pulmonary pressure, and Right Ventricular Systolic Pressure (RVSP).

	Pressure	Saturation
Left ventricle	120/0–10	95
Right ventricle	95/0–7	70
PAP	95/40	85
Ascending aorta	120/80	95
Descending aorta	120/80	95

LV injection showed severe LV enlargement and mild systolic dysfunction, moderate MR. Large PDA seen in aortic isthmus injection, normal coronary artery

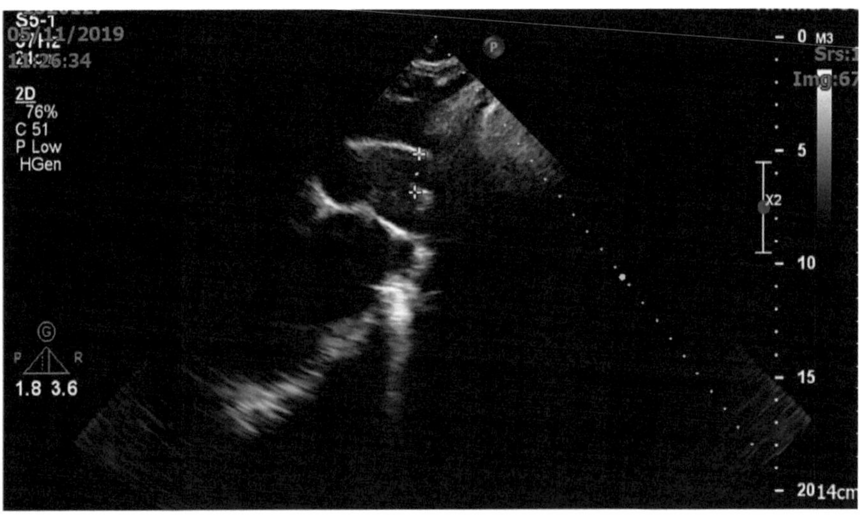

Fig. 52.1 Suprasternal view showed large PDA

system, and no AI in aortic root injection revealed. After 20-min vasoreactivity test by oxygen 100%, we noticed a significant decline in the mean of PAP.

Management Regarding evidence of significant left to right shunt via PDA, vasoreactivity, and moderate regurgitation of MV, we think that closure of PDA could postponed surgical procedure of MV repair and also declined pulmonary artery pressure to lowering surgical risk in future.

Cefazolin IV 1000 mg was administered and guidewire was advanced through catheter from the femoral vein to IVC, RA, and RV to LPA and then across the PDA to descending aorta. The stiff wire then passed through the catheter. The venous sheath and catheter were then removed and an introducer sheath was advanced over the stiff guidewire to the descending aorta, the guidewire was removed. Next, a muscular VSD occluder 18 (occlutech) was mounted on a delivery cable, advanced through the introducer sheath across the PDA to the aorta, and first aortic disc opened and waist of the device deployed on the duct gently and finally the pulmonic disc opened. Then the deployment place checked by a gentle push and pulling maneuver and device released. Then descending aorta angiography demonstrated the proper position of device.

The Day After Device Closure

One day later, echocardiography performed but the device was not on the duct and turbulent flow of PDA was seen, after interrogation, we found the device in right pulmonary artery that confirmed by fluoroscopy. So, the patient transferred to the operating room, the device was removed from RPA, the PDA and mitral valve were repaired and the patient transferred uneventfully from operating room to ICU. During follow-up echocardiography 1 month later there is a significant decline in PAP(SPAP = 50 mmHg) and trace residual MR (Fig. 52.2).

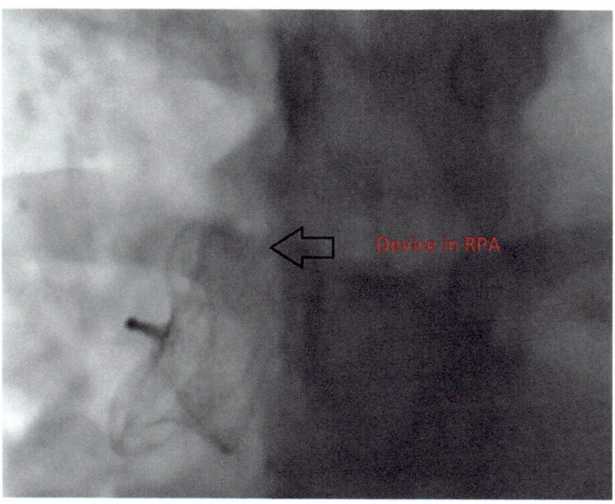

Fig. 52.2 Fluoroscopy showed the device in RPA

Discussion Patent ductus arteriosus is a structure that resulted of persistence of the distal portion of the left sixth aortic arch [1]. This duct has a necessary role in embryonic blood circulation and after birth closed during the first 48–72 h. Patency of the duct after birth could have harmful effects on cardiovascular and pulmonary artery systems and it depends on the size and the flow through the duct. The volume load causes left cardiac enlargement and failure, and also inducing pulmonary artery hypertension [2]. It also had the chance of endarteritis that it could be seen in small size PDA. This defect should be closed in all cases except silent PDA and large cases that caused Eisenmenger syndrome. In most cases, percutaneous catheter intervention can be done unless complex shape or active endarteritis [3]. Especially in adults, percutaneous intervention is preferred to surgery due to the calcification of the duct, fragile aorta, and higher pulmonary artery pressure. The devices that approved for PDA closure are ADO I, ADO II, and some type of coils [4]. But the variety in shape and size of the duct in some cases makes it less possible to be closed by current devices, so another devices like vascular plug, muscular VSD, and ASD device can be used off-label [5]. Muscular VSD occluder devices had a higher waist-to-disk ratio and also larger maximum waist diameter, so it can be used in larger PDA with a diameter of more than 14 mm. The position of the waist on the duct, relation of retention disk to duct and aorta and appropriate size of the device are important factors in not embolizing the device. The larger size of the duct relation to the chosen device size in our case and position of the retention disk in the aorta were the factors of the device displacement.

References

1. Schneider DJ, Moore JW. Patent ductus arteriosus. Circulation. 2006;114:1873–82.
2. Campbell M. Patent ductus arteriosus: some notes on prognosis and on pulmonary hypertension. Br Heart J. 1955;17:511–33.
3. Meadows J, Landzberg MJ. Advances in transcatheter interventions in adults with congenital heart disease. Prog Cardiovasc Dis. 2011;53:265–73.
4. Krichenko A, Benson LN, Burrows P, et al. Angiographic classification of the isolated, persistently patent ductus arteriosus and implications for percutaneous catheter occlusion. Am J Cardiol. 1989;63:877–80.
5. Fernando R, Koranne K, Loyalka P, Kar B, Gregoric I. Patent ductus arteriosus closure using an Amplatzer™ ventricular septal defect closure device. Exp Clin Cardiol. 2013;18(1):e50–4.

Chapter 53
Total Anomalous Pulmonary Veins Return in a Young Lady

Zahra Khajali

Abstract A 27-year-old lady referred to us with cyanosis and history of one miscarriage at 9 weeks of pregnancy. She did not have any workup before, and this the first time that workup performed for her. In physical examination, electrocardiogram and echocardiography we suspect to TAPVR that this diagnosis confirmed by CT angiography. For exact hemodynamic evaluation catheterization performed and by evaluation of all data, finally surgical repair was done uneventfully. Systemic saturation returned to normal level and the patient feels well after one-year follow-up.

History and Clinical Presentation

A 27-year-old lady presented for evaluation of cyanosis and also, she had one miscarriage that had occurred at 9 weeks' gestational age. She had mild dyspnea during exercise.

The patient had not been diagnosed with a cardiac abnormality or heart murmur in childhood and had not undergone prior cardiac evaluation.

Physical Examination

Blood Pressure: 100/70 mmHg, **Heart Rate**: 70 beats per minute, **Oxygen Saturation**: 78% in the air room.

Electronic Supplementary Material The online version of this chapter (https://doi.org/10.1007/978-1-4471-7496-7_53) contains supplementary material, which is available to authorized users.

Z. Khajali (✉)
Rajaei Cardiovascular Medical and Research Center, Iran University of Medical Sciences, Tehran, Iran

M. Maleki, A. Alizadehasl (eds.), *Case-Based Clinical Cardiology*,
https://doi.org/10.1007/978-1-4471-7496-7_53

General appearance: On examination, the patient was well developed. The nailbeds, lips, and mucous membranes were cyanotic and digital clubbing was noted, there was not any respiratory distress at rest.

Lung/chest: No deformity of the chest wall, the lungs were clear.

Heart: Cardiac auscultation revealed a normal first heart sound but wide splitting and loud second heart sound and a grade II/VI systolic murmur at the upper left sternal border, with no diastolic murmur or gallop. The rhythm was regular.

Abdomen: The abdomen was soft with normal sounds, and also the abdominal examination showed that the liver was on the right side with a normal span.

Extremities: There was no peripheral edema, but there was a digital clubbing. The pulses were regular and symmetric.

Electrocardiogram

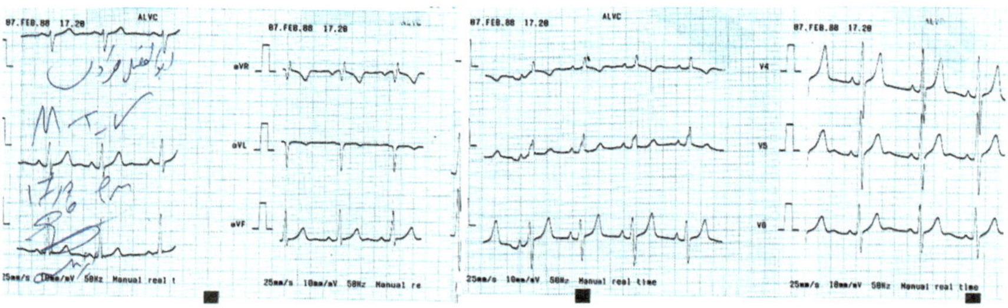

Twelve lead standard electrocardiogram

Normal sinus rhythm

Heart Rate: 64 beats per minute, regular

Right axis deviation

Normal PR interval

Peaked P in leads II, III, aVF suggesting Right Atrium overload

qR in V1 and deep S in V5, V6 in favor of RV volume and pressure overload

Normal QRS duration

Chest X-Ray

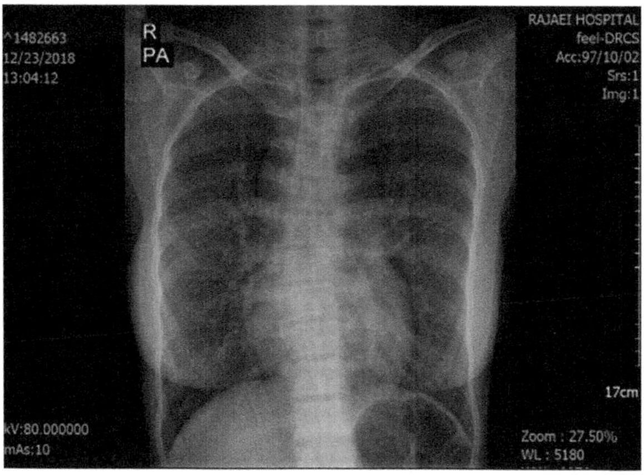

Posteroanterior projection, full inspiration

Levocardia (apex orientation to the left), situs solitus (The gastric bubble is seen in the left)

Left aortic arch

Increased cardiothoracic ratio (RV and RA enlargement)

Increased pulmonary vascularity

Small aortic knob

Dilated SVC at right and vertical vein at the left border all of the features resemble the figure of eight or snowman consistent with diagnosis of TAPVR.

Echocardiography

- Normal left ventricle size with normal systolic function (left ventricle ejection fraction = 55%).
- Dilated right ventricle and right atrium with mild systolic dysfunction.
- Large interatrial septal defect with right to left shunt.
- Normal mitral valve leaflets, no mitral stenosis, no mitral regurgitation.
- Normal tricuspid aortic valve, no aortic stenosis, no aortic insufficiency.
- Normal tricuspid valve leaflets, no tricuspid valve stenosis, mild tricuspid valve regurgitation (tricuspid regurgitation gradient = 45 mmHg, moderate PAH,PAP = 50 mmHg).
- Normal pulmonary valve, no pulmonary stenosis, mild pulmonary insufficiency.
- No pulmonary veins drained to LA.
- In suprasternal view a large vein was seen that drained to innominate vein and SVC with pulmonary veins doppler (Fig. 53.1).

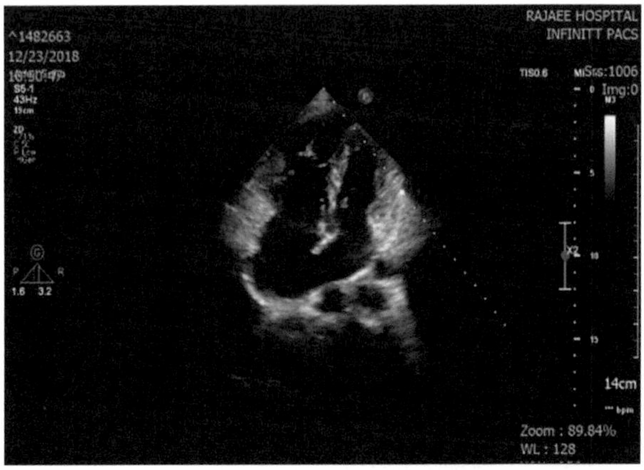

Fig. 53.1 In 4 chamber view dilated RV and RA was seen and there was no pulmonary veins at LA border, large ASD

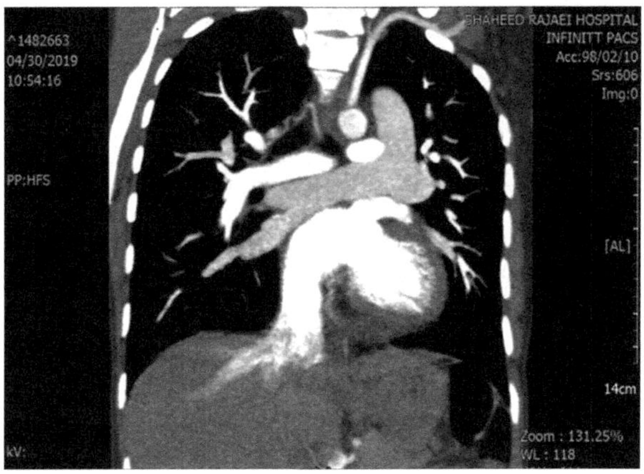

Fig. 53.2 All pulmonary veins drained to vertical vein

Congenital CT Angiography

Normal epicardial coronary arteries. Cardiomegaly and large atrial septal defect with severe RA and RV enlargement are noted. No pulmonary veins drained to LA and all of them connected to a large chamber that drains to vertical vein and innominate vein and superior vena cava. Dilated SVC and vertical vein noted (Fig. 53.2).

Catheterization

- Hemodynamic and pressure study showed evidence of the right to left shunt, normal Right Atrium Pressure, and Right Ventricular End Diastolic Pressure (RVEDP) that they were about 6 mmHg. Pulmonary arterial pressure was moderate to severely elevated (55/20/33 mmHg).

- Pulmonary artery injection in levophase showed all pulmonary veins drain to vertical vein, then innominate vein and superior vena cava.
- After all these diagnostic modalities the patient became a candidate for surgical procedure.

Management

Common pulmonary vein opened to LA and vertical vein closed from the site of innominate vein insertion. Then atrial septal defect repaired by pericardial patch.

The patient had a normal course in ICU with oxygen saturation about 96–98%.

Post-op echocardiography showed no residual atrial septal defect with no stenosis at the opening site of common pulmonary veins to the left atrium, and there was no flow in the vertical vein.

Discussion Total anomalous pulmonary veins drainage or return is a rare cyanotic congenital heart disease that in this anomaly all pulmonary veins drained to another chamber or veins except left atrium [1].

This anomaly classified into four types:

(1) Supra cardiac (2) cardiac (3) Infra cardiac and (4) mixed type [2].

This anomaly presented in infancy with cyanosis and rarely it is detected in adulthood. The severity of symptoms depends on the size of interatrial septal defect, obstruction of pulmonary veins, and also pulmonary artery pressure [3].

If the interatrial septal defect is restricted the infant would have severe cyanosis and could not tolerate the symptoms, but with large interatrial defect, the patients may be reached to adulthood [4].

The definite treatment is surgery and these patients will have acceptable survival if operation was done in the early months of the birth date.

The patient whom reached adolescence and adulthood usually has pulmonary arterial hypertension, but if the pulmonary vascular bed is reactive for this age group also surgery is a definite procedure.

References

1. Michielon G, Di Donato RM, Pasquini L, Giannico S, Brancaccio G, Mazzera E, Squitieri C, et al. Total anomalous pulmonary venous connection: long-term appraisal with evolving technical solutions. Eur J Cardiothorac Surg. 2002;22(2):184–91. https://doi.org/10.1016/S1010-7940(02)00247-6.
2. Sano S, Brawn WJ, Mee RB. Total anomalous pulmonary venous drainage. J Thorac Cardiovasc Surg. 1989;97(6):886–92.
3. Wang JK, Lue HC, Wu MH, Young ML, Wu FF, Wu JM. Obstructed total anomalous pulmonary venous connection. Pediatr Cardiol. 1993;14(1):28–32.
4. Karamlou T, Gurofsky R, Al Sukhni E, Coles JG, Williams WG, Caldarone CA, Van Arsdell GS, et al. Factors associated with mortality and reoperation in 377 children with total anomalous pulmonary venous connection. Circulation. 2007;115(12):1591–8.

Chapter 54
Coarctation of Aorta Associated with Large Patent Ductus Arteriosus and Severe Pulmonary Artery Hypertension

Zahra Khajali

Abstract A 19-year-old lady referred to us with ascites and dyspnea functional class III. She had history of known congenital heart disease but no procedure or management performed her. In physical examination we noticed differential cyanosis, ascites, peripheral edema. In ECG had evidence of bi-ventricular hypertrophy. In echocardiography and CT angiography the patient had large PDA, large VSD, severe coarctation of aorta, severe PAH and severe LV dysfunction. In cardiac catheterization we resulted evidence of left to right shunt via VSD, and pulmonary artery vasoreactivity, so we decided to perform staged intervention, first for coarctation of aorta and PDA. So, we closed PDA and opened the coarctation by a CP covered stent. PDA only had mild residual flow and coarctation gradient completely eliminated. In follow-up LVEF improved significantly and patient symptoms alleviated.

History and Clinical Presentation

A 19 years old female, known case of congenital heart disease but on irregular follow-up came to our clinic with ascites and severe dyspnea. She was admitted to our Hospital. The patient did not receive any drug or management before.

Electronic Supplementary Material The online version of this chapter (https://doi.org/10.1007/978-1-4471-7496-7_54) contains supplementary material, which is available to authorized users.

Z. Khajali (✉)
Rajaei Cardiovascular Medical and Research Center, Iran University of Medical Sciences, Tehran, Iran

M. Maleki, A. Alizadehasl (eds.), *Case-Based Clinical Cardiology*,
https://doi.org/10.1007/978-1-4471-7496-7_54

Physical Examination

Blood Pressure: 150/80 mmHg, **Heart Rate**: 110 beats per minute, **Oxygen Saturation**: 91% in finger and 83% in toes in the air room.

General Appearance: On examination, the patient was well developed. The nailbeds, lips, and mucous membranes were mildly cyanotic, and mild digital clubbing was noted especially in toes, there was respiratory distress at rest.

Lung/Chest: No deformity of the chest wall, the lungs had fine rales at the base of both lungs.

Heart: Cardiac auscultation revealed a normal first heart sound, increased pulmonary component of second heart sound, and a grade III/VI systolic murmur at the left sternal border. The rhythm was irregular.

Abdomen: The abdomen was generalized distended, and also the abdominal examination showed fluctuant sensation in pulsation and also dullness in flanks.

Extremities: There was lower limb peripheral edema. The pulses were irregular and very weak in femoral and non-palpable in dorsalis pedis.

Laboratory Data

Hemoglobin	14.5 gr/dl
Hematocrit	43.5%
White Blood Count	5000 cells/mm3
Platelet	245,000 cells/mm3
Creatinine	0.7 mg/dl
Blood urea nitrogen	13 mg/dl
Cholesterol	115 mg/dl
Triglyceride	86 mg/dl
ALT (Alanine transaminase)	49 IU/L
AST (Aspartate transaminase)	53 IU/L
TSH (Thyroid stimulating hormone)	1.7 micro IU/ml

Electrocardiogram

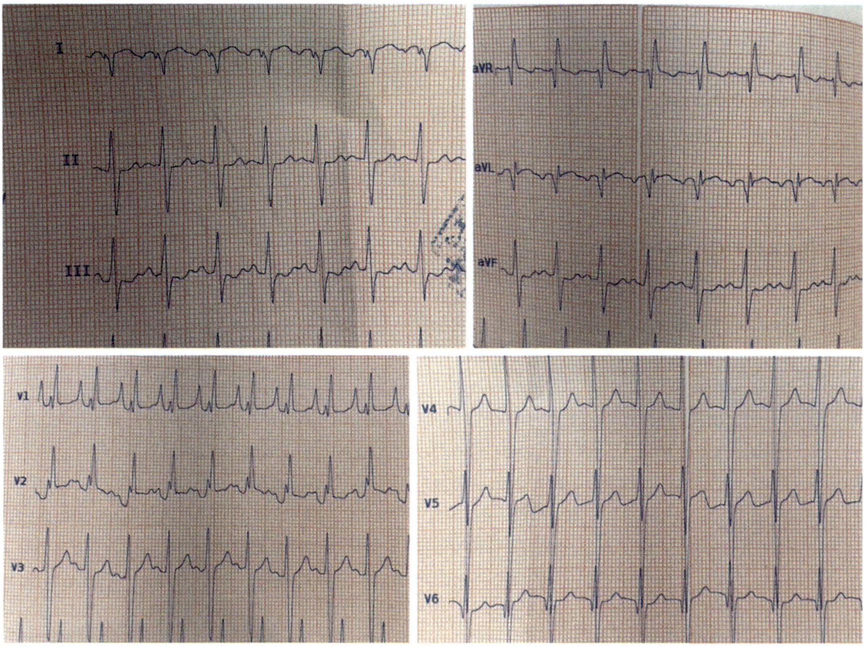

Twelve lead standard electrocardiogram

sinus tachycardia

Heart Rate: 115 beats per minute, regular

Right axis deviation

Tall R in VI, deep S in V5, V6 in favor of RVH and deep S in V3, V4 in favor of LVH, Diphasic V3 and V4 in favor of BVH

Chest X-Ray

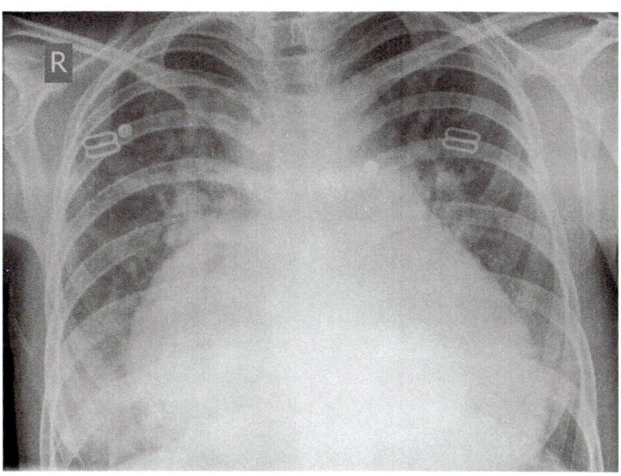

Posteroanterior projection, full inspiration

Levocardia (apex orientation to the left), situs solitus (the gastric bubble is seen in the left)

Left aortic arch

Increased cardiothoracic ratio and severe cardiomegaly

Increased pulmonary vascularity

Dilated PA border

Echocardiography

- Moderate left ventricle enlargement with severe systolic dysfunction (left ventricle ejection fraction = 30%), LVH
- Bi-atrial enlargement
- Moderate enlargement of right ventricle with moderate systolic dysfunction
- No mitral stenosis, mild to moderate mitral regurgitation
- Normal tricuspid aortic valve, no aortic stenosis, no aortic insufficiency
- Normal tricuspid valve leaflets, no tricuspid valve stenosis, moderate tricuspid valve regurgitation (tricuspid regurgitation gradient = 85 mmHg, severe PAH)
- Normal pulmonary valve, no pulmonary stenosis, moderate pulmonary insufficiency
- Large size PDA with bidirectional shunt (size: 14 mm)
- Large VSD restricted to some extent by TV septal leaflet with left to right shunt
- Severe narrowing after left subclavian artery consistent with coarctation of the aorta
- Mild pericardial effusion (Figs. 54.1, 54.2, and 54.3)

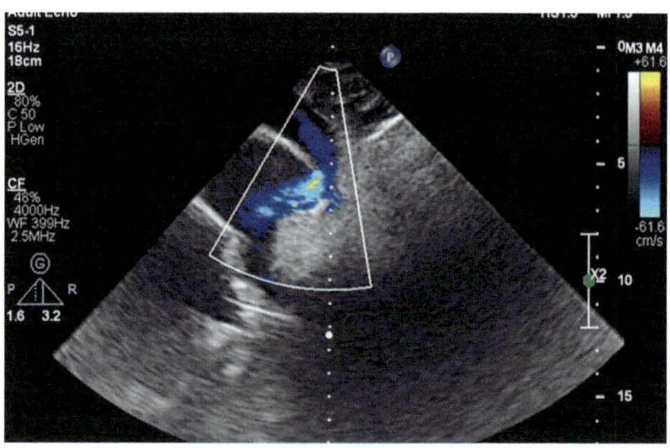

Fig. 54.1 Suprasternal view showed large PDA with right to left shunt and narrowing of aorta after PDA

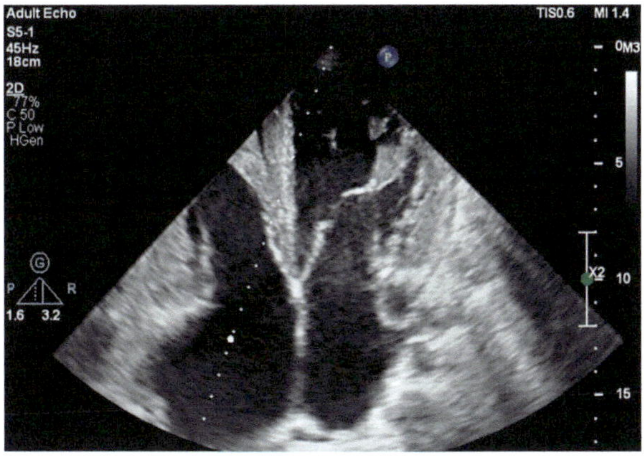

Fig. 54.2 4 chamber view showed LVH and enlarged LA and RA

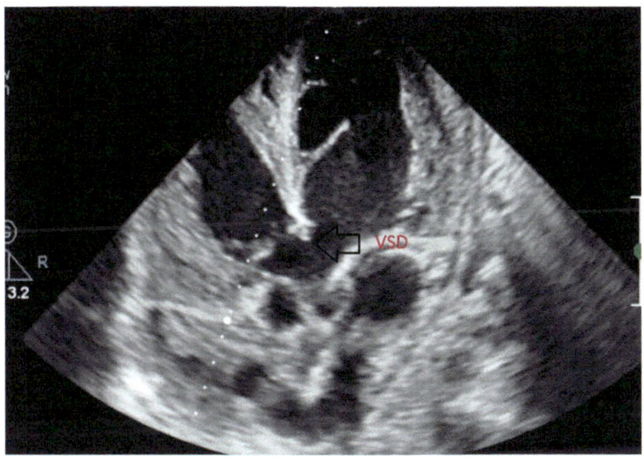

Fig. 54.3 5 chamber view showed large VSD restricted by TV septal leaflet

Congenital CT Angiography

Cardiomegaly and large Ventricular Septal Defect and a large patent ductus arteriosus with LV and RV enlargement are noted. Severe narrowing after left subclavian artery and before PDA was seen and it seems to flow from pulmonary artery via PDA filled descending aorta (Fig. 54.4).

Cardiac Catheterization

- Hemodynamic and pressure study showed evidence of bidirectional shunt via PDA and left to right shunt via VSD, elevated pulmonary Pressure, and Right Ventricular systolic Pressure (RVSP) that they were about 10 mmHg.

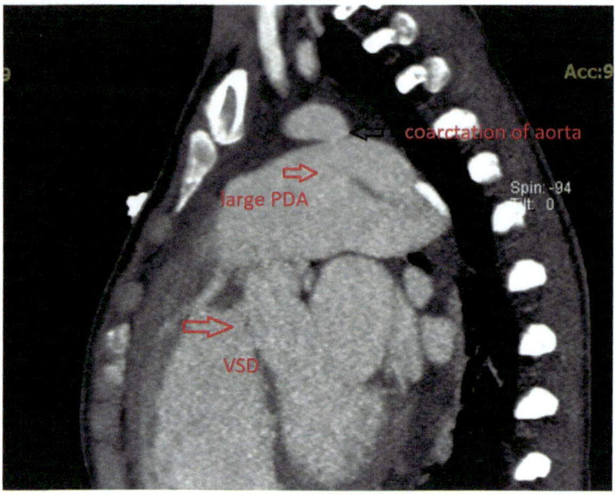

Fig. 54.4 CT angiography showed a large PDA and significant pre-ductal coarctation of the aorta

	Pressure	Saturation
Left ventricle	140/0–14	93
Right ventricle	95/0–10	62
PAP	95/65	73
Ascending aorta	140/70	93
Descending aorta	95/60	88

- Left Ventricle injection showed severely enlarged and severe systolic dysfunction, large perimembranous ventricular septal defect.
- Ascending aorta injection showed severe coarctation of the aorta and large PDA.
- Pulmonary vasodilator test performed by 100% O_2, and after 20 min the mean of PAP decreased from 75 to 60 mmHg.

Management

- Regarding evidence of sub-systemic PAP, vasoreactivity of pulmonary artery, left to right shunt via VSD and eligible anatomy for stenting a covered stent CP 45 mm 8 zig mounted on BIB 22 × 45 mm deployed on coarctation site that opened the stenosis site and covered most part of ductus arteriosus. Gradient though coarctation improved completely and pulmonary artery pressure declined to 75/35 mmHg.

Post-Procedure Echocardiography The day after procedure echocardiography showed significant improvement in LVEF, and small residual flow through PDA, the position of the stent was appropriate with no significant gradient (Fig. 54.5).

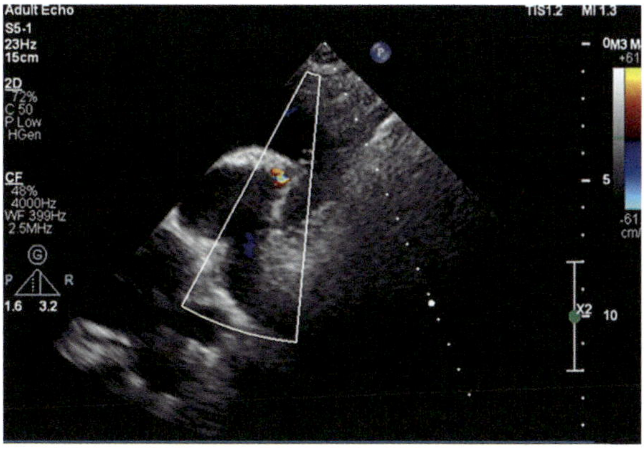

Fig. 54.5 Post-intervention echo showed the position of stent and mild PDA residual flow

Discussion PDA is a common congenital heart disease that is seen in 8–10% of CHD anomalies. This abnormality is more common in premature neonate. Coarctation of the aorta is the fifth common CHD and associated with bicuspid aortic valve in 40–50% of cases [1]. Association of coarctation of aorta and PDA especially in the adult is rare. There are two types of co-acreation of aorta in relation to the position of the duct: pre-ductal and post-ductal. The pre-ductal or infantile type has seen in neonate and infant, in this type coarctation site is before the duct and flow of descending aorta is from pulmonary artery via a duct, so the closure of the duct could worsen the patient condition. In this anomaly differential cyanosis is evident and rarely the patient reached adulthood, but in post-ductal or adult-type coarctation is after duct position and the patient is not dependent on ductal flow, this type dominantly in an adult could be seen. Management of pre-ductal type is more complicated especially in adulthood because of the size of the duct and associated pulmonary artery hypertension. Surgical repair could be done but because of the high-risk condition of these patients catheter intervention [2] is more logical and it could be performed in one stage or sequentially.

References

1. Khajali Z, Ali Basiri H, Maleki M. Persistent fifth aortic arch associated with coarctation of aorta: a case report. Congenit Heart Dis. 2011;6(6):650–2.
2. Khajali Z, Sanati HR, Pouraliakbar H, Mohebbi B, Aeinfar K, Zolfaghari R. Self-expandable stent for repairing coarctation of the left-circumferential aortic arch with right-sided descending aorta and aberrant right subclavian artery with Kommerell's Aneurysm. Ann Vasc Surg. 2017;38:318.e7–318.e10.

Chapter 55
Paravalvular Leakage of Bioprosthetic Pulmonary Valve

Zahra Khajali

Abstract The patient is 27 year-old-male whom had history of two times surgery. First at 1-year-old undergone total correction of tetralogy of Fallot. The second surgery was at 17 years-old, that pulmonary valve replaced with a bioprosthetic valve. During follow-up echocardiography the patient had progressive paravalvular regurgitation of pulmonary valve. Because of the patient refused redo PVR, we performed paravalvular leakage closure by ADO device 14*18mm. The procedure was successful and no complication was seen early and at 6 months follow-up.

History and Clinical Presentation

Our patient is a 27-year-old man and known case of Tetralogy of Fallot with a history of total correction operation (TFTC) 26 years ago and bioprosthetic PVR with a 27-mm PORCINE EPIC bioprosthetic valve 10 years ago. He had also history of Permanent Pacemaker implantation 26 years ago after the first operation. He complained of dyspnea on exertion function class II that begin from 6 months ago. He had paravalvular regurgitation with moderate severity in the previous echocardiography report.

Electronic Supplementary Material The online version of this chapter (https://doi.org/10.1007/978-1-4471-7496-7_55) contains supplementary material, which is available to authorized users.

Z. Khajali (✉)
Rajaei Cardiovascular Medical and Research Center, Iran University of Medical Sciences, Tehran, Iran

M. Maleki, A. Alizadehasl (eds.), *Case-Based Clinical Cardiology*,
https://doi.org/10.1007/978-1-4471-7496-7_55

Physical Examination

Blood Pressure: 110/60 mmHg, Heart Rate: 72 beats per minute, Oxygen Saturation: 95% in the air room.

General appearance: On examination, the patient was well developed.

Lung/chest: No deformity of the chest wall, the lungs were clear.

Heart: Cardiac auscultation revealed a normal first and second heart sound, ejection systolic murmur grade III/VI at the left sternal border, with short diastolic murmur on that area. The rhythm was regular.

Abdomen: The abdomen was soft with normal sounds, and also the abdominal examination showed that the liver was on the right side with a normal span.

Extremities: There was no peripheral edema. The pulses were regular and symmetric.

Electrocardiogram

Electrocardiogram showed pace rhythm with acceptable rate.

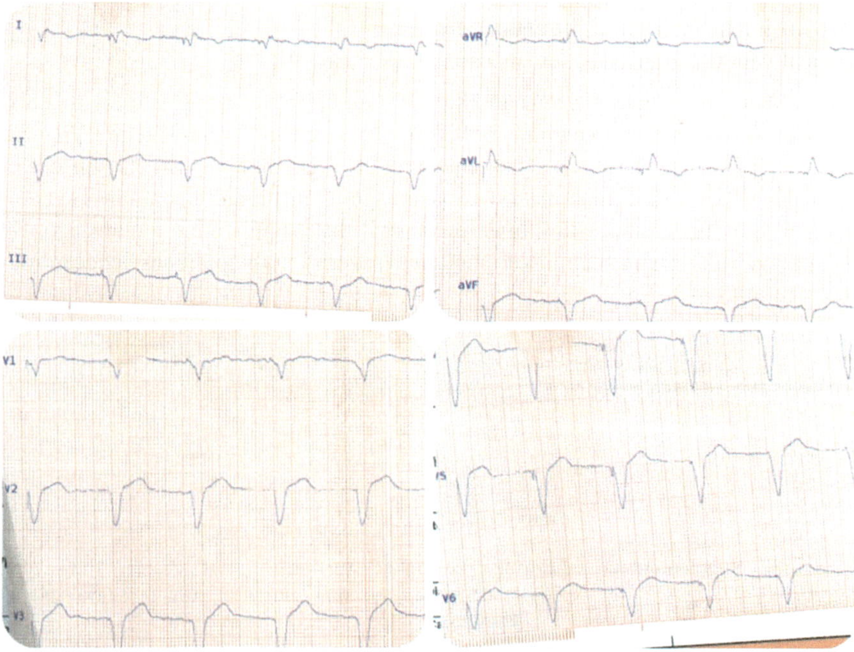

Chest X-Ray

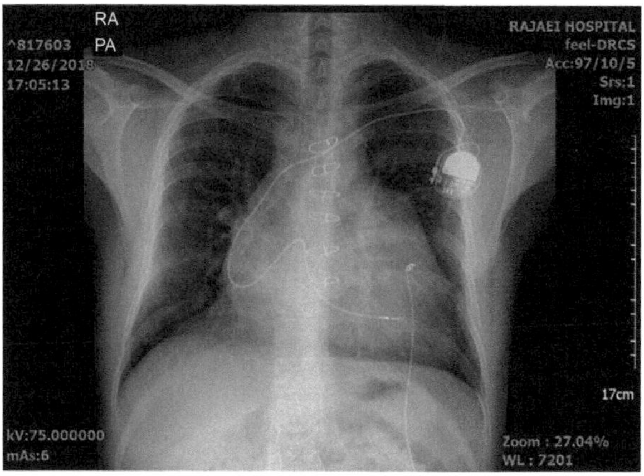

Posteroanterior projection, full inspiration

Levocardia (apex orientation to the left), situs solitus (the gastric bubble is seen in the left)

Left aortic arch

Increased cardiothoracic ratio

Sternal wire

Swing ring of the prosthetic valve was seen in the pulmonary position

Decreased pulmonary vascularity

Aneurysmal RVOT

PPM (single chamber) and its lead in RV apex was seen

Another epicardial lead was seen on the right ventricle

Echocardiography

- Mild left ventricular enlargement with moderate systolic dysfunction, (LVEF:35–40%).
- Severe right ventricular enlargement with moderate to severe systolic dysfunction, and aneurysmal dilation right ventricle outflow tract (RVOT).
- Interrupted IVC.
- Mild to moderate TR.
- No residual VSD.
- Tricuspid Aortic Valve, no aortic stenosis, no aortic insufficiency.
- No bioprosthetic pulmonary valve stenosis but a hole in medial side of the prosthetic valve and severe paravalvular leakage (Fig. 55.1).

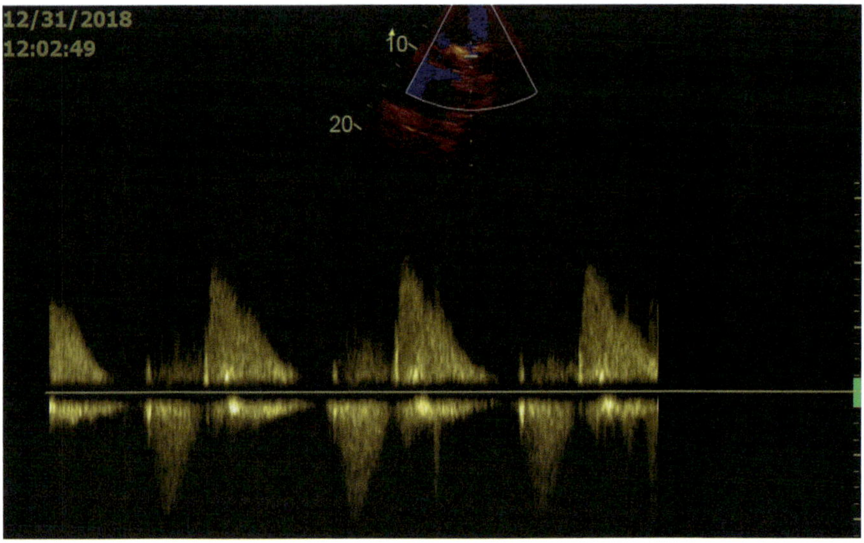

Fig. 55.1 PW doppler showed severe PI jet with short PHT and long NFT

Management and Procedure

The family was reluctant for a third operation, so the patient was scheduled for catheterization and possible closure of the paravalvular leak. The precise etiology of the PVL was unknown, but there was no evidence to suggest endocarditis as a cause.

A hematological evaluation did not reveal any evidence of hemolysis. The patient was referred to the cardiac catheterization laboratory for percutaneous closure of the bioprosthetic paravalvular leak.

A dilator was placed in the right femoral artery for standard hemodynamic monitoring and a sheath was placed in the right femoral vein. Hemodynamic and angiographic data obtained prior to the planned intervention demonstrated mild LV enlargement and mild systolic dysfunction, severe RV enlargement, and moderate systolic dysfunction, bioprosthetic PV in RVOT with severe paravalvular leakage, normal coronary artery system and no residual VSD, interrupted IVC with azygos continuity to SVC, the aneurysmal dilation of the main pulmonary artery and the branch pulmonary arteries. Pulmonary artery angiography demonstrated severe pulmonary bioprosthetic paravalvular leak, also transesophageal echocardiography (TEE) in Cath lab was done and it showed severe pulmonary paravalvular leakage from the posteromedial side of sewing ring with diameter 20 × 14 mm. Cefazolin IV 1000 mg was administered and guidewire was advanced through catheter from azygos pathway to SVC and then across the paravalvular leak. The venous sheath and catheter were then removed and an introducer sheath was advanced over the guidewire to the level of the leak and the guidewire was removed. Next, a PDA occluder 14/18 (occlutech) was mounted on a delivery cable, advanced through the introducer sheath across the paravalvular leak, and deployed without difficulty. Then Pulmonary artery angiography demonstrating mild residual pulmonary paravalvular leak.

- The patient recovered from the procedure without complication. A hematological evaluation did not reveal any evidence of post-procedure hemolysis. Outpatient follow-up revealed his dyspnea resolved. Echocardiography performed one day following the interventional procedure revealed the paravalvular occlude device in proper position with no clot on it and no compressive effects on adjacent sites and two mild to moderate jets of paravalvular leaks were seen from posteromedial side of sewing ring.

Follow-Up Echocardiography The echocardiography a day after closure showed a significant decline in paravalvular leakage severity.

Discussion

Paravalvular leak following prosthetic valve surgery has a reported incidence of 2–3% and typically results from suture dehiscence between the sewing ring and native tissue [1]. These leaks are usually small and follow a benign course; however, they have the potential to cause serious complications such as anemia secondary to hemolysis and congestive heart failure if the resultant regurgitation is significant enough. When symptomatic, these defects are increasingly being closed using the percutaneous catheter technique. Bioprosthetic valves (BPV) are increasingly used for surgical pulmonary valve replacement (PVR) in patients with repaired congenital heart defects, and with mounting evidence about the long-term consequences of chronic pulmonary regurgitation (PR), it seems that an increasing number of patients are undergoing PVR for postoperative PR [2]. Clinically significant paravalvular leaks (PVL) are uncommon after PVR and may be more complex anatomically than left-sided PVL due to the variability in implant location and technique in the trabeculated and often dilated right ventricular outflow tract (RVOT).

Given the anatomic complexity of the RVOT and the variability of the PVR implant site and orientation, transcatheter treatment of pulmonary PVLs is likely to differ from the closure of other PVLs in respect. Also, the relationship of the defect to the coronary arteries, which may be aberrant in the forms of congenital heart disease (CHD) most likely to be treated with PVR (e.g., tetralogy of Fallot), can also be an important consideration and should be evaluated angiographically before device delivery. Also, the procedure was very difficult due to the presence of PPM leads in the right atrium and right ventricle.

The transcatheter devices typically used for PVL closure are not specifically designed for occlusion of these defects, and certainly not for pulmonary leaks [3]. With the complexity and variability of pulmonary PVL, it may be difficult to determine the best device.

The patient tolerated the procedure well and there was no evidence of valve leaflet obstruction, device migration, or hemolysis, only Mild to moderate pulmonary valve insufficiency by echocardiography.

Although percutaneous closure of paravalvular leaks has the potential of avoiding reoperation following valve replacement surgery, it is not without risks. These risks include impingement and impairment of the prosthetic valve leaflet motion, device dislodgement and embolization, and hemolysis [4]. Our limited experience to close a prosthetic pulmonary need more cases and more experience, but it appears as though this technique may represent a useful alternative to reoperation in this population.

References

1. Pate GE, Al Zubaidi A, Chandavimol M, Thompson CR, Munt BI, Webb JG. Percutaneous closure of prosthetic paravalvular leaks: case series and review. Catheter Cardiovasc Interv. 2006;68:528–33.
2. Sadeghpour A, Javani B, Peighambari M, Kyavar M, Khajali Z. Mid-term follow-up of pulmonary valve bioprostheses in adults with congenital heart disease. Anadolu Kardiyol Derg. 2012;12(5):434–6.
3. Shapira Y, Hirsch R, Kornowski R, et al. Percutaneous closure of perivalvular leaks with Amplatzer occluders: feasibility, safety, and short term results. J Heart Valve Dis. 2007;16:305–13.
4. Lasorda DM, Mohsin JC. Percutaneous closure of perivalvular mitral regurgitation with an Amplatzer occluder device in a patient with both prosthetic mitral and aortic valves. J Interv Cardiol. 2008;21:190–5.

Chapter 56
Complicated Aortic Paravalvular Leakage with Aneurysmal Tunnel Formation in a Young Man

Zahra Khajali

Abstract The patient is 23 year-old-male whom had history of coarctation of aorta angioplasty and subaortic web resection at childhood. In follow-up echocardiography he had severe aortic stenosis and bicuspid aortic valve, so surgical AVR performed uneventfully. During follow-up echocardiography one month later, the patient had large round formation mass on surgical patch in LA roof and mild paravalvular regurgitation. With suspicious to IE antibiotic therapy started and because of no decline in the size of mass and progressive paravalvular regurgitation of AV surgery performed and patient had massive stroke at post-operative period. Finally, after one month he discharged but with mild paravalvular regurgitation of AV. 2 months later in follow-up echocardiography he had severe paravalvular regurgitation. Regarding to the patient condition we decided to catheter intervention. We performed paravalvular leakage closure by muscular VSD device 10 mm. The procedure was successful and no complication was seen early and at 6 months follow-up.

History and Clinical Presentation

A 23-year-old man with a history of coarctation of aorta balloon angioplasty and sub-Arctic web resection at childhood presented to the adult congenital heart disease clinic for follow-up. He complained of dyspnea on exertion (NYHA FC II–III) and atypical chest pain. On physical examination, there was an III/VI systolic murmur on the left sternal border.

Electronic Supplementary Material The online version of this chapter (https://doi.org/10.1007/978-1-4471-7496-7_56) contains supplementary material, which is available to authorized users.

Z. Khajali (✉)
Rajaei Cardiovascular Medical and Research Center, Iran University of Medical Sciences, Tehran, Iran

M. Maleki, A. Alizadehasl (eds.), *Case-Based Clinical Cardiology*,
https://doi.org/10.1007/978-1-4471-7496-7_56

Echocardiography evaluation revealed Bicuspid aortic valves with severe valvular AS (AVPG:124 mmHg, AVMG:83 mmHg, AVA by 3D:0.4 cm), mild to moderate AI.

According to patient symptom and echocardiographic data surgical consult was done and because of small annulus of aorta, aortoplasty, and then insertion of mechanical AVR (Top hat:25) was accomplished.

After about 1 month and during follow-up the patient presented with low-grade fever and no other symptom. For better evaluation of prosthetic valve echocardiography TTE then TEE was done and a large round formation mass on surgical patch in LA roof suggestive for endocarditis or hematoma formation and mild to moderate paravalvular leakage was detected. Infectious disease specialist consult was performed and antibiotic treatment was started and because of progressive paravalvular regurgitation the patient was referred to a surgeon and further surgery for mass removal and paravalvular leakage repair was done. We should express that all blood culture was negative and ESR, CRP was not so high (ESR = 40, CRP = 6).

Surgeon replaced the valve with a new prosthetic valve (top hat 25) and drained the hematoma but affirmed there was not any vegetation and the only hematoma was seen.

After surgery and during the hospital course the patient suffered from an embolic stroke. The patient finished the antibiotic course and discharged with the acceptable condition but, during echocardiographic follow-up, progressive paravalvular leakage with aneurismal tunnel formation was detected. At this time there was no evidence of vegetation.

Physical Examination at Lost Admission

Blood Pressure: 110/60 mmHg, Heart Rate: regular and 95 beats per minute, Oxygen Saturation: 96% in the air room.

General appearance: On examination, the patient was well developed. The nailbeds, lips, and mucous membranes were normal.

Heart: the good metallic sound was heard.

Abdomen: The abdomen was soft with normal sounds, and also the abdominal examination showed that the liver was on the right side with a normal span.

Laboratory Data

Hemoglobin	12.5 gr/dl
White Blood Count	4500 cells/mm^3
Platelet	215,000 cells/mm^3
Creatinine	0.8 mg/dl
Blood urea nitrogen	18 mg/dl

Cholesterol	105 mg/dl
Triglyceride	125 mg/dl
ESR	30 mm
CRP	Negative

Electrocardiogram

Electrocardiography showed a sinus rhythm with a heart rate of 100 beats per minute, a normal axis deviation, and a strain pattern in the lateral leads.

Chest X-Ray

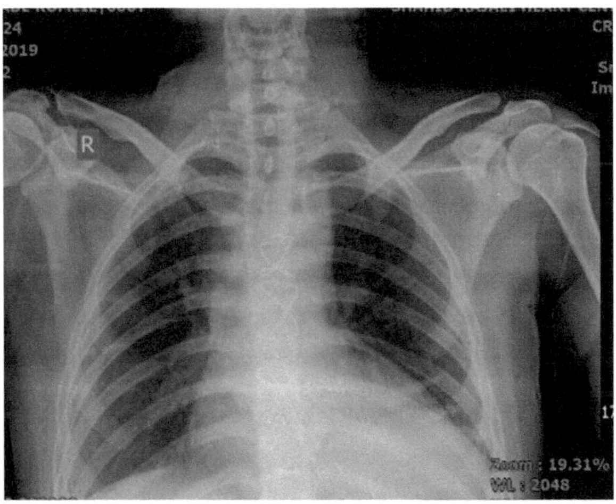

Posteroanterior projection, full inspiration

Levocardia (apex orientation to the left), situs solitus (the gastric bubble is seen in the left)

Left aortic arch

Increased cardiothoracic ratio

Normal pulmonary vascularity

Sternal wire

Mechanical aortic valve

Echocardiography at Lost Admission

- Mild left ventricular enlargement with preserved systolic function (LVEF: 50–55%).
- Normal RV size and systolic function.
- Mild TR.
- No ASD, VSD.
- Mechanical aortic valve with normal both leaflet motion and mild increased transvalvular gradient, but there is a hole around swing ring of aortic valve with severe paravalvular regurgitation, also there is aneurysm formation around LVOT that extended to the left ventricle.
- No pulmonary valve stenosis and regurgitation.

The patient had advanced symptom of dyspnea and orthopnea, admitted again and surgical consult for paravalvular leakage closure was done but the surgeon refused surgery because of very high-risk patient.

Procedure

After heart team consults and patient preference, the paravalvular leak was closed with a VSD occluder device 10 mm with an acceptable result. After 1 month follow-up the patient feels good and paravalvular leak decreased significantly (Figs. 56.1 and 56.2).

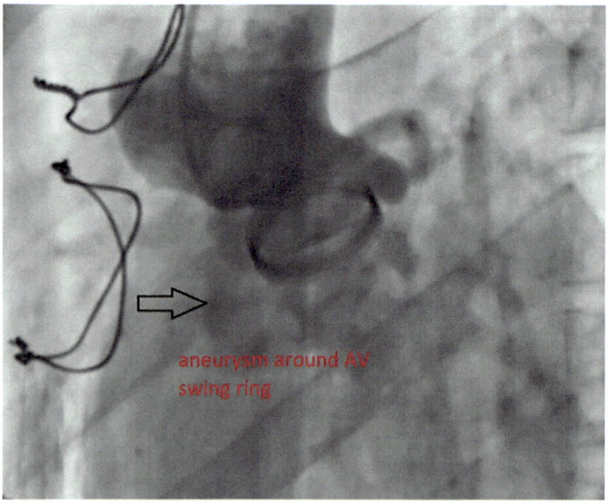

Fig. 56.1 Aortic root injection showed aneurysm at LVOT around swing ring and severe paravalvular regurgitation

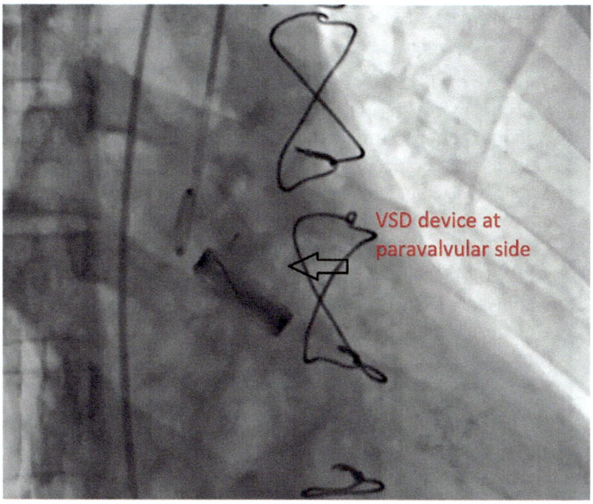

Fig. 56.2 Post-intervention aortogram showed the position of VSD device to mechanical AV

Discussion

One of the important complications after surgical valve replacement is a paravalvular leak which is a challenging problem. The prevalence of PVL for mitral valve replacement is 7% to 17% and for Aortic valve replacement is 5% to 10%. because the tissues around PVL are eager and brittle, repeat surgery is very high risk and leaks may recur [1]. Conservative management of significant leaks also has adverse outcomes because the leaks deteriorate over time and lead to congestive heart failure, hemolytic anemia, and endocarditis [2].

Mild PVLs are nonsignificant hemodynamic effect but large leakage can cause heart failure and increased risk of endocarditis. Hemolytic anemia is more common in mild PVL. Predisposing factors for PVLs are technical parameters, severe annulus calcification, and endocarditis. The indication for closure is congestive heart failure with dyspnea on exertion NYHA functional class II–III or greater despite optimal medical therapy and hemolytic anemia which needs blood transfusion to maintain hemoglobin level above 10 mg/dl [3]. Diagnosis of paravalvular leakage is challenging. Transthoracic echocardiography (TTE) often cannot diagnosis PVL truly, using transesophageal echocardiography (TEE) which is able to also detect small, nonsignificant jets, is crucial in this situation. The shape of PVLs is often crescent and has a serpiginous track from the downstream to the upstream chamber.

Surgical repair is a treatment of choice for PVLs, but it has significant mortality and morbidity, nowadays there is interest in minimally invasive percutaneous techniques, which has not sternotomy and is a successful treatment. Percutaneous device closure of PVL is a complex procedure with varying success rates. There is not a specific device for closure of PVLs [4].

In this case with two times aortic valve replacement and severe paravalvular leakage with aneurismal tunnel and very high-risk surgery, device paravalvular leakage closure with VSD occluder device 10 mm, was done safely with improvement in clinical and echocardiographic parameters.

References

1. Taramasso M, Maisano F, Denti P, Guidotti A, Sticchi A, Pozzoli A, Buzzatti N, De Bonis M, La Canna G, Alfieri O. Surgical treatment of paravalvular leak: Long-term results in a single-center experience (up to 14 years). J Thorac Cardiovasc Surg. 2015;149:1270–5.
2. Genoni M, Franzen D, Vogt P, Seifert B, Jenni R, Künzli A, Niederhäuser U, Turina M. Paravalvular leakage after mitral valve replacement: improved long-term survival with aggressive surgery? Eur J Cardiothorac Surg. 2000;17:14–9.
3. Cruz-Gonzalez I, Rama-Merchan JC, Rodríguez-Collado J, Martín-Moreiras J, Diego-Nieto A, Barreiro-Pérez M, Sánchez PL. Transcatheter closure of paravalvular leaks: state of the art. Neth Heart J. 2017;25(2):116–24.
4. Grzegorz Smolka, Wojciech Wojakowski. Paravalvular leak – important complication after implantation of prosthetic valve. An article from the E-Journal of the ESC Council for Cardiology Practice, Vol. 9, N° 8, 08 Nov 2010.

Chapter 57
Total Correction of Tetralogy of Fallot in a 45 Years Old Man With Dextrocardia

Zahra Khajali

Abstract A 45-year-old gentleman referred to us with cyanosis. He had history of tetralogy of Fallot but the parents and also the patient refused surgery because of fearing of the risk of surgery. In physical examination, electrocardiogram and echocardiography he had dextrocardia and tetralogy of Fallot with well-developed pulmonary artery branches. For exact evaluation of the breadth and size of collaterals and pulmonary artery anatomy and pressure catheterization performed and by evaluation of all data, finally surgical repair was done uneventfully. Systemic saturation returned to normal level and the patient is very well after 5-years follow-up.

History and Clinical Presentation

A 45 years old man referred to our ACHD clinic by severe cyanosis. He had a history of known CHD and catheterization in 8 years old but his parents refused surgical repair. He admitted with aggravation of dyspnea functional class III, and also one-episode hemoptysis.

Physical Examination

Blood Pressure: 100/70 mmHg, **Heart Rate**: 70 beats per minute, **Oxygen Saturation**: 82% in the air room.

Electronic Supplementary Material The online version of this chapter (https://doi.org/10.1007/978-1-4471-7496-7_57) contains supplementary material, which is available to authorized users.

Z. Khajali (✉)
Rajaei Cardiovascular Medical and Research Center, Iran University of Medical Sciences, Tehran, Iran

M. Maleki, A. Alizadehasl (eds.), *Case-Based Clinical Cardiology*,
https://doi.org/10.1007/978-1-4471-7496-7_57

General appearance: On examination, the patient was well developed. The nailbeds, lips, and mucous membranes were cyanotic and digital clubbing was noted, there was not respiratory distress at rest.

Lung/chest: No deformity of the chest wall, the lungs were clear.

Heart: Cardiac auscultation at the right side of the chest revealed a normal first sound and single S2 and a grade IV/VI systolic murmur associated by thrill at the upper part of the sternum, with no diastolic murmur or gallop. The rhythm was regular.

Abdomen: The abdomen was soft with normal sounds, and also the abdominal examination showed that the liver was on the right side with a normal span.

Extremities: There was no peripheral edema, but there was a digital clubbing. The pulses were regular and symmetric.

Laboratory Data

Hemoglobin	18.5 gr/dl
Hematocrit	54.5%
White Blood Count	5300 cells/mm^3
Platelet	216,000 cells/mm^3
Creatinine	0.7 mg/dl
Blood urea nitrogen	13 mg/dl
ABG:	PH:7.43 PO2:45 PCO2:40

Electrocardiogram

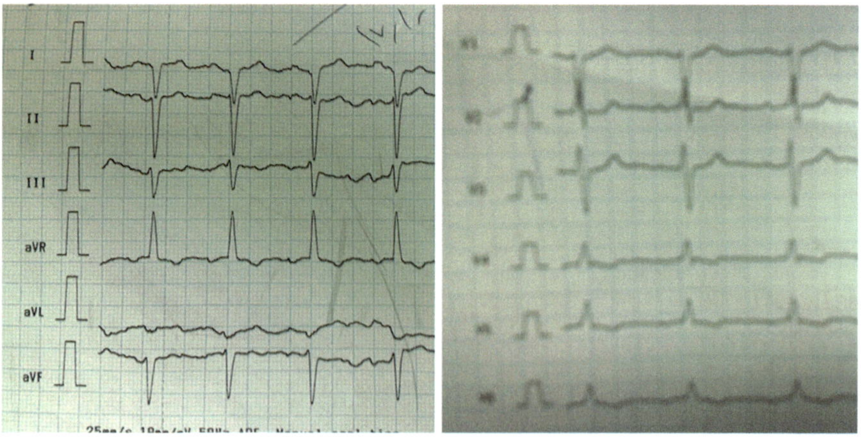

Twelve lead standard electrocardiogram
Normal sinus rhythm
Heart Rate: 65 beats per minute, regular
Extreme axis deviation
Normal PR interval
Negative P in aVR and positive in I and aVL in favor of atrial situs solitus
Poor R progression in favor of dextrocardia
Normal QRS duration

Chest X-Ray

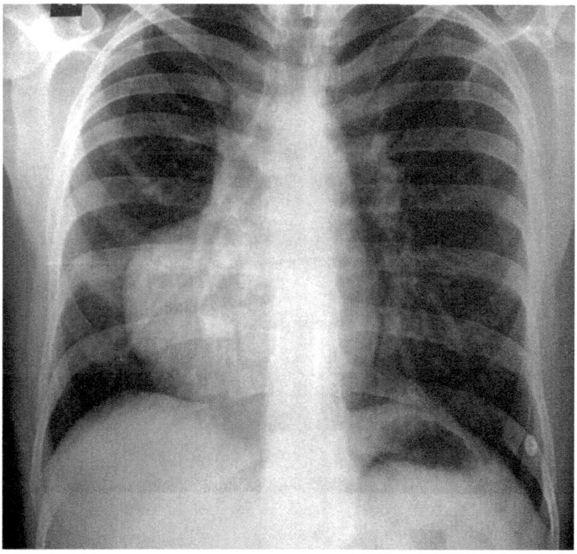

Posteroanterior projection, full inspiration

Dextrocardia (apex orientation to the right), situs solitus (the gastric bubble is seen in the left)

Right aortic arch

Normal cardiothoracic ratio

Decreased pulmonary vascularity

Concave shape of right border and boot-shaped appearance in favor of tetralogy of Fallot

Echocardiography

- Normal left ventricle size with normal systolic function (left ventricle ejection fraction = 55%)
- Mild enlarged right ventricle with mild systolic dysfunction, severe RVH
- Large subaortic ventricular septal defect with bidirectional shunt
- Overriding of aorta
- Normal mitral valve leaflets, no mitral stenosis, no mitral regurgitation
- Normal tricuspid aortic valve, no aortic stenosis, no aortic insufficiency, dilated aortic root, and ascending aorta
- Normal tricuspid valve leaflets, no tricuspid valve stenosis, mild tricuspid valve regurgitation (tricuspid regurgitation gradient = 95 mmHg)
- Thickened pulmonary leaflets and hypoplastic PV annulus, good size of main of pulmonary artery, and branches (Fig. 57.1)

Congenital CT Angiography

Normal epicardial coronary arteries. Dextrocardia and large ventricular septal defect with severe RV hypertrophy are noted. Confluent and well-developed pulmonary arteries branches were seen.

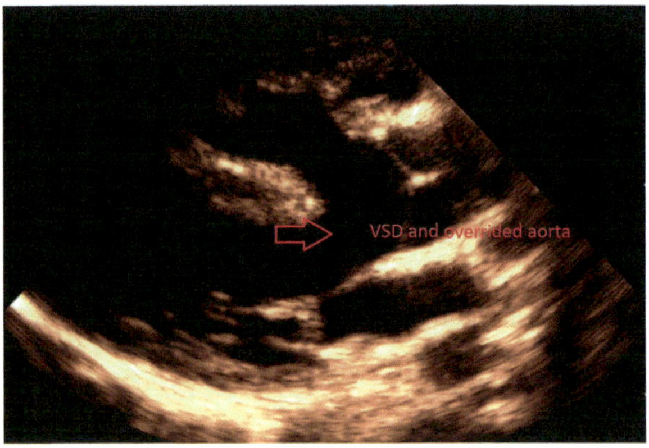

Fig. 57.1 In parasternal long-axis view large subaortic VSD and overriding of the aorta was seen

Catheterization

- Hemodynamic and pressure study showed evidence of mildly elevated Right Atrium Pressure and Right Ventricular End Diastolic Pressure (RVEDP) and normal LVEDP. PA pressure was 20/12/15 mmHg. RVSP and LVSP are the same and about 110 mmHg. There is 90 mmHg gradient at pulmonary and RVOT level.
- RV injection showed large subaortic VSD, severe RVOT obstruction, thickened pulmonary leaflets but the acceptable size of MPA and PA branches. Selective coronary angiography showed a normal course of coronary arteries.

Management

Regarding acceptable size and confluency of PA branches and the good function of both ventricles we decided to perform the surgical repair for the patient. Patient undergone total correction by the closure of VSD and resection of RVOT muscles and valvotomy of the pulmonary valve. The procedure was successful and the patient became off from cardiopulmonary pump easily, the course of ICU was uneventful, cyanosis eliminated and the patient felt good at follow-ups.

Discussion Tetralogy of Fallot is a tetrad of abnormality that consisted of large subaortic VSD, RVOT obstruction, RVH, and overriding of aorta [1]. All these abnormalities are due to anterocephalad deviation of outlet septum and malalignment with a trabecular septum that created subaortic VSD and overriding aorta. This congenital abnormality presented after birth by cyanosis, and the degree of cyanosis depends on RVOT obstruction severity. Most of the cases are amenable to total correction at the neonatal period [2]. The cases that were not appropriate for total correction had very small or nonconfluent pulmonary artery branches. The age was not a limitation for surgical repair and at the presence of appropriate biventricular function and well-developed pulmonary artery branches the repair would be possible at any age [3]. The prognosis after total correction is good and 20 years survival is about 90% [4]. In surgery, RVOT obstruction is alleviated by muscle resection and VSD repaired by the patch [5]. Pulmonary valve stenosis repaired by valvotomy but in the adults, this is preferable to pulmonary valve replacement instead of repair [6]. Sometimes the strategy of palliative shunt before total correction for improving cyanosis degree and decreasing the risk of the surgery recommended.

References

1. Khajali Z. Tetralogy of Fallot, Chapter 28. Practical cardiology, pp. 485–487.
2. Pozzi M, Trivedi DB, Kitchiner D, et al. Tetralogy of Fallot: what operation, at what age. Eur J Cardiothorac Surg. 2000;17(6):631–6.
3. Atik FA, Atik E, da Cunha CR, et al. Long-term results of correction of tetralogy of Fallot in adulthood. EJCTS. 2004;25:250–5.
4. Murphy JG, Gersh BJ, Mair DD, et al. Long-term outcome in patients undergoing surgical repair of tetralogy of Fallot. N Engl J Med. 1993;329:593–9.
5. Kirklin John W. Barratt-Boyes. Cardiac Surgery. In Ventricular septal defect and pulmonary stenosis or atresia. New York: Churchill Livingston; 1993. p. 861–1012.
6. Katz NM, Blackstone EH, Kirklin JW, et al. Late survival and symptoms after repair of tetralogy of Fallot. Circulation. 1982;65:403–10.

Chapter 58
Waterston Shunt and Unilateral Pulmonary Artery Hypertension in a Case of Tetralogy of Fallot

Zahra Khajali

Abstract A 25-year-old gentleman referred to us with cyanosis and dyspnea He had a history of Waterstone shunt in 1991 and catheterization in 1996 and 2002, when he was candidate for total correction. But the surgeon deemed the patient inoperable after sternotomy. In physical examination, electrocardiogram and echocardiography he had tetralogy of Fallot with well-developed pulmonary artery branches and patent Waterston shunt. In cardiac MRI there was significant stenosis at proximal of LPA and dilated branch after stenosis. For hemodynamic evaluation catheterization performed and we found LPA normal pressure, moderately elevated MPA pressure but severe pulmonary hypertension in RPA. Regarding to unilateral pulmonary hypertension and the anatomy of PABs, we found the patient inoperable, so medical treatment continued for him.

History and Clinical Presentation

A 25-year-old man presented as a case of TOF. He had a history of Waterston shunt in 1991 and catheterization in 1996 and 2002, when he was a candidate for total correction. After sternotomy, the surgeon deemed the patient inoperable due to the size and anatomy of PABs.

He had dyspnea functional class III that aggravated during the last months.

Electronic Supplementary Material The online version of this chapter (https://doi.org/10.1007/978-1-4471-7496-7_58) contains supplementary material, which is available to authorized users.

Z. Khajali (✉)
Rajaei Cardiovascular Medical and Research Center, Iran University of Medical Sciences, Tehran, Iran

M. Maleki, A. Alizadehasl (eds.), *Case-Based Clinical Cardiology*,
https://doi.org/10.1007/978-1-4471-7496-7_58

Physical Examination

Blood Pressure: 100/70 mmHg, **Heart Rate**: 70 beats per minute, **Oxygen Saturation**: 86% in the air room.

General appearance: On examination, the patient was well developed. The nailbeds, lips, and mucous membranes were cyanotic and digital clubbing was noted, there was no respiratory distress at rest.

Heart: Cardiac auscultation revealed a normal S1 and loud S2 and a grade III/VI systolic murmur at the upper left sternal border, with no diastolic murmur or gallop. The rhythm was regular.

Extremities: There was no peripheral edema, but there was a digital clubbing. The pulses were regular and symmetric.

Laboratory Data

Hemoglobin	19 gr/dl
Hematocrit	57.5%
White Blood Count	5300 cells/mm^3
Platelet	152,000 cells/mm^3
Creatinine	1.1 mg/dl

Electrocardiogram

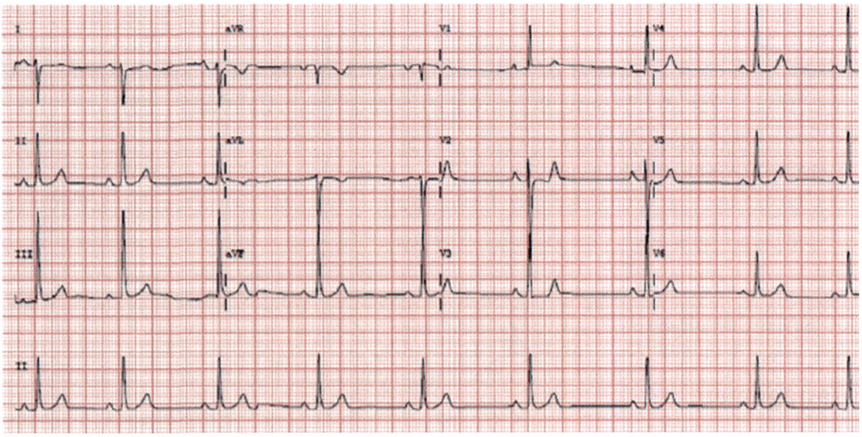

Twelve lead standard electrocardiogram
Normal sinus rhythm
Heart Rate: 54 beats per minute, regular
Right axis deviation
Normal PR interval
R in V1 and deep S in V5, V6 in favor of RVH
Transition of tall in V1 to deep S in V2 is highly suggestive of TOF
Normal QRS duration

Chest X-Ray

Increased cardiothoracic ratio and increased vascularity at the right lung was seen.

Echocardiography

- Normal left ventricle size with normal systolic function (left ventricle ejection fraction = 55%)
- Moderate enlarged right ventricle with mild systolic dysfunction, severe RVH
- Large subaortic ventricular septal defect with bidirectional shunt
- Overriding of aorta
- Normal mitral valve leaflets, no mitral stenosis, no mitral regurgitation
- Normal tricuspid aortic valve, no aortic stenosis, mild aortic insufficiency, dilated aortic root and ascending aorta
- Normal tricuspid valve leaflets, no tricuspid valve stenosis, mild tricuspid valve regurgitation (tricuspid regurgitation gradient = 105 mmHg)
- Thickened pulmonary leaflets and hypoplastic PV annulus, good size of main of pulmonary artery and branches
- Waterston shunt was seen between ascending aorta and right pulmonary artery with continuous but the decreased velocity of flow (Fig. 58.1).

Congenital Cardiac MRI

Normal LV volume and EF, with a moderate increased in RV volume, were noted. Large subaortic VSD and overriding of aorta was seen. There was patent side by side shunt between ascending aorta and RPA. Proximal of LPA had severe stenosis and after stenosis, there was dilated pulmonary artery (Figs. 58.2 and 58.3).

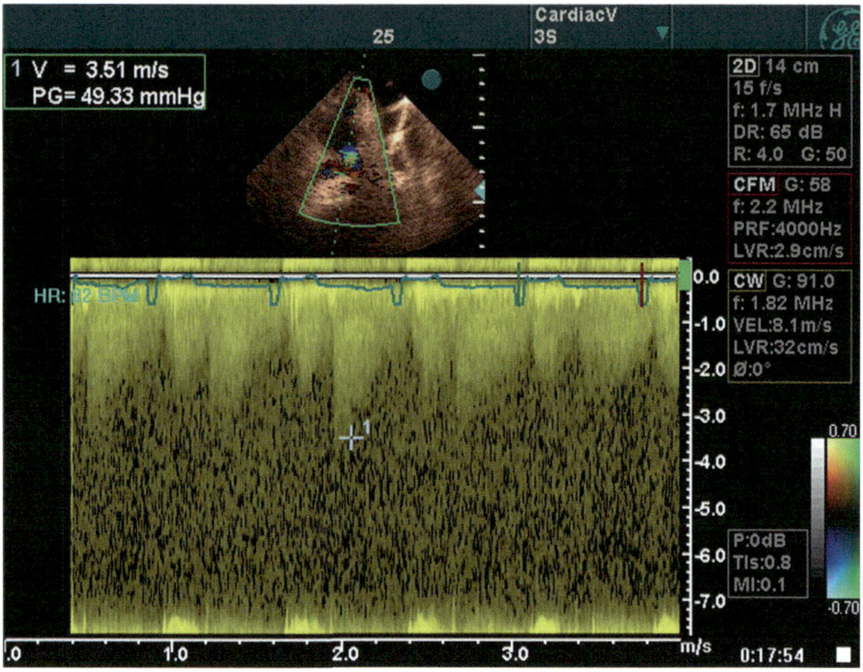

Fig. 58.1 Continuous doppler flow from Waterston shunt flow in suprasternal view

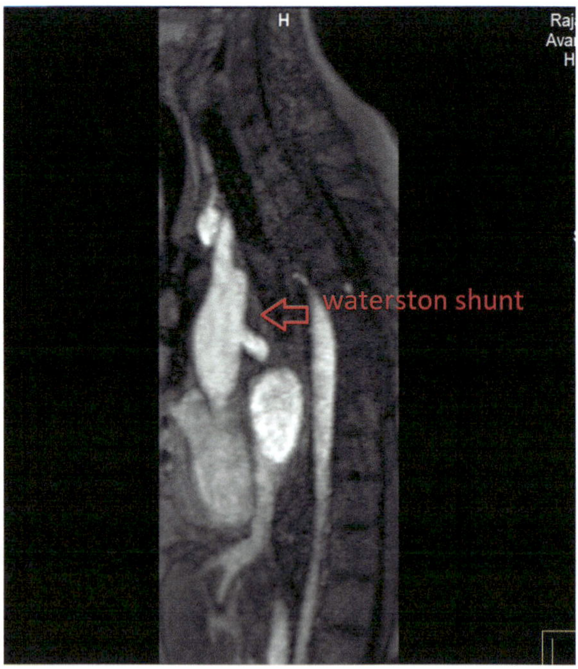

Fig. 58.2 cardiac MR showed Waterston shunt

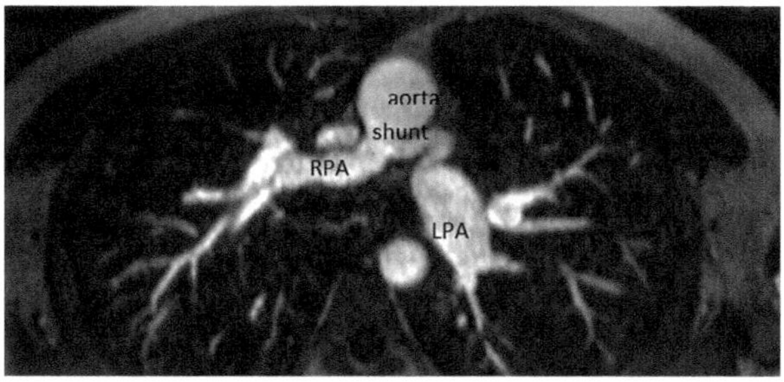

Fig. 58.3 CMR showed stenosis at proximal of LPA, dilated LPA after stenosis, patent shunt between ascending aorta and RPA

Catheterization

- Hemodynamic and pressure study showed evidence of mildly elevated right atrium pressure and Right Ventricular End Diastolic Pressure (RVEDP) and normal LVEDP. MPA pressure was 65/45 mmHg, LPA pressure was 20/5 mmHg and RPA pressure was 95/45 mmHg. RVSP and LVSP are the same and about 105 mmHg. There is 40 mmHg gradient at pulmonary and RVOT level and 45 mmHg gradient between MPA and LPA, RPA that filled dominantly via Waterston shunt had a high pressure a bit fewer than systemic aorta pressure.

  RV injection showed large subaortic VSD, severe RVOT obstruction, thickened pulmonary leaflets, near-normal MPA size, severe LPA stenosis, and dilated LPA after stenosis. RPA was not seen in RV injection. Aortic injection showed a normal course of coronary arteries. RPA filled via palliative shunt and ascending aorta with normal size and good arborization. There is no response to the oxygen vasodilator test.

Management

Regarding unilateral pulmonary artery hypertension, long stenosis at proximal of LPA, and one history of sternotomy that surgical note underlined the patient inoperable, we started sildenafil and bosentan for unilateral pulmonary hypertension, and decided to follow the patient periodically, If the PAH responded to pulmonary vasodilator therapy, maybe he become a candidate for surgical repair in the future.

Discussion Tetralogy of Fallot is a tetrad of abnormality that consisted of large subaortic VSD, RVOT obstruction, RVH, and overriding of aorta [1]. This congenital abnormality presented after birth by cyanosis, and the degree of cyanosis depends on RVOT obstruction severity. Most of the cases are amenable to total correction at the neonatal period. The cases that were not appropriate for total correction had very small or nonconfluent pulmonary artery branches [2]. If the size of the PA branches was not appropriate for total correction, in the neonatal period palliative arterial shunts were applied to improving the cyanosis and also to helping the growth of pulmonary artery branches [3]. The first palliative shunts that performed was side to side anastomosis of ascending aorta to RPA(Waterston), descending aorta to LPA (Pott's shunt), and end to side anastomose of the subclavian artery to ipsilateral PA branch (classic BT shunt) [4]. Because of the chance of dilating these shunts and inducing severe PAH, these palliative shunts extinct. After that, the modified BT shunt was done that a Gortex tube with specified diameter anastomosed between subclavian artery and ipsilateral PA branch [5]. These modified shunts do not increase the PAP but after a while, these break the pulmonary artery branches anatomy and integrity. So, these palliative shunts are temporary solutions and total correction must be done at the right time.

References

1. Khajali Z. Tetralogy of Fallot, Chapter 28. Practical cardiology, pp. 485–487.
2. Joffs C, Sade RM. Congenital Heart Surgery Nomenclature and Database Project: palliation, correction or repair? Ann Thorac Surg. 2000;69:S369–72.
3. Moulton AL, Brenner JI, Ringel R, et al. Classic versus modified Blalock-Taussig's shunts in neonates and infants. Circulation. 1985;72:II35–44.
4. Karpawich PP, Bush CP, Antillon JR, Amato JJ, Marbey ML, Agarwal KC. Modified Blalock-Taussig's shunt in infants and young children. Clinical and catheterization assessment. J Thorac Cardiovasc Surg. 1985;89:275–9.
5. Godart F, Qureshi SA, Simha A, et al. Effects of modified and classic Blalock-Taussig's shunts on the pulmonary arterial tree. Ann Thorac Surg. 1998;66:512–7.

Chapter 59
Intervention in Multiple Pulmonary Arteriovenous Malformation in an Adult

Zahra Khajali

Abstract The patient is a 29-year-old woman that came to ACHD clinic by severe cyanosis. After complete work-up we diagnosed her as a case of multiple pulmonary arteriovenous fistula. We decided to manage her by catheter intervention. Three occlude devices that include two ADOs and one muscular VSD device applied, cyanosis improved significantly and no complication occurred during procedure.

History and Clinical Presentation

A 29-year-old lady referred to our clinic by deep cyanosis. She had dyspnea functional class II. The patient had not undergone prior cardiac evaluation but she declared an increase in cyanosis during last years. The family history was nonremarkable.

Physical Examination

Blood Pressure: 110/70 mmHg, **Heart Rate**: 76 beats per minute, **Oxygen Saturation**: 75% in the air room.

General appearance: On examination, the patient was well developed. The nailbeds, lips, and mucous membranes were cyanotic and digital clubbing was noted, there was not any respiratory distress at rest.

Lung/chest: No deformity of the chest wall, the lungs were clear.

Electronic Supplementary Material The online version of this chapter (https://doi.org/10.1007/978-1-4471-7496-7_59) contains supplementary material, which is available to authorized users.

Z. Khajali (✉)
Rajaei Cardiovascular Medical and Research Center, Iran University of Medical Sciences, Tehran, Iran

M. Maleki, A. Alizadehasl (eds.), *Case-Based Clinical Cardiology*,
https://doi.org/10.1007/978-1-4471-7496-7_59

Heart: Cardiac auscultation revealed a normal first heart sound and second heart sound and no systolic and diastolic murmur was heard. The rhythm was regular.

Abdomen: The abdomen was soft with normal sounds, and also the abdominal examination showed that the liver was on the right side with a normal span.

Extremities: There was no peripheral edema, but there was a digital clubbing. The pulses were regular and symmetric.

Laboratory Data

Hemoglobin	20 gr/dl
Hematocrit	63%
White Blood Count	5500 cells/mm^3
Platelet	297,000 cells/mm^3
Creatinine	0.7 mg/dl
Blood urea nitrogen	13 mg/dl
ALT	25 U/L
AST	35 U/L
Bilirubin	3 mg/dl

Electrocardiogram

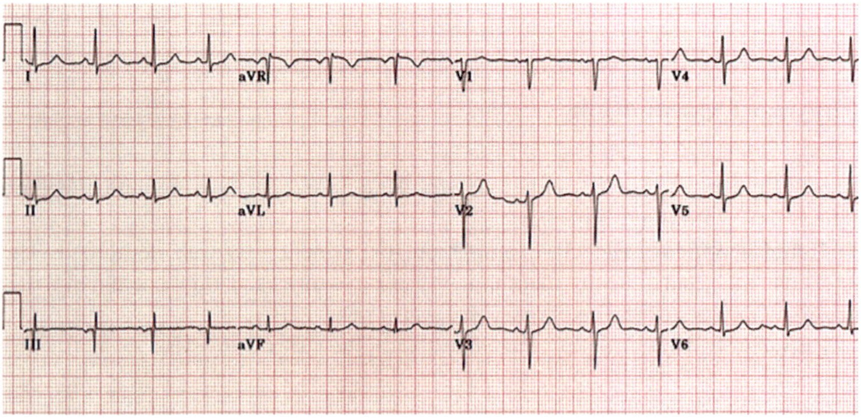

Twelve lead standard electrocardiogram

Normal sinus rhythm

Heart Rate: 76 beats per minute, regular

Normal axis deviation

Normal PR interval

Normal QRS duration
No ST-T changes

Chest X-Ray

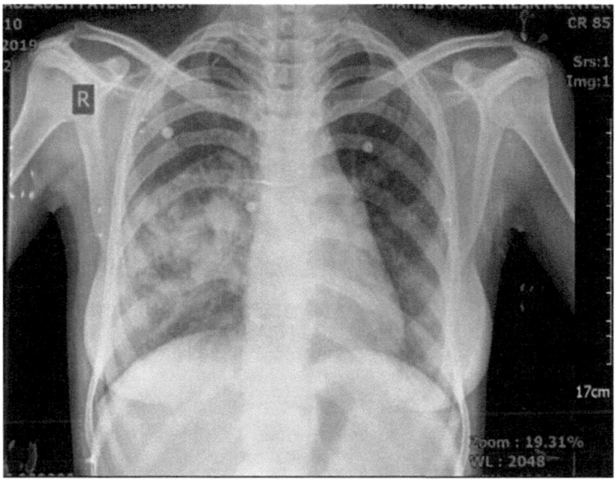

Posteroanterior projection, full inspiration

Levocardia (apex orientation to the left), situs solitus (the gastric bubble is seen in the left)

Left aortic arch

Normal cardiothoracic ratio

Normal pulmonary parenchyma and vascularity at the left lung

Multiple vascular type round density at right lung especially at middle and lower lobes

Echocardiography

- Normal left ventricle size with normal systolic function (left ventricle ejection fraction = 55%)
- No atrial and ventricular septal defect
- Normal right ventricle size and normal systolic function
- Normal mitral valve leaflets, no mitral stenosis, mild mitral regurgitation
- Normal tricuspid aortic valve, no aortic stenosis, no aortic insufficiency
- Normal tricuspid valve leaflets, no tricuspid valve stenosis, mild tricuspid valve regurgitation (tricuspid regurgitation gradient = 22 mmHg)

- Normal pulmonary valve, no pulmonary stenosis, mild to moderate pulmonary insufficiency
- Contrast injection showed filling of left heart chambers after three cycles of injection (Fig. 59.1)

Congenital CT Angiography

Normal epicardial coronary arteries. heart size is normal. diffuse segmental smooth dilatation of branch pulmonary arteries and veins, with tortuosity. Aneurysmal dilation on the venous side of the right lower pulmonary vein. Multiple feeding arteries and veins were seen (Fig. 59.2).

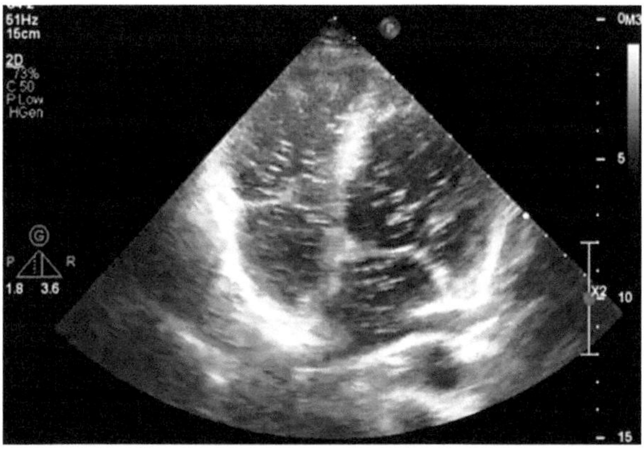

Fig. 59.1 All chambers filled during contrast injection

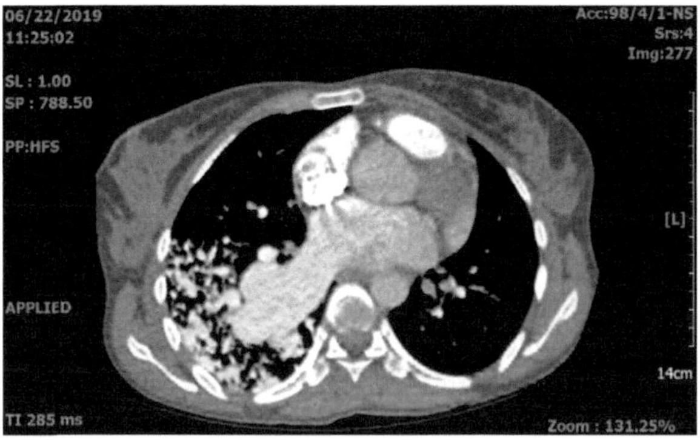

Fig. 59.2 Multiple round homogenous mass and dilated right pulmonary vein was seen

Catheterization

- Hemodynamic and pressure study showed normal RA and RV and pulmonary artery pressure. Desaturation of arterial sample was revealed.
- RPA injection showed multiple pulmonary AV fistula or aneurysm between the lower branch of the right pulmonary artery and right lower pulmonary vein with multiple feeding arteries.
- Cefazolin IV 1000 mg was administered and guidewire was advanced through catheter from femoral vein to IVC, RA, and RV to RPA. The stiff wire then passed through the catheter. The venous sheath and catheter were then removed and an introducer sheath was advanced over the stiff guidewire to the RPA, the guidewire was removed. Next, a muscular VSD occluder 8 mm (occlutech) was mounted on a delivery cable, advanced through the introducer sheath, and released in one of aneurysmal formation site. This procedure was repeated with two other devices (2 Amplatzer ADO type I 6 × 8 mm).
- Finally, RPA injection showed a significant decline in aneurysmal formation, feeding arteries and systemic saturation of the patient increased from 75% to 88%.
- So, the procedure was terminated and closure of the rest of the lesions postponed to another session (Fig. 59.3).

Discussion Pulmonary arteriovenous malformation or fistula is a low resistance high flow abnormal vascular structure that bypasses the pulmonary capillary system and, in this abnormality, the arterial system directly connected to the venous system [1], so it caused an intrapulmonary right to left shunt [2]. In most cases this abnormality is congenital, and acquired cases are very rare. Some cases are sporadic but in about 80% of the cases, hereditary hemangioma telangiectasia (HHT) was seen [3]. The clinical manifestation depends on the degree of right to left shunt, and it maybe asymptomatic in the mild form to deep cyanosis, fatigue, and hypoxemia in severe cases [4]. In this abnormality the patients are susceptible to paradoxical emboli, CVA, and brain abscess, these consequences especially seen in larger aneu-

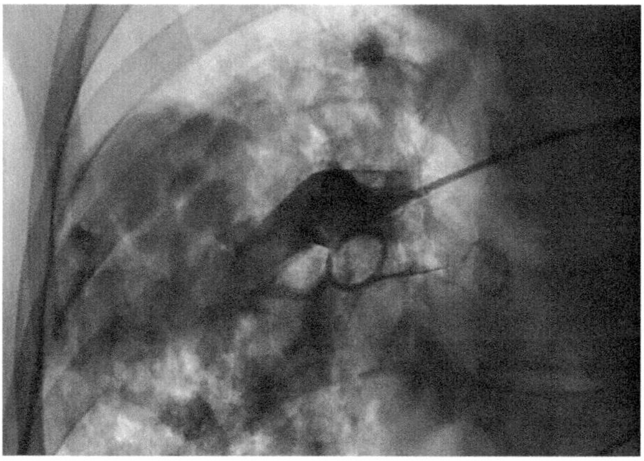

Fig. 59.3 RPA injection showed multiple fistula ad feeding arteries that connected to the right lower pulmonary vein

rysm with feeding artery diameter more than 3 mm and multiple lesions and feeding arteries [5]. Pulmonary artery hypertension was seen in patients with HHT.

In cases with cyanosis, intervention is mandatory for the elimination of cyanosis and the risk of paradoxical emboli. This abnormality could be managed by percutaneous interventional occlusion of aneurysmal lesions by coil, vascular plugs, or ADO devices.

Sometimes in multiple and complex surgical removals of involved lobe of the lung is the only option [6].

References

1. Churton T. Multiple aneurysms of pulmonary artery. Br Med J. 1897;1:1223.
2. Burke CM, Safai C, Nelson DP, et al. Pulmonary arteriovenous malformations: a critical update. Am Rev Respir Dis. 1986;134:334–9.
3. Gill SS, Roddie ME, Shovlin CL, et al. Pulmonary arteriovenous malformations and their mimics. Clin Radiol. 2015;70:96–110. https://doi.org/10.1016/j.crad.2014.09.003.
4. Moussouttas M, Fayad P, Rosenblatt M, et al. Pulmonary arteriovenous malformations: cerebral ischemia and neurologic manifestations. Neurology. 2000;55:959–64. https://doi.org/10.1212/WNL.55.7.959.
5. Bosher LH Jr, Blake DA, Byrd BR. An analysis of the pathologic anatomy of pulmonary arteriovenous aneurysms with particular reference to the applicability of local excision. Surgery. 1959;45:91–104.
6. Saboo SS, Chamarthy M, Bhalla S, Park H, Sutphin P, Kay F, Battaile J, Kalva SP. Pulmonary arteriovenous malformations: diagnosis. Cardiovasc Diagn Ther. 2018;8(3):325–37.

Chapter 60
Abnormal Origin of Right Coronary Artery from Pulmonary Artery in a Healthy Woman

Zahra Khajali

Abstract The patient is a 31-year-old lady whom complained of atypical chest pain, she had no family history of coronary artery disease. Her physical examination was nonremarkable. In electrocardiogram only nonspecific ST-T change was seen in inferior leads. In echocardiography abnormal turbulent coronary flow was seen, so coronary CT angiography and then coronary angiography performed. After these imaging we reached to ARCAPA diagnosis. We scheduled patient for surgical procedure, but she refused.

History and Clinical Presentation

A 31-year-old lady presented for evaluation of atypical chest pain in the past 2 months ago. She had mild dyspnea during exercise. The patient had not any risk factors for coronary artery disease.

Physical Examination

Blood Pressure: 100/70 mmHg, **Heart Rate**: 78 beats per minute, **Oxygen Saturation**: 97% in the air room.

General appearance: On examination, the patient was well developed. The nailbeds, lips, and mucous membranes were normal.

Lung/chest: No deformity of the chest wall, the lungs were clear.

Electronic Supplementary Material The online version of this chapter (https://doi.org/10.1007/978-1-4471-7496-7_60) contains supplementary material, which is available to authorized users.

Z. Khajali (✉)
Rajaei Cardiovascular Medical and Research Center, Iran University of Medical Sciences, Tehran, Iran

M. Maleki, A. Alizadehasl (eds.), *Case-Based Clinical Cardiology*,
https://doi.org/10.1007/978-1-4471-7496-7_60

Heart: Cardiac auscultation was unremarkable. The rhythm was regular.

Abdomen: The abdomen was soft with normal sounds, and also the abdominal examination showed that the liver was on the right side with a normal span.

Extremities: There was no peripheral edema. The pulses were regular and symmetric.

Electrocardiogram

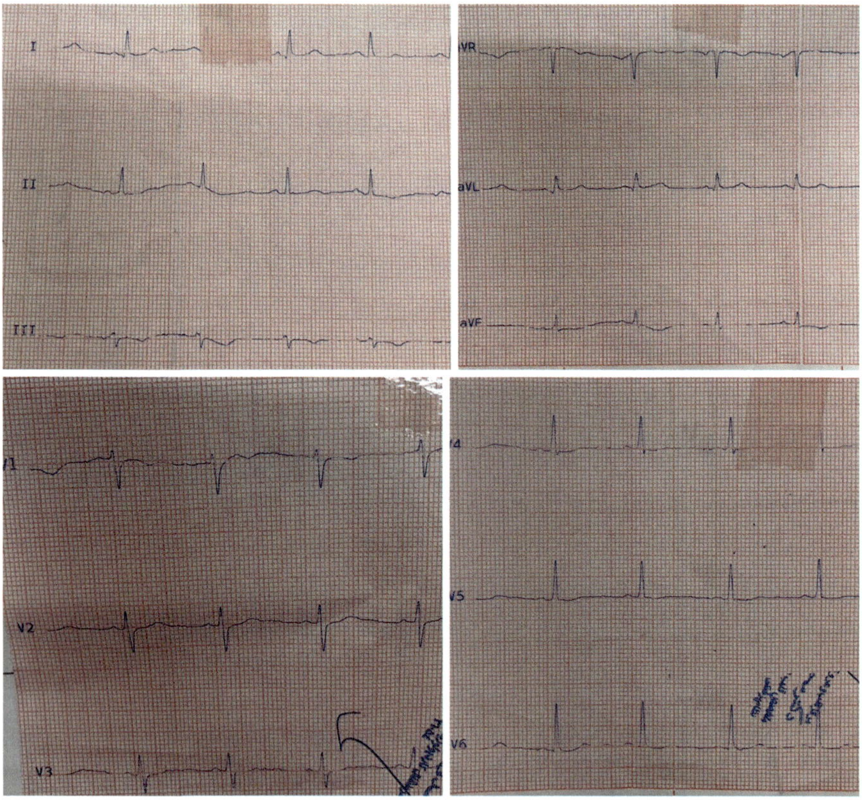

Twelve lead standard electrocardiogram

Normal sinus rhythm

Heart Rate: 78 beats per minute, regular

Normal axis deviation

Normal PR interval

Normal QRS duration

Mild ST-T changes in inferior leads (Invert T in III and aVF)

Chest X-Ray

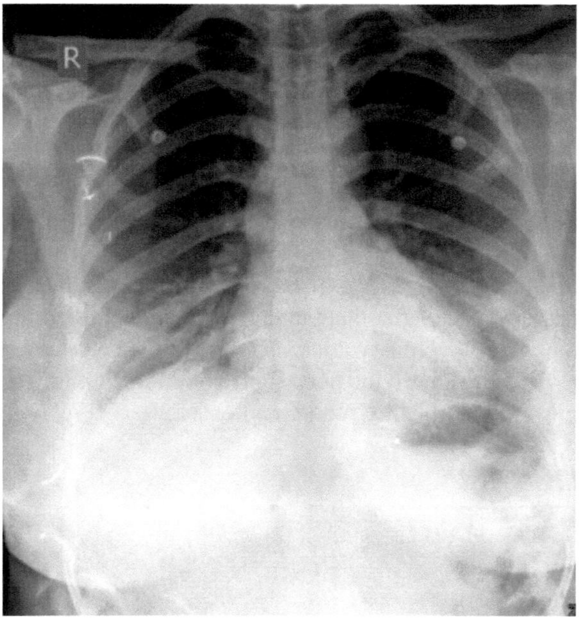

Posteroanterior projection, full inspiration

Levocardia (apex orientation to the left), situs solitus (the gastric bubble is seen in the left)

Left aortic arch

Normal cardiothoracic ratio

Normal pulmonary vascularity

Echocardiography

- Normal left ventricle size with normal systolic function (left ventricle ejection fraction = 55%)
- Normal right ventricle and right atrium size with normal systolic function
- No septal defect
- Normal mitral valve leaflets, no mitral stenosis, no mitral regurgitation
- Normal tricuspid aortic valve, no aortic stenosis, no aortic insufficiency
- Normal tricuspid valve leaflets, no tricuspid valve stenosis, mild tricuspid valve regurgitation (tricuspid regurgitation gradient = 25 mmHg)
- Normal pulmonary valve, no pulmonary stenosis, mild pulmonary insufficiency
- Dilated and tortoise vessel was seen adjacent to the right ventricle and also septum that terminated to pulmonary artery suggestive to coronary fistula to PA

Coronary CT Angiography

In coronary CT angiography, the left main artery had normal origin but it is dilated especially LAD, and the right coronary artery originated from the pulmonary artery and also dilated (Fig. 60.1).

Coronary Angiography

- Left main originated from left Valsalva sinus and dilated and via collaterals filled right coronary artery and after that pulmonary artery appeared in the late phase.
- No origin for the right coronary artery from aorta was detected.
- Aortic root injection showed the normal origin of left coronary arteries, dilated, and tortoise LAD that filled RCA and pulmonary artery (Fig. 60.2).

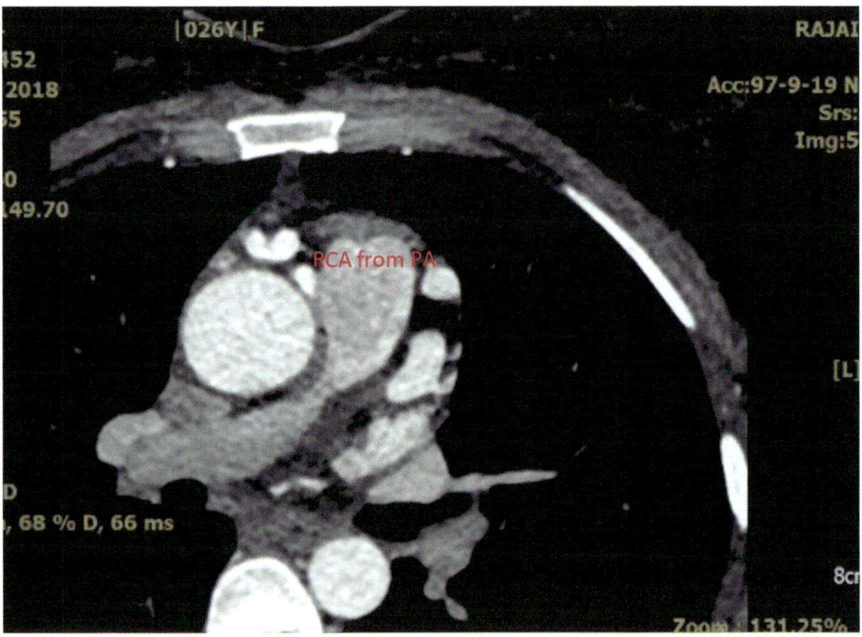

Fig. 60.1 Origin of RCA from PA in CT angiography

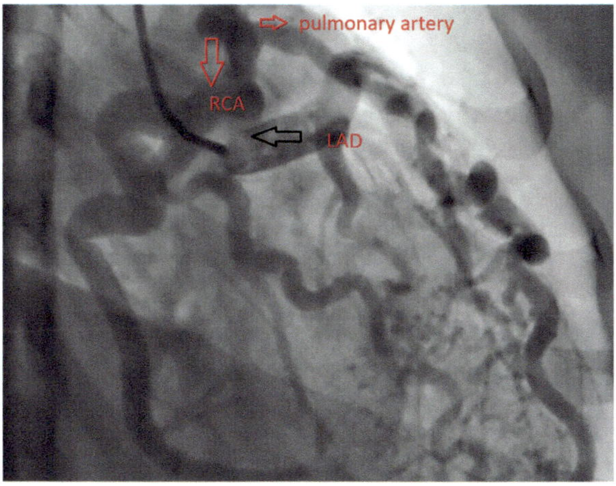

Fig. 60.2 Dilated LAD and RCA, filling of pa from RCA

Management

After this modality imaging, we performed an MPI scan for evaluation of the severity of ischemia. The patient had moderate ischemia at the territory of RCA. Regarding this degree of ischemia and also the nature of the disease, we decided to perform surgery for the patient but she refused.

Discussion ARCAPA is a rare anomaly on that right coronary artery originated from the pulmonary trunk, the prevalence estimated about 2 in 100,000 population [1]. In most situation, this anomaly is detected incidentally but sometimes may cause myocardial ischemia and even sudden cardiac arrest [2].

The age of the patients was variable and it occurred from neonate to elderly patients [3].

The severity of ischemia depends on the shunt size, collateral circulation, and myocardial oxygen demands [4]. Because the right ventricle needs less oxygen than the left ventricle, ARCAPA has a mild form of ischemia than ALCAPA. Also, in patients with left dominant system ARCAPA has mild ischemia than the patients with right dominancy.

Regarding multiple studies all cases of ARCAPA should be undergone surgery because of the progression of ischemia and prevention of the risk of sudden cardiac death [5].

References

1. Li RJ, Yang Y, Li ZA, Xie JJ, Zhang XS. Right coronary artery arising from the main pulmonary artery: evaluation with 2-dimensional transthoracic echocardiography and multislice computed tomography. Tex Heart Inst J. 2010;37:376–7.
2. Choi E, Park JJ, Yoon TJ, Kim YH, Ko JK, Park IS, et al. Anomalous origin of the right coronary artery from the pulmonary artery. Korean J Thorac Cardiovasc Surg. 2002;35:894–7.
3. Park CS, Kim W, Hong SB, Hwang SH, Kim W, An BH. Anomalous origin of the right coronary artery from the main pulmonary artery presenting as angina pectoris in an adult. Korean Circ J. 2008;38:627–9.
4. Gupta R, Marwah A, Shrivastva S. Anomalous origin of right coronary artery from pulmonary artery. Ann Pediatr Cardiol. 2012;5:95–6.
5. Al-Dairy A, Rezaei Y, Pouraliakbar H, Mahdavi M, Bayati P, Gholampour-Dehaki M. Surgical repair for anomalous origin of the right coronary artery from the pulmonary artery. Korean Circ J. 2017;47(1):144–7.

Chapter 61
Thrombolytic Therapy in Fontan Circuit Thrombosis

Zahra Khajali

Abstract A 21-year-old gentleman with history of Fontan surgery at 15 years ago referred to us with frequent episodes of palpitation. His basal rhythm was atrial fibrillation but he had some episodes of non-sustained VT, so he admitted for VT ablation. He was on anticoagulation therapy by warfarin in the last 4 years. In echocardiography, a mobile linear clot was seen on fenestration that closed the fenestration completely and protruded to atrium. Because of patient condition and high-risk surgery, we started thrombolytic treatment. After 25 hours very slow infusion regime the clot resolved completely and fenestration flow was seen in follow-up echocardiography.

History and Clinical Presentation

A 21-year-old gentleman with a history of Fontan operation and frequent episodes of non-sustained VT which did not respond to medical therapy was admitted to our hospital for VT ablation. The patient had history of frequent palpitations and hospitalization due to intolerable arrythmia. The patient was on warfarin for many years and his INR was 1.8 on admission (under expected range).

Physical Examination

Blood Pressure: 90/60 mmHg, **Heart Rate**: irregular and 110 beats per minute, **Oxygen Saturation**: 88% in the air room.

Electronic Supplementary Material The online version of this chapter (https://doi.org/10.1007/978-1-4471-7496-7_61) contains supplementary material, which is available to authorized users.

Z. Khajali (✉)
Rajaei Cardiovascular Medical and Research Center, Iran University of Medical Sciences, Tehran, Iran

M. Maleki, A. Alizadehasl (eds.), *Case-Based Clinical Cardiology*,
https://doi.org/10.1007/978-1-4471-7496-7_61

General appearance: On examination, the patient was well developed. The nailbeds, lips, and mucous membranes were mildly cyanotic.

Heart: Normal S1, and single S2 was heard, harsh diastolic murmurs of grade 3/6 on the right sternal border were heard.

Abdomen: The abdomen was soft with normal sounds, and also the abdominal examination showed that the liver was on the right side with increased span.

Laboratory Data

Hemoglobin	17.5 gr/dl
White Blood Count	4500 cells/mm^3
Platelet	215,000 cells/mm^3
Creatinine	0.8 mg/dl
Blood urea nitrogen	18 mg/dl
Cholesterol	105 mg/dl
Triglyceride	125 mg/dl
ALT	55 U/L
AST	65 U/L
Bilirubin	6 mg/dl

Electrocardiogram

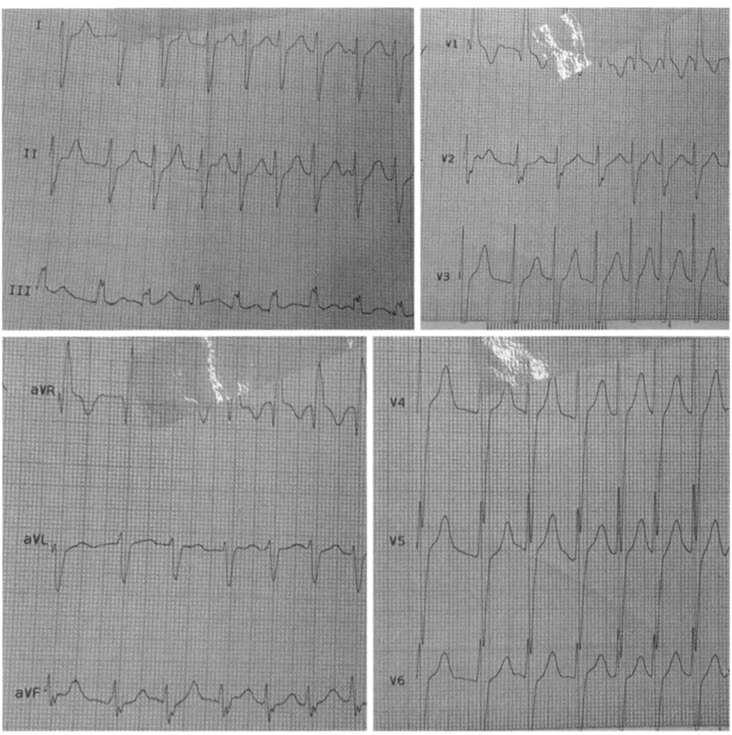

Electrocardiography showed an AF rhythm with a heart rate of 115 beats per minute, a right axis deviation, and tall R in V1 and deep S in V5, V6 with loss of LV force was in favor of single ventricle with RV morphology or TGA.

Chest X-Ray

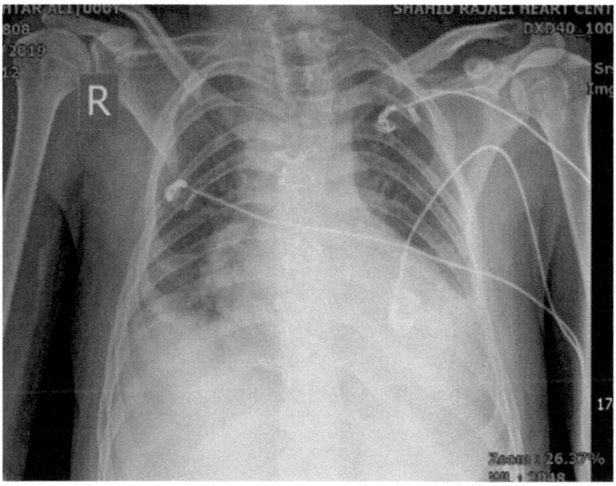

Posteroanterior projection, full inspiration

Levocardia (apex orientation to the left), situs solitus (the gastric bubble is seen in the left)

Left aortic arch

Increased cardiothoracic ratio

Decreased pulmonary vascularity

Sternal wires

Dilated ascending aorta

Echocardiography

- Moderate systemic ventricle with RV morphology enlargement and severe systolic dysfunction (RVEF = 35%).
- Hypoplastic left ventricle.
- Both AV valves committed to RV(DIRV).
- No left-sided AV valve Stenosis with mild regurgitation.
- Moderate right-sided AV valve regurgitation.
- Tricuspid aortic valve, no aortic stenosis, moderate to severe aortic insufficiency.

- Pulmonary artery closed surgically.
- Both great arteries arose RV(DORV).
- The fresh clot was seen on Fontan fenestration with no flow through fenestration (Fig. 61.1).

Management Then the low dose alteplase (1 mg/h) was infused for the patient, after 25 h the clot was resolved completely without any complication. Then electrophysiology consult was done and because of the patient's condition ICD was implanted (Fig. 61.2).

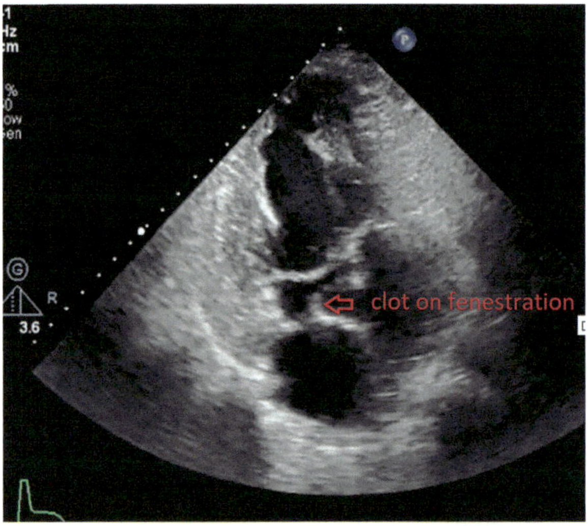

Fig. 61.1 The linear clot on conduit fenestration was seen

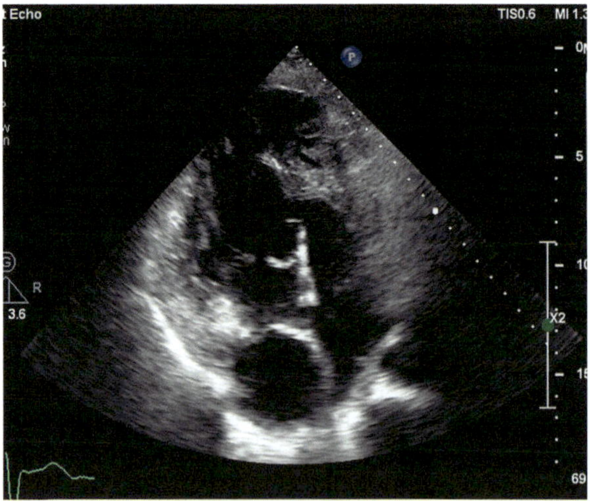

Fig. 61.2 Post-thrombolytic therapy showed a complete resolved clot

Discussion

The Fontan procedure is an operation that bypasses a right ventricle and diverts a systemic venous blood to the pulmonary arteries [1]. It is a palliative treatment for many complex congenital heart diseases with single ventricle morphology of functionally single ventricle. There are different types of Fontan circulation. (A) Atriopulmonary connection; (B) intracardiac total Cavo pulmonary connection (lateral tunnel or intracardiac conduit); (C) extracardiac total Cavo pulmonary connection. Patients who have undergone the Fontan operation are at a high risk for thromboembolism and the majority of these events are "silent," without any symptoms [2]. The incidence of thromboembolism is highest in the first year after Fontan surgery but remains a persistent risk several years later [3]. Fibrinolytic therapy, also known as thrombolytic therapy, is used in the treatment of a ST segment elevation myocardial infarction (STEMI), acute stroke, and other less common indications such as pulmonary embolism, acute deep venous thrombosis and some mechanical valve thrombosis [4, 5]. Low dose very slow infusion fibrinolytic (alteplase 1 mg/h) is a safe regime and in high-risk patients like those whom had history of Fontan surgery should be considered. For the patients with history of Fontan surgery who had the rhythm except for sinus, anticoagulation with close monitoring recommended.

References

1. Maleki M, Alizadehasl A, Haghjoo M. Practical cardiology, Chapter 28. Fontan operation, pp. 496–498.
2. Literature Review (PDF Available) in Heart (British Cardiac Society) 96(12):911-6 June 2010 with 1,643 Reads. doi: https://doi.org/10.1136/hrt.2010.193912
3. Rosenthal DN, Friedman AH, Kleinman CS, Kopf GS, Rosenfeld LE, Hellenbrand WE. Thromboembolic complications after Fontan operations. Circulation. 1995;92:287–93.
4. Khajali Z, Mohammadzadeh S, Maleki M, Peighambari MM, Sadeghpoor A, Ghavidel A, Elahi B, Mirzaaghayan M. Fibrinolytic therapy for mechanical pulmonary valve thrombosis. Pediatr Cardiol. 2015;36(1):171–6.
5. Sadeghpour A, Kyavar M, Javani B, Bakhshandeh H, Maleki M, Khajali Z, et al. Mid-term outcome of mechanical pulmonary valve prostheses: The importance of anticoagulation. J Cardiovasc Thorac Res. 2014;6(3):163.

Chapter 62
Stenting of Fontan Pathway at Anastomose of Conduit to Pulmonary Artery

Zahra Khajali

Abstract A 23-year-old lady with history of Fontan surgery at 12 years ago referred to us with ascites and lower limb edema. She also declared loss of appetite and fatigue in the last 2 months ago. In physical examination and echocardiography, we suspect to stenosis at fontan pathways that this diagnosis confirmed by CT angiography, for hemodynamic evaluation and also intervention catheterization performed and stenosis at conduit to pulmonary artery confirmed. stenting of the stenotic area performed without complication. The symptoms of the patient alleviated at 2 days after procedure.

History and Clinical Presentation

A 23-year-old lady with history of Fontan surgery 12 years ago came to the ACHD clinic by fatigue, loss of appetite, abdominal swelling, and limb edema for the last 2 months. She did not return for follow-up examination from 2 years ago.

She declared that she did not any symptoms after surgery until 2 months ago.

In surgical report, she had undergone TCPC operation by an extracardiac conduit and Glenn shunt.

Physical Examination

Blood Pressure: 90/60 mmHg, **Heart Rate**: 75 beats per minute, **Oxygen Saturation**: 89% in the air room.

Electronic Supplementary Material The online version of this chapter (https://doi.org/10.1007/978-1-4471-7496-7_62) contains supplementary material, which is available to authorized users.

Z. Khajali (✉)
Rajaei Cardiovascular Medical and Research Center, Iran University of Medical Sciences, Tehran, Iran

M. Maleki, A. Alizadehasl (eds.), *Case-Based Clinical Cardiology*, https://doi.org/10.1007/978-1-4471-7496-7_62

General appearance: On examination, the patient was well developed. The nailbeds, lips, and mucous membranes were mildly cyanotic and digital clubbing was noted, there was not any respiratory distress at rest. The eyes and skin are icteric.

Lung/chest: No deformity of the chest wall, the lungs were clear.

Heart: Cardiac auscultation revealed a normal first and second heart sounds. No systolic and diastolic murmur or gallop was heard. The rhythm was regular.

Abdomen: The abdomen was generalized distended, and also the abdominal examination showed fluctuant sensation in pulsation and also dullness in flanks.

Extremities: There was lower limb peripheral edema. The pulses were regular and symmetric but weak.

Laboratory Data

Hemoglobin	16.5 gr/dl
Hematocrit	48.5%
White Blood Count	5300 cells/mm^3
Platelet	216,000 cells/mm^3
Creatinine	0.7 mg/dl
Blood urea nitrogen	13 mg/dl
Cholesterol	115 mg/dl
Triglyceride	86 mg/dl
ALT (Alanine transaminase)	62 IU/L
AST (Aspartate transaminase)	71 IU/L
TSH (Thyroid stimulating hormone)	3.2 micro IU/ml
HIV-Ab	Negative
HBS-Ag	Negative
HCV-Ab	Negative
Bilirubin	7 mg/dl

Electrocardiogram

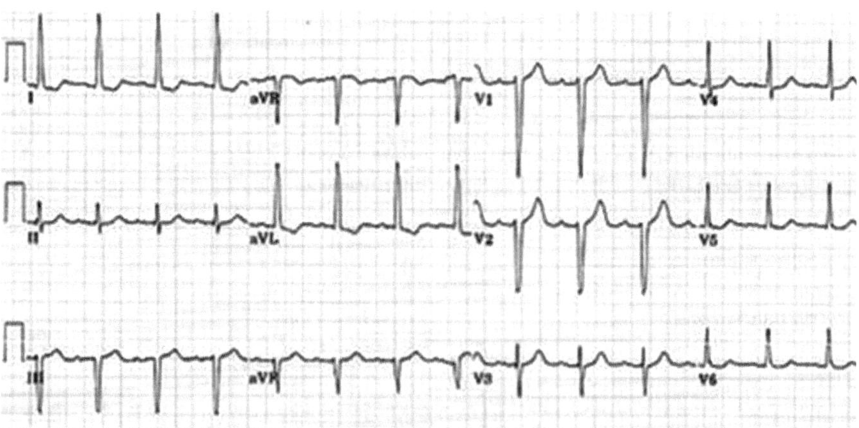

Twelve lead standard electrocardiogram
Normal sinus rhythm
Heart Rate: 90 beats per minute, regular
Normal QRS duration
Left axis deviation
Normal PR interval
Loss of RV forces suggested tricuspid atresia or DILV in a cyanotic patient

Chest X-Ray

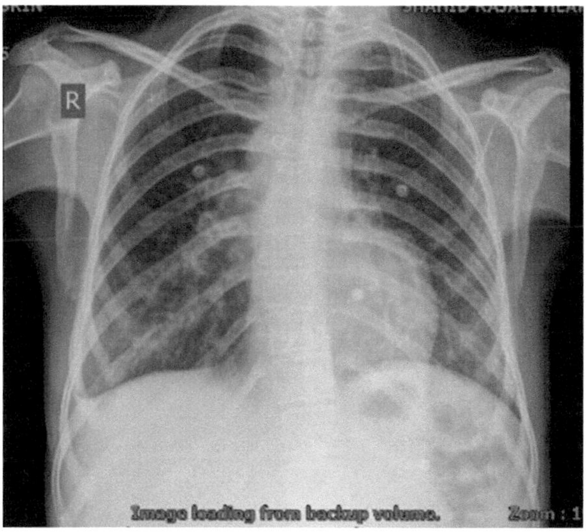

Posteroanterior projection, full inspiration
Levocardia (apex orientation to the left), situs solitus (the gastric bubble is seen in the left)
Left aortic arch
Straight border of the right silhouette in favor of tricuspid atresia
Decreased pulmonary vascularity
Narrow mediastinum in favor of TGA

Echocardiography

- Enlarged systemic left ventricle with preserved systolic function (left ventricle ejection fraction = 50%)
- Hypoplastic RV (Video 62.1)

- Large interatrial septal defect
- Normal mitral valve leaflets, no mitral stenosis, mild mitral regurgitation
- Normal tricuspid aortic valve, no aortic stenosis, no aortic insufficiency
- Atretic tricuspid valve
- Pulmonary artery closed surgically
- Extracardiac conduit was seen with an increased gradient of fenestration(10 mmHg) and turbulent flow with 8 mmHg gradient was seen between the conduit and right pulmonary artery (Video 62.2)
- -Normal laminar flow through Glenn shunt

Congenital CT Angiography

Normal epicardial coronary arteries. Tricuspid atresia and hypoplastic RV was seen. Severe stenosis at conduit insertion to the pulmonary artery was noted (Fig. 62.1).

Catheterization

- Hemodynamic and pressure study showed evidence of elevated pressure in IVC and conduit (20 mmHg), and normal pressure in PA and SVC (12 mmHg).
- Conduit injection showed severe stenosis at conduit anastomose to right pulmonary artery (Fig. 62.2).

Management

- After conduit injection, we decided to stent the stenosis area. Cefazolin IV 1000 mg was administered and guidewire was advanced through catheter from the femoral vein to IVC, conduit, and RPA. The stiff wire then passed through

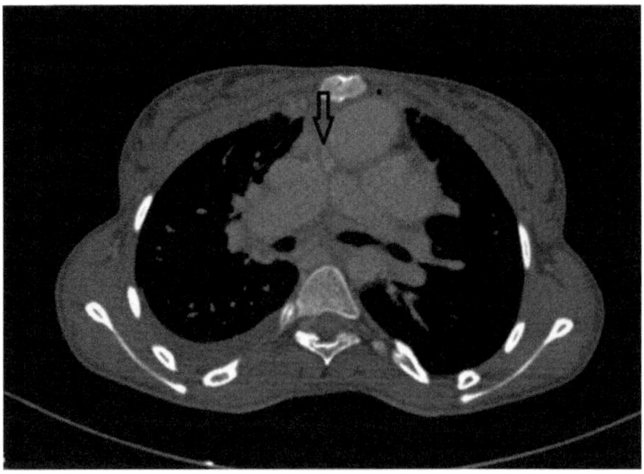

Fig. 62.1 Ct Angio showed Severe stenosis at conduit insertion to the right pulmonary artery

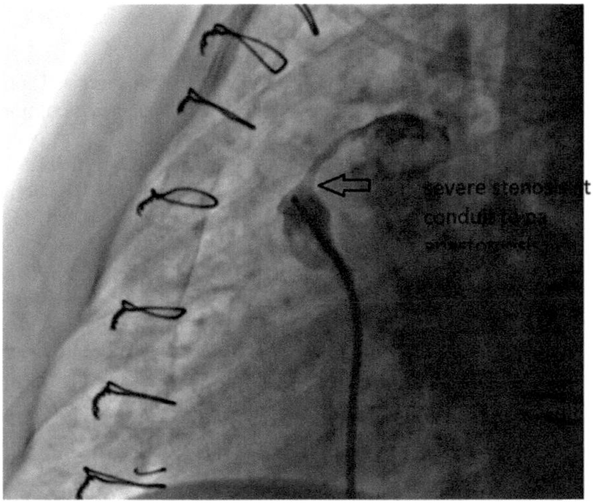

Fig. 62.2 Severe stenosis at conduit insertion to RPA

the catheter. The venous sheath and catheter were then removed and an introducer sheath was advanced over the stiff guidewire to the RPA, the guidewire was removed. Next, a Palmaz Genesis stent 28 mm mounted on Balloon 30 × 10 mm, advanced through the introducer sheath and inflated at the anastomosis site. Then post-dilation performed by balloon 16 × 30 mm and gradient eliminated completely.

- During some days after the procedure the ascites and icterus alleviated and after 1 month patient feels completely healthy condition. She had under treatment with warfarin and clopidogrel. After 3 months clopidogrel discontinued and warfarin continued.

Discussion The Fontan procedure is an operation that bypasses a right ventricle and diverts a systemic venous blood to the pulmonary arteries [1]. It is a palliative treatment for many complex congenital heart diseases that biventricular repair is impossible or more challenging. There are different types of Fontan circulation. (1) Atriopulmonary connection that is historical and not performed nowadays; (2) intracardiac total Cavo pulmonary connection (lateral tunnel or intracardiac conduit); (3) extracardiac total Cavo pulmonary connection [2].

The patients who undergone Fontan procedure may have many complications during follow-up. One of the complications is obstruction at Fontan circuit and it may be focal or diffuse and can happen at IVC anastomosis to conduit or conduit anastomosis to the pulmonary artery or at through the conduit length [3]. This obstruction may be due to technical surgical problems with less probability, multiple thrombosis formation at the circuit, or more likely stretching of the conduit during child growth. Most of this stenosis amenable for catheter intervention [4] and symptoms of the patient and NYHA functional class improved after the intervention.

References

1. Fontan F, Baudet E. Surgical repair of tricuspid atresia. Thorax. 1971;26:240–8.
2. de Leval MR, Kilner P, Gewillig M, Bull C. Total cavopulmonary connection: a logical alternative to atriopulmonary connection for complex Fontan operations. Experimental studies and early clinical experience. J Thorac Cardiovasc Surg. 1988;96:682–95.
3. Hagler DJ, Mirand WR, Haggerty BJ, Anderson JH, Johnson JN, Cetta F, et al. Fate of the Fontan connection: mechanisms of stenosis and Management. Congenit Heart Dis J. 2019;14(4):571–81.
4. Mets JM, Bergersen L, Mayer JE Jr, et al. Outcomes of stent implantation for obstruction of intracardiac laterl tunnel Fontan pathways. Circ Cardiovasc Interv. 2013;6:92–100.
5. Maleki M, Alizadehasl A, Haghjoo M. Practical Cardiology book. Chapter 28. Fontan operation. P. 496–8.

Chapter 63
Transcatheter Secundum ASD Device Closure

Ata Firouzi and Zahra Hosseini

Abstract ASD secundum is the most congenital heart disease in adults which usually being symptomatic in third or fourth decade of life. The common symptoms are exertional dyspnea, palpitation and rarely systemic thromboembolism. If left to right shunt in right heart catheterization (RHC) be $\geq$ 1.5 or any evidence of RV volume overload would occur, the patient is candidate for ASD closure. Nowadays, the choice of closure is trans-catheter approach if in trans-esophageal echocardiography (TEE) the defect being suitable with adequate rims. The success rate is more than 95%. The long term outcome of these patients is comparable to surgical closure with lesser complications. Regular follow-up by echocardiography, post closure is mandatory to evaluate the residual shunt and rarely catastrophic complications.

History

The patient was a 32 years old lady who was referred with complaints of exertional dyspnea and occasional episodes of palpitation since one year ago. In diagnostic work-up she had a large secundum ASD which was suitable for percutaneous closure.

ASD in Adulthoswod

The most common congenital heart disease (CHD) in adults is ASD (Atrial Septal Defect) after Bicuspid Aortic Valve. In adults, it accounts for 7–10% of all CHD and between 20 and 40% of all newly diagnosed CHD [1]. Secundum ASD is the commonest form of ASDs (75%) which frequently diagnosed in adulthood. With continuous left-to-right shunt depending on the defect size and RV volume overload

A. Firouzi (✉) · Z. Hosseini
Interventional Cardiology, Cardiovascular Intervention Research Center, Rajaie Cardiovascular Medical and Research Center, Iran University of Medical Sciences, Tehran, Iran

M. Maleki, A. Alizadehasl (eds.), *Case-Based Clinical Cardiology*,
https://doi.org/10.1007/978-1-4471-7496-7_63

and consequently with reduced the compliance of left side chambers with aging, patients with secundum ASD usually remain asymptomatic till the third or fourth decade [2]. Common initial symptoms are exertional dyspnea, fatigue, paradoxical systemic thromboembolism, and palpitation (PSVT) especially in those over 40 years. Without correction of the defect and long-standing left to right shunting, RV pressure eventually increased and this may result in decrease of left to right shunt, mild-to-moderate Pulmonary Artery Hypertension (PAH) and finally RV failure. Severe PAH rarely happens in this type of ASD and concomitant diseases should be considered.

Diagnostic Work-Up

The key findings in physical examination are RV heave and fixed S2 splitting. The ECG usually shows right axis deviation, rsR' in right precordial leads suggestive of RV volume over load, and sometimes crochetage sign in Inferior leads. TTE (Trans Thoracic Echocardiography) is the first imaging modality for detecting the defect and its hemodynamic effects and any other anomalies. Finally, TEE and recently 3D-TEE is the most sensitive imaging tool for detection of the defect and any other concomitant fenestrations, PFO, or anomalies like PAPVCs, evaluation of the defect size, surrounding rims and structures, total interatrial length or any septal aneurysm (ISA), the direction of the shunt and eventuality the suitability of the ASD for device closure.

Indications and Contraindications of ASD Closure

Any patients with hemodynamically significant shunt (Qp/Qs ratio > 1.5 Wood Units), RV volume overload, or paradoxical thromboembolism irrespective of symptoms or age should be considered for closure unless, in RHC, PVR (Pulmonary Vascular Resistance) be more than 5 Wood Units. Even in such circumstances, if the net shunt direction be left to right and PAP or PVR be less than 2/3 of systemic level or be reactive to vasoreactive test, closure can be valuable [3].

RHC (Right Heart Catheterization)

- Qp/Qs: 3
- PVR: 1.5 WU
- SVR: 120 WU
- PAP: 35/15 mm Hg
- So2: 98%

Procedural Technique

Only secundum type ASDs are suitable for transcatheter device closure. It has similar efficacy with less complications compared with surgical closure. In defects >38 mm or those with no suitable rims especially posteroinferior rims deficient (the least important is anterosuperior rims deficiency), surgical closure is recommended [4].

In our case, who was loaded with ASA 325 mg and Clopidogrel 600 mg (which must continue ASA 80 mg for at least 6 months and Clopidogrel 75 mg for one month until fully device endothelialization), after arterial and venous short sheaths (6F) insertion and RHC, under general anesthesia and supervision by a skilled technician, fully assessments of the defect with TEE probe by dedicated profession was performed, which showed, non-stretch 26 mm round secundum type ASD defect (Anterosuperior floppy rim: 2 mm, Posterior rim: 6 mm, Inferior rim: 5 mm and Anteroinferior rim: 4 mm) with no any fenestrations, PFO, or PAPVCs. The net shunt was left to right.

After completing IV Heparin with the goal of ACT > 200 s and crossing the defect with Multipurpose catheter which its tip was positioned in the LUPV, a floppy tip Amplatzer Superstiff guide-wire was placed in the LUPV. After prepping and de-airing of Sizing Balloon (SB) 35 (it has been recommended as an essential step of the procedure) under TEE, the balloon was inflated with diluted contrast until the Stop Flow Diameter (SFD) was reported by the Echo-man and also according to the shape of the balloon in the fluoroscopy. Sometimes it is difficult for stabilizing the sizing balloon due to melon-seeding in large defects with deficient rims.

Stop-flow technique: The sizing balloon is placed across the ASD and inflated until there is no flow across the defect on Color-Flow imaging. The maximum width of the balloon is then measured by TEE/ICE as well as fluoroscopy [5].

Waist measurement technique: The sizing balloon is placed across the ASD and inflated until there is a waist formation noted along both the margins of the balloon on fluoroscopy. This waist is then measured on fluoroscopy (Fig. 63.1) [5].

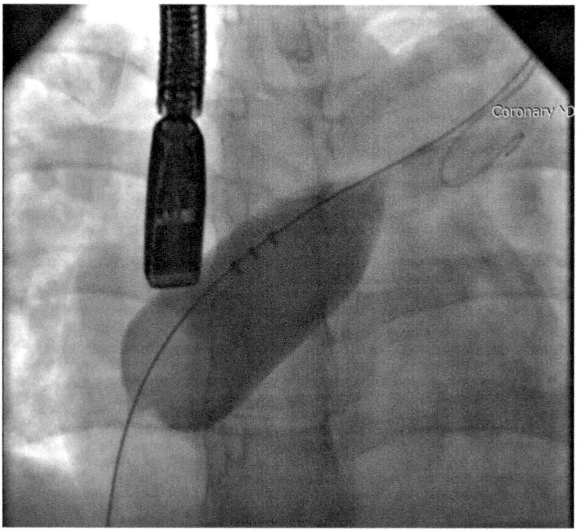

Fig. 63.1 Waist measurement technique: The sizing balloon is placed across the ASD and inflated until there is a waist formation noted along both the margins of the balloon on fluoroscopy. This waist is then measured on fluoroscopy

The SFD was 30 mm. Because of anterosuperior rim deficiency, Occlutech Figulla FlexII 33 mm was chosen.

After flushed and de-airing of all the segments of the delivery sheath (COOK 12F) and positioning the sheath in the IVC-RA junction, dilator was removed to allow back bleed and prevent air embolism. Thereafter the delivery sheath was advanced in the left atrium just outside of the LUPV.

After loading the delivery cable and connecting the cable to the hub of RA disk and retraction of the whole device to the loader (slenderized the device) and fully flushed with heparinized saline, the loader was connected to the delivery sheath and the device was being passed through the delivery sheath. Left atrial disk of the device was being extruded in the left atrium and after fully extruded the left disk (Fig. 63.2a), all the system was pulled back all together under TEE guidance (for

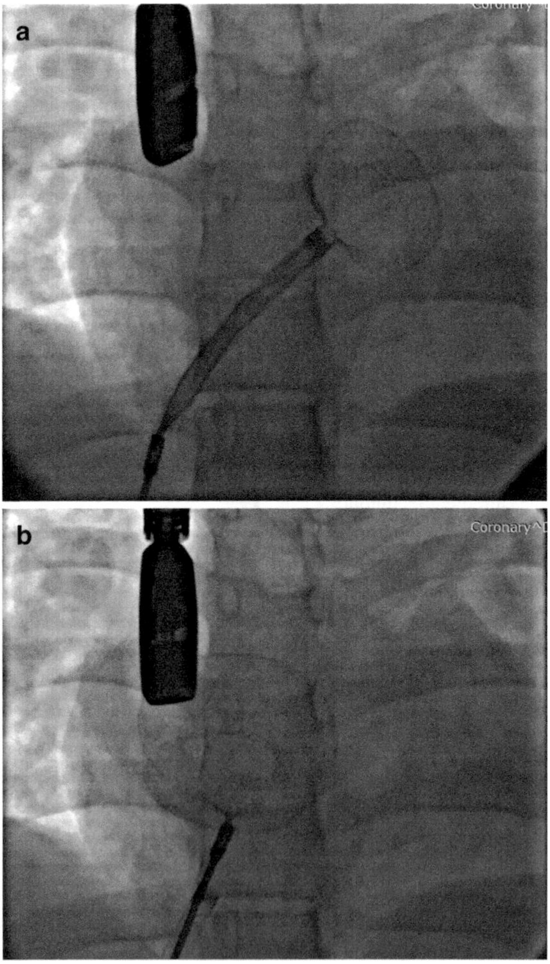

Fig. 63.2 (**a**, **b**) Left atrial disk of the device was being extruded in the left atrium and after fully extruded the left disk, all the system was pulled back all together under TEE guidance (for evaluation of alignment). After being sure about the optimal position of the device, the waist and RA disk was fully extruded too

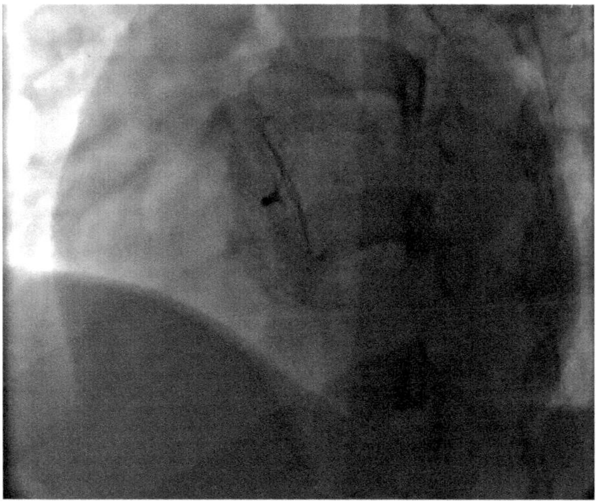

Fig. 63.3 After complete evaluation of all the surrounding rims with no encroachment of the device on the nearby cardiac structures and stable position of the device, the device was released

evaluation of alignment) and finally after being sure about the optimal position of the device, the waist, and RA disk was fully extruded too (Fig. 63.2b).

After complete evaluation of all the surrounding rims with no encroachment of the device on the nearby cardiac structures and stable position of the device by Echocardiographist and Minnesota maneuvers (which is controversy about this maneuver), the device was released (Fig. 63.3).

Conclusion

Currently, transcatheter secundum ASD closure is the default strategy for most ones with a success rate more than 95% in the hands of expert interventionist with less than 1% complications such as: device embolization, device erosion, arrhythmia, and … [6], but by selecting the most appropriate cases and new devices design, these events rarely happened even less than the past.

References

1. Wiktor DM, Carroll JD. ASD closure in structural heart disease. Curr Cardiol Rep. 2018;20:37.
2. Yong G, Khairy P, Guise PD, et al. Pulmonary arterial hypertension in patients with transcatheter closure of secundum atrial septal defects a longitudinal study. Circ Cardiovasc Interv. 2009;2:455–62.
3. Warnes CA, Williams RG, Bashore TM, et al. ACC/AHA 2008 guidelines for the management of adults with congenital heart disease: a report of the American College of Cardiology/American Heart Association Task Force on Practice Guidelines (Writing Committee to Develop Guidelines on the Management of Adults With Congenital Heart Disease). Developed in Collaboration With the American Society of Echocardiography, Heart Rhythm Society,

International Society for Adult Congenital Heart Disease, Society for Cardiovascular Angiography and Interventions, and Society of Thoracic Surgeons. J Am Coll Cardiol. 2008;52:e143–263.
4. Podnar T, Martanovic P, Gavora P, Masura J. Morphological variations of secundum-type atrial septal defects: feasibility for percutaneous closure using Amplatzer septal occluders. Catheter Cardiovasc Interv J Soc Card Angiogr Interv. 2001;53:386–91.
5. Jain SA, Dalvi BV, et al. Atrial septal defect: step-by-step catheter closure. J Struct Heart Dis. 2016;2(1):15–32.
6. Majunke N, Bialkowski J, Wilson N, et al. Closure of atrial septal defect with the Amplatzer septal occluder in adults. Am J Cardiol. 2009;103:550–4.

Chapter 64
Transcatheter PFO Device Closure

Ata Firouzi and Zahra Hosseini

Abstract Persistent PFO prevalence is estimated to be 20-25% in general population. Frequently, detected incidentally in adults. In patients with cryptogenic stroke (40% of all ischemic strokes), there is conflict between neurologist and cardiologist about the role of PFO as the underlying cause. Recent trials are in favor of PFO closure in those with high risk feature PFO in TEE. Trans-catheter closure is the choice strategy with high success rate and no major complications.

History

The patient was a 30 years old man, who was referred with two episodes of TIA within recent 6 months. Despite of several neurogical work-up and ASA therapy, no underlying cause was detected. In TEE for rulling out the source of emboli, a PFO was detected.

PFO closure is one of the most challenging topics in the field of cardiology. The controversy about PFO pathology has consequently prompted a paradigm shift of research interest from medical therapy with antiplatelets or anticoagulants to percutaneous transcatheter closure for secondary prevention (Close, RESPECT, GORE-REDUCE, and DEFENSE trials) [1]. PFO is a tunnel-like passage in the interatrial septum formed by the failure of postnatal fusion of the septum primum and secundum. Persistent PFO is estimated to occur in approximately 20–25% of the adult population. Over the years, PFO has been implicated in multiple clinical conditions for which closure has been proposed, including cryptogenic stroke, migraine, decompression sickness, platypnea-orthodeoxia syndrome, and paradoxical cardio-systemic embolization. In a PFO, the overlapping anatomy of the primum and secundum atrial septa forms a flap valve that usually only opens when the right

A. Firouzi (✉) · Z. Hosseini
Interventional Cardiology, Cardiovascular Intervention Research Center, Rajaie Cardiovascular Medical and Research Center, Iran University of Medical Sciences, Tehran, Iran

M. Maleki, A. Alizadehasl (eds.), *Case-Based Clinical Cardiology*,
https://doi.org/10.1007/978-1-4471-7496-7_64

atrial pressure exceeds the left atrial pressure. However, since the right atrial pressure is usually less than the left atrial pressure, PFOs are functionally closed most of the time. However, this pressure gradient can be reversed by maneuvers that change the intra-thoracic pressure (e.g. coughing, sneezing, or straining to defecate), thereby allowing the PFO to open and for blood, thrombus, or any other substances to pass from the right to the left atrium.

Diagnostic Work-Up in Cryptogenic Stroke (CS) (Table 64.1)

There are no gold standard tools for diagnosing of PFO. A combination of transthoracic echocardiography (TTE), (TEE), and Trans-Cranial Doppler (TCD) may be required. If TTE is positive, pursue TEE for corroboration, An atrial septal aneurysm, moderate-to-severe shunt, and atrial septal hypermobility have been strongly associated with a causal role of PFO in cryptogenic stroke. If TCD is positive, pursue TEE for corroboration. If TTE is negative or equivocal, pursue TCD, and if TCD is negative, stop investigation. To rule out causes other than PFO, patients with left circulation embolism and PFO should undergo 12-leads ECG and either inpatient telemetry or 24-h Holter monitoring to detect any atrial fibrillation (AF). Patients ≥65 years or patients between 55 and 64 years with AF risk factors should undergo 6 months of AF monitoring with an implantable cardiac monitor [2]. The risk of

Table 64.1 Cryptogenic stroke evaluation

Condition	Recommended testing
Hypercoagulable disorder	CBC (hemoglobin and platelet count); factor V Leiden protein C, protein S, antithrombin III, and homocysteine levels; prothrombin G20210A mutation, antiphospholipid antibodies
Paroxysmal atrial fibrillation	A 30-day continuous cardiac monitoring
Cardiac thrombus, vegetation, or tumor; mitral stenosis	TTE followed by TEE (if TTE is normal); cardiac CT or MRI can be considered if high suspicion
Carotid atherosclerotic disease	Carotid duplex ultrasound, CTA or MRA of the neck and head
Cerebral vascular atherosclerotic disease	CTA or MRA of the head
Aortic arch atheroma	TEE of CTA of the chest
Arterial dissection	CTA of the chest and neck (TEE can see proximal dissection)
Cerebral venous sinus thrombosis	Brain MRV
May-Thurner syndrome	Pelvic MRV

Table 64.2 RoPE score calculator

Characteristic	Points	Score
No history of hypertension	1	
No history of diabetes	1	
No history of stroke or TIA	1	
Nonsmoker	1	
Cortical infarct on imaging	1	
Age (years)		
18–29	5	
30–39	4	
40–49	3	
50–59	2	
60–139	1	
≥70	0	
Total score (sum of individual points)		
Maximum score (a patient <30 years without vascular risk factors, no history of stroke or TIA, and. cortical infarct)		10
Minimum score (a patient ≥70 years with vascular risk factors, prior stroke, and no cortical infarct)		0

paradoxical embolism (RoPE) score (Table 64.2) attempts to predict how likely a PFO is causal in the setting of a cryptogenic stroke. The RoPE score can be used to guide management decisions. High RoPE scores identify younger patients without conventional vascular risk factors and with infarcts located superficially in the brain (more likely embolic); low RoPE scores identify older patients with deep infarcts and multiple conventional risk factors. The RoPE score successfully disaggregates CS patients into a stratum with a PFO prevalence that matches the background population (23%, RoPE score 0–3), which then increases in a linear fashion to the highest RoPE score with a very high prevalence of PFO (73%, RoPE score 9–10), but should be used in conjunction with other parameters, such as the presence of atrial septal aneurysm or deep venous thrombosis/pulmonary embolism [3].

Indications for PFO Closure in 2019 Guideline

Interdisciplinary collaboration with an interventional cardiologist and a relevant specialist (e.g., neurologist) and active collaboration with the patient are key in decision-making regarding PFO management. Patients ages 18–65 years with a confirmed cryptogenic stroke, transient ischemic attack, or systemic embolism with a high probability of a causal role of their PFO should undergo percutaneous PFO closure (Figs. 64.1 and 64.2) [2].

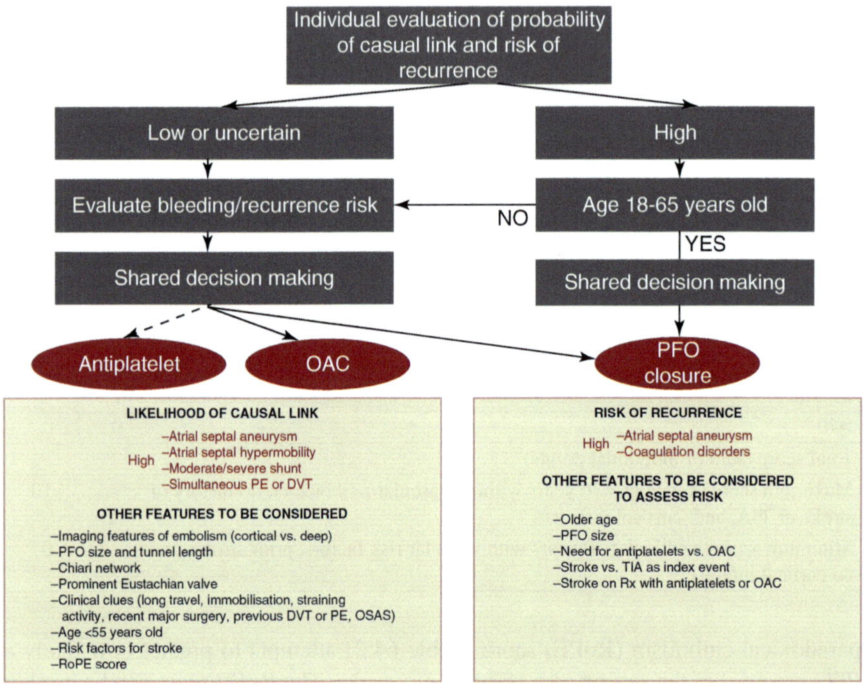

Fig. 64.1 Treatment algorithm for secondary prevention of left circulation cryptogenic thromboembolism

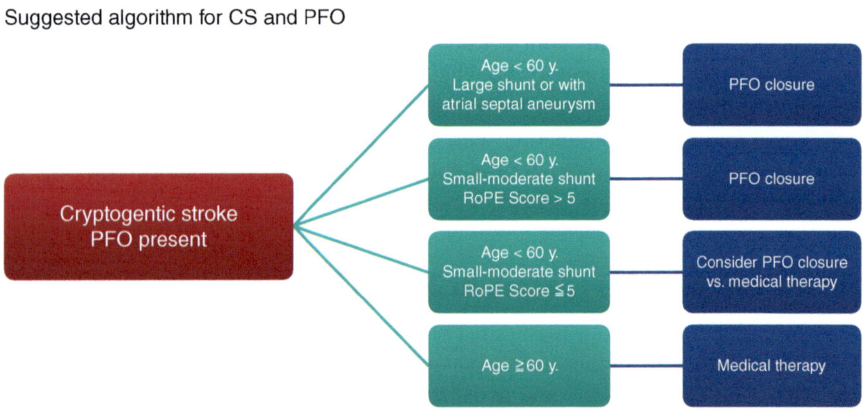

Fig. 64.2 Approach to the PFO closure in patients with cryptogenic stroke

Procedural Technique

After loading ASA 325 mg and Clopidogrel 600 mg, under local anesthesia, right femoral artery and vein sheaths (6F) was inserted. IV Heparin injected to achieve ACT >200 s. Crossing the PFO with 0.035 inch j tip wire and the Multipurpose catheter was performed which its tip was in LUPV (in our center, during the procedure, TEE is not obligatory except in especial ones, like those with suspicious concomitant fenestrations or large aneurysmal IAS; also sizing balloon is not use). After exchanging the wire with Amplatzer Superstiff wire, the delivery sheath (Occlutech 10F) was passed over the wire into the mid LA, after that, the dilator was removed to allow back bleed. According to the previous TEE data (large PFO-5 mm with ASA and tunnel length of 10 m), Occlutech Figulla II 31/35 was chosen. After loading the device and connecting to the delivery cable and fully de-aired, the device was passed through the delivery sheath to reach the tip of the sheath, then by retracting the sheath, the Left Disk (LD) was deployed, after that, the whole system was pulled back against the septum and finally, the Right Disk (RD) was deployed (Fig. 64.3). In fluoroscopy, Pacman sign (septum secundum must be between LD and RD- the cranial halves of the left and right atrial disks should appear like open jaws biting into the thick septum secundum) is confirming for the correct position of the device before release (Figs. 64.4 and 64.5).

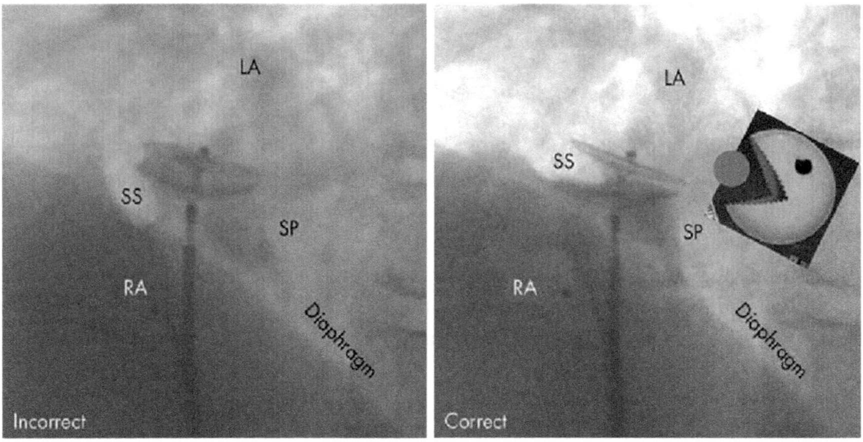

Fig. 64.3 Pacman sign

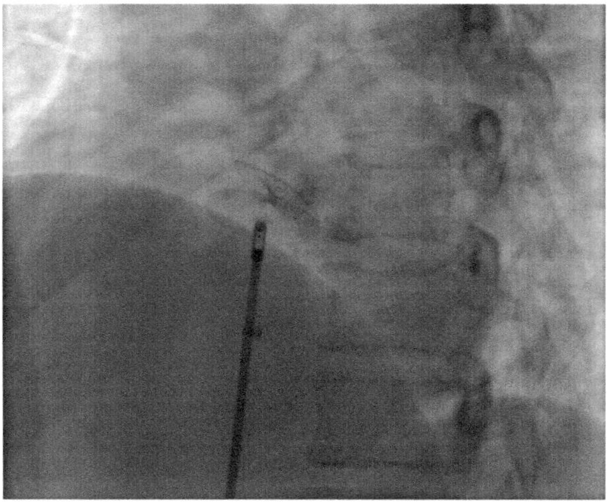

Fig. 64.4 After wiring the PFO, the device was deployed just like ASD closure

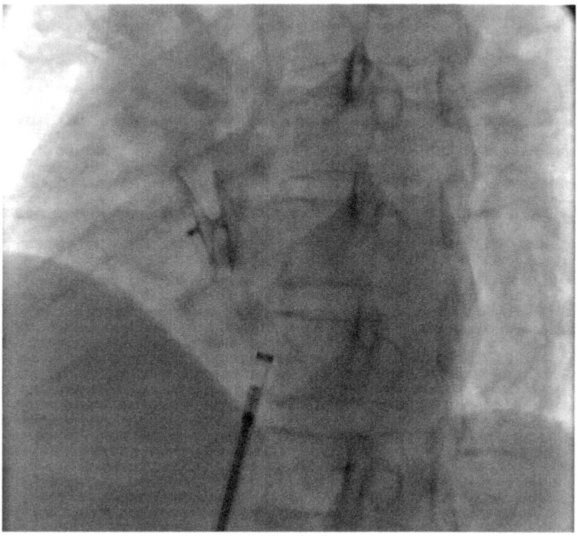

Fig. 64.5 The Occlutech (Figulla flex II). After releasing the device, Pacman sign is visualized

Conclusion

The pathophysiological link between PFO and neurological events is confused and contradictory and should be searched with great attention. It is certainly possible that some patients might benefit from PFO closure, but there is scant evidence to justify extensive PFO closure. A careful examination of clinical and anatomical risk factors for neurological recurrence is mandatory. In the absence of a clear scientific mandate, young patients with large PFO and recurrent CS and who are extensively worked up by a neurologist are the groups that is most likely to benefit from PFO closure [4]. Primary technical closure success approaches 100% and complete closure is seen in 93–96% at 1 year. The use of larger devices has a higher risk of residual shunts, the AMPLATZER™ PFO Occluder may have lower residual shunt rates than other devices. In on meta-analysis of RCTs with an average 3.8 years of follow-up, the incidence of recurrent stroke was 2% in the closure arms, and the number needed to treat (NNT) with PFO closure to prevent one stroke overall was 37 and 21 in patients with high-risk and low-risk PFO features [2]. Procedural complications had a 2.6% incidence in RCTs. The most frequent late complication is device thrombosis, which is seen in 1.0–2.0%. Device embolism is a serious event and occurs at a rate of 0.9–1.3%. Atrial wall erosions are serious events that have been reported anecdotally [2] (Table 64.3).

Table 64.3 PFO closure devices with CE MARK

Company name	Device name	Size (right/left disk)	Material
Abbott vascular	Amplatzer PFO occluder	18 mm (18/18 mm)/8 F 25 mm (25/18 mm}/8 F 30 mm (30/30 mm)/9 F 35 mm (35/25 mm)/9 F	Nitinol and polyester construction, recapturable and repositionable, self-centering
	Amplatzer multifenestrated septal occluder-Cribriform	18 mm (18/18 mm)/8 F 25 mm (25/25 mm)/8 F 30 mm (30/30 mm)/8 F 35 mm (35/25 mm)/9 F 40 mm (40/40 mm)/10 F	Nitinol and polyester construction; thin waist offers optimal fit and occlusion of the multifenestrated atrial septal defect
Cardia, Inc.	Ultrasept PFO occlude	20 mm/10 F 25 mm/10 F 30 mm/11 F 35 mm/11 F	Two ivalon (polyvinyl alcohol) discs supported by nitinol struts
Corned BV	Hyperion PFO occlude	18–18 mm/10 F 24–18 mm/10 F 28–22 mm/12 F 34–25 mm/12 F	Self-expandable PFO double occluder device made of 72 precocidized nitinol wires. Available with and without hub using an asymmetric and symmetric design
Gore & Associates	Cardioform septal occluder	20 mm (20/20 mm)/10 F 25 mm (25/25 mm)/10 F 30 mm (30/30 mm)/10 F	Minimal wire nitinol frame; thromboresistant ePTFE membrane allows tissue ingrowth; soft conformable design to reduce wall injury; folly retrievable even after tension-free assessment
Kiewei Rising	Amender PFO occluder	18–18, 25–18, 30–30 mm/5 F 35–25 mm/9 F	Nitinol wire polyester fabrics
Lepu Medial	MemoPart PFO ocduder	18–18, 18–24 mm/10 F 22–22, 25–34 mm/12 F	Self-expanding nitinol mesh double disc device
Lifetech Scientific	CeraFlex PFO occluder	18–18 mm/9 F 25–18 mm/10 F 25–25 mm/10 F 30–25 mm/12 F 30–30 mm/12 F 35–25 mm/14 F	Self-expandable PFO occluder device; all metallic structures are plated with titanium nitride

(continued)

Table 64.3 (continued)

Company name	Device name	Size (right/left disk)	Material
Nobles Medical Technologies II, Inc.	Noblestitch EL P, EL S, KwiKnot	1 size/12 F	Three devices provided in a single sterile kit for the release and attachment of suture in polypropylene 4-0 nonabsorbable
Occlutech International AB	Figulla Flex II	18/18 mm/7 F 23/25 mm/9 F 27/30 mm/9 F 31/55 mm/11 F	Double disc made of self-expandable nitinol wire covered by a ceramic titanium oxidate surface

References

1. Kent DM, Dahabreh IJ, Ruthazer R, et al. Device closure of patent foramen ovale after stroke: pooled analysis of completed randomized trials. J Am Coll Cardiol. 2016;67:907–17.
2. Christian P, Horst S, Fabrizio D, et al. European position paper on the management of patients with patent foramen ovale. General approach and left circulation thromboembolism. Eur Heart J. 2019;40(38):3182–95.
3. Kent DM, Ruthazer R, Weimar C, et al. An index to identify stroke-related vs incidental patent foramen ovale in cryptogenic stroke. Neurology. 2013;81:619–25.
4. Gabriella F, Scipione C, et al. How to understand patent foramen ovale clinical significant – Part II: therapeutic strategies in cryptogenic stroke. J Cardiovasc Ecgogr. 2015;25(2):46–53.

Chapter 65
Transcatheter Patent Ductus Arteriosus (PDA) Device Closure

Ata Firouzi and Zahra Hosseini

Abstract PDA is accounts for 5-10% of all congenital heart disease. If detected in adulthood usually present with LV volume overload or Eisenmenger syndrome. If, there is no contraindication for closure and anatomically be suitable, trans-catheter device closure is the preferred option. The success rate is high and actually residual shunt would disappear within weeks to months.

History

The patient was a 21 years old lady (the known case of CHD with no follow-up) who was referred with complaint of exertional dyspnea and palpitation since 2 years ago. In TTE a large PDA was detected, so she was scheduled for RHC and device closure if it was suitable.

In children who were born at term, the incidence of PDA has been reported to be ≈1 in 2000 births. This accounts for ≈5–10% of all congenital heart disease. However, if we include children with "silent" PDA, the incidence has been estimated to be as high as 1 in 500. The female to male ratio is ≈2:1 in most reports. The ductus arteriosus connects the left pulmonary artery near its origin to the descending aorta just after the left subclavian artery origin. The PDA may persist in a wide variety of sizes and configurations (Fig. 65.1). Usually, the aortic end of the PDA is larger than the pulmonary artery end, which results in a somewhat conical configuration. The size, configuration, and relationship to the adjacent structures are important with respect to determine the resistance to blood flow (an important determinant in the degree of shunt) and also have important implications with regard to interventional closure [1].

Left-to-right shunt through the PDA results in pulmonary over-circulation and left heart volume overload. Increased pulmonary flow from the ductal shunting

A. Firouzi (✉) · Z. Hosseini
Interventional Cardiology, Cardiovascular Intervention Research Center, Rajaie Cardiovascular Medical and Research Center, Iran University of Medical Sciences, Tehran, Iran

M. Maleki, A. Alizadehasl (eds.), *Case-Based Clinical Cardiology*,
https://doi.org/10.1007/978-1-4471-7496-7_65

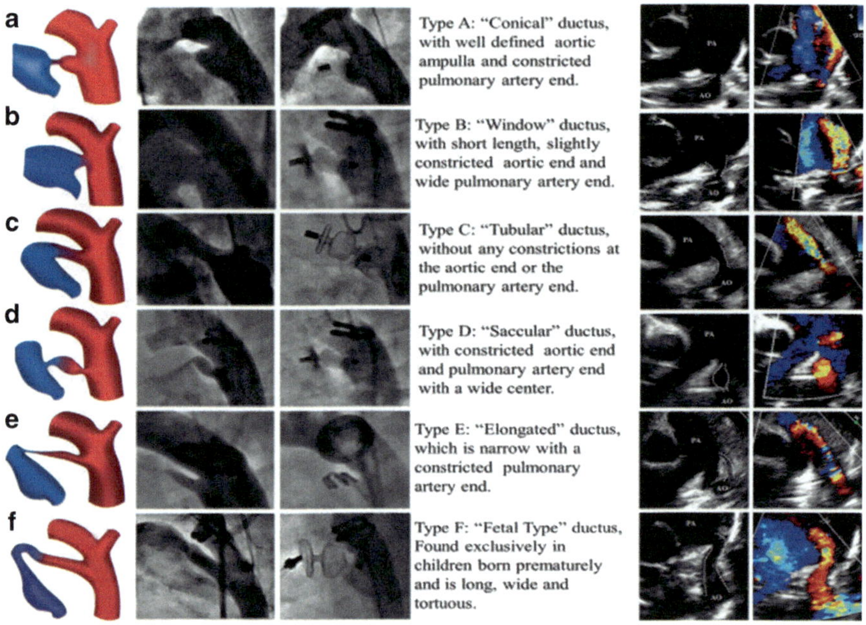

Fig. 65.1 Classification of PDAs based on their morphologies

leads to increase pulmonary fluid volume, and in patients with moderate or large shunts, this causes decreased lung compliance. With long-standing left-to-right shunt, exposure of the pulmonary artery system to high-pressure and increased flow leads to progressive morphological changes in the pulmonary vasculature and result in a progressive increase in pulmonary vascular resistance. When pulmonary vascular resistance approaches and exceeds systemic vascular resistance, ductal shunting reverses and becomes right to left. Most patients are asymptomatic and incidentally detected by TTE or typical murmur but some have congestive symptoms, endarteritis, arrhythmia, or Eisenmenger signs when presenting in adulthood.

Diagnostic Work-Up

The halmark finding in physical examination of these patients is continues machinery murmur at the upper LSB usually with trill and wide pulse pressure. Those with Eisenmenger syndrome are cyanotic with differential cyanosis, minimal murmur, loud P2 sound, RV heave, and sometimes TR or PI murmur. ECG in moderate size PDA shows LVH and strain pattern and in those with Eisenmenger syndrome, right axis deviation and biventricular hypertrophy are seen. TTE is the first diagnostic modality that can detect silent, small, moderate, and large ones, hemodynamic effects, the direction of the shunt, LV and RV sizes and functions and PAP. In those with elevated PVR, the detection of PDA with color Doppler even in large types could be difficult. Fully assessment for the detection of other concomitant anomalies should be performed.

Indications and Contraindications for PDA Closure [2]

ACC-AHA Guideline 2018

COR	LOE	Recommendations
Diagnostic		
I	C-EO	1. Measurement of oxygen saturation should be performed in feet and both hands in adults with a PDA to assess for the presence of right-to-left shunting.
IIa	C-EO	2. In addition to the standard diagnostic tools, cardiac catheterization can be useful in patients with PDA and suspected pulmonary hypertension (Section 3.5).
Therapeutic		
I	C-LD	3. PDA closure in adults is recommended if left atrial or LV enlargement is present and attributable to PDA with net left-to-right shunt, PA systolic pressure less than 50% systemic and pulmonary vascular resistance less than one third systemic.[54.1.5-1-54.1.5.3]
IIb	B-NR	4. PDA closure in adults may be considered in the presence of a net left-to-right shunt if PA systolic pressure is 50% or greater systemic, and/or pulmonary vascular resistance is greater than one third systemic.[54.1.5-3-54.1.5.4]
III: Harm	C-LD	5. PDA closure should not be performed in adults with a net right-to-left shunt and PA systolic pressure greater than two thirds systemic or pulmonary vascular resistance greater than two thirds systemic.[54.1.5-5]

RHC

- Qp/Qs: 2.7
- PVR: 3 WU
- SVR: 110 WU
- BP: 110/50 mm Hg
- PAP: 60/30 mm Hg
- PCWP: 20 mm Hg
- mRAP: 12 mm Hg

Procedural Technique

After right femoral artery and vein sheaths (6F) insertion and IV Heparin injection to achieve ACT > 200 s, angiography of LV (Fig. 65.2), Ascending and descending aorta in RAO and Lateral projections was done to estimate the size and shape of the PDA (in this case, it was window type with pulmonary end size about 18 mm, Figs. 65.2, 65.3 and 65.4). After crossing the PDA from the pulmonary end with straight 0.035 inch guide-wire and Multipurpose catheter (Figs. 65.5 and 65.6), the wire exchanged with long Amplatzer Superstiff wire. Under fluoroscopy the long delivery sheath (Cook 12) was advanced to the descending aorta, the dilator was removed and allowed back bleed. According to the shape and the size of the PDA,

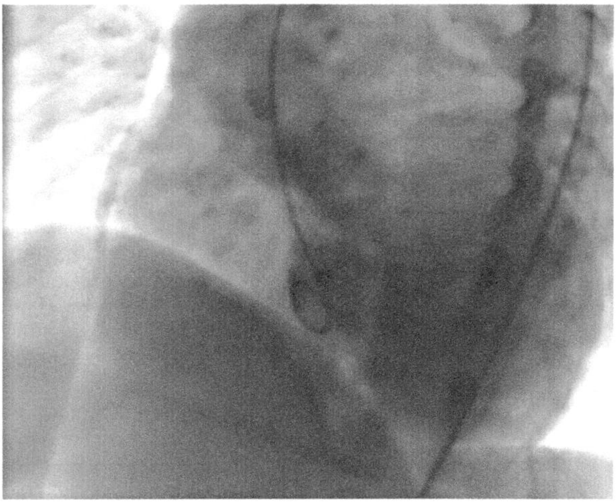

Fig. 65.2 LV injection showed: moderate LV enlargement, no VSD

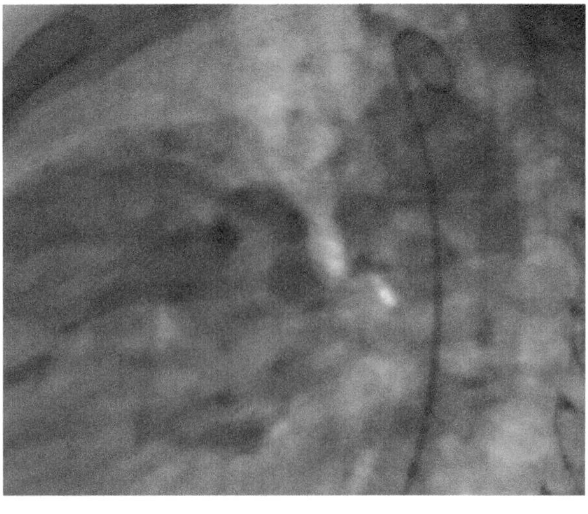

Fig. 65.3 During descending aorta injection in lateral projection, a large window type PDA with PA contrast opacification is noticeable

Muscular VSD 20 mm (Occlutech device Fig. 65.7) was chosen, (although in most cases, ductal occluder devices such as Occlutech or Amplatzer designs are chosen-Fig. 65.8a, b). After loading the delivery cable and connecting the cable to the hub and retraction of the whole device to the loader (slenderized the device) and fully flushed with heparinized saline, the loader was connected to the delivery sheath and the device was being passed through the delivery sheath. In the descending aorta, the delivery sheath was retraced slowly to expose the Left Disk (LD) then whole the system as a unit was pulled back slowly to reach the defect (under fluoroscopy with aortic injection in LAO, Fig. 65.9), when the correct position of LD was confirmed,

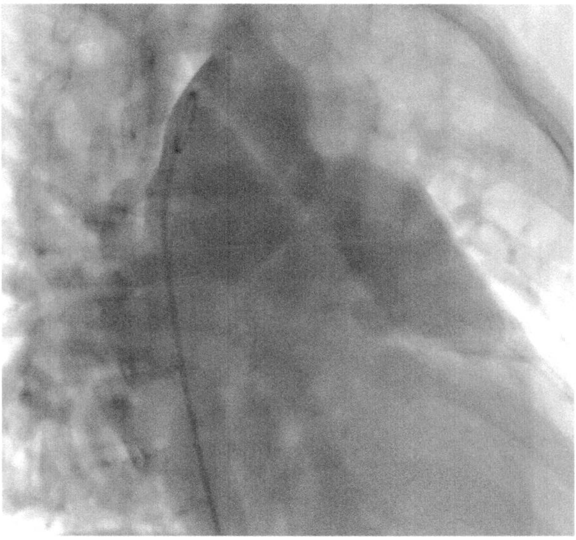

Fig. 65.4 Descending aorta injection in RAO, confirmed the shape and size of the PDA

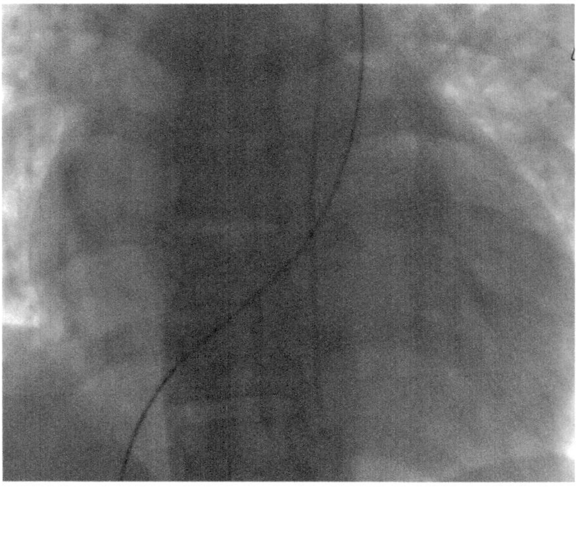

Fig. 65.5 Catheterization coarse: Right FV → IVC → RA → RV → PA → PDA → Descending aorta

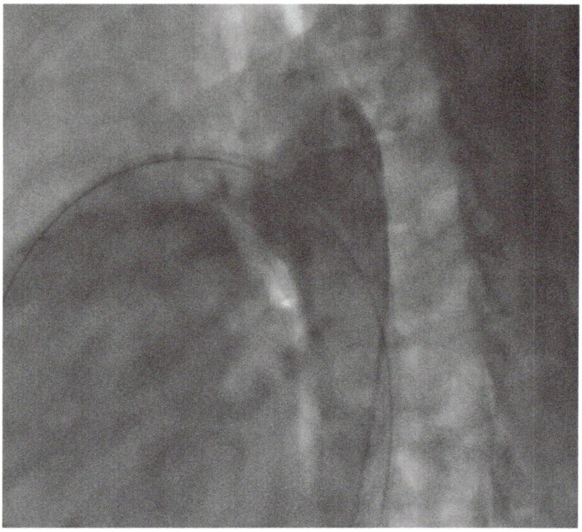

Fig. 65.6 After the passage of the long sheath through the PDA and aortic injection, the shape and the size of the PDA were estimated and the Muscular VSD device 20 mm Occlutech occluder was chosen

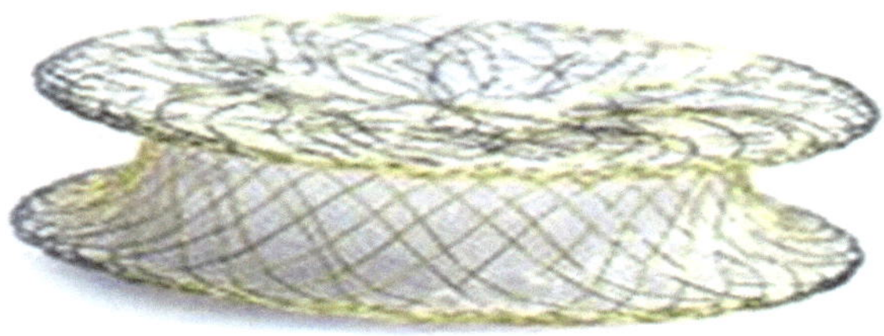

Fig. 65.7 Muscular VSD occluder device for window types PDA

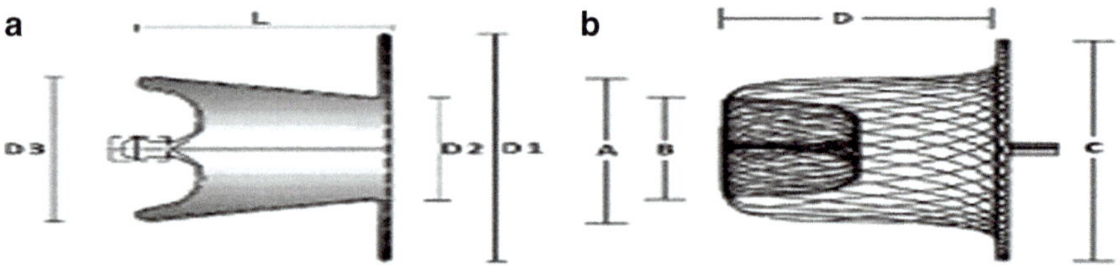

Fig. 65.8 Ductal occluder device for conical types PDA (**a**: Occlutech design, **b**: Amplatzer design)

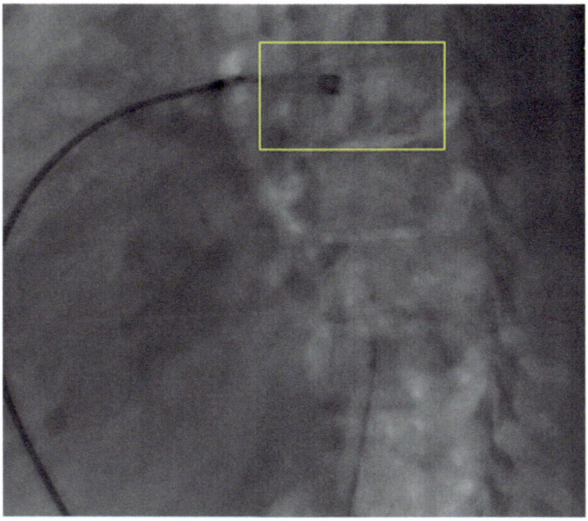

Fig. 65.9 In the descending aorta, the delivery sheath is retracted slowly to expose the Left Disk (LD) then whole the system as a unit was pulled back slowly to reach the defect (under fluoroscopy with aortic injection)

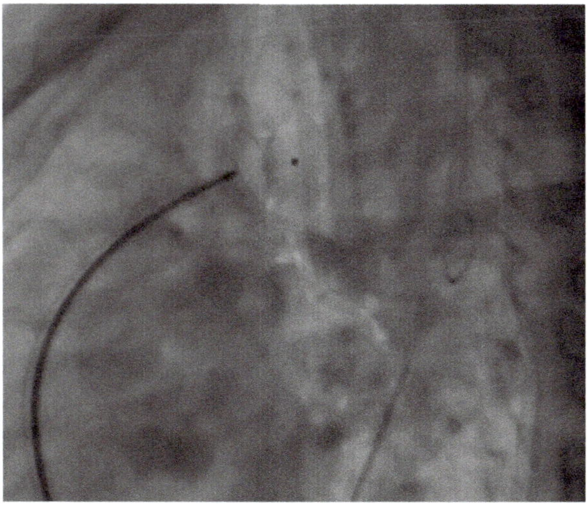

Fig. 65.10 When the correct position of LD was confirmed, delivery sheath was retracted to deploy the waist and finally the Right Disk (RD)

the delivery sheath was retracted to deploy the waist and finally the Right Disk (RD) (Fig. 65.10). After multiple injections in LAO and RAO views and being sure about the stable position of the device, the device was released (Fig. 65.11). Final injection showed mild residual shunt (Fig. 65.12).

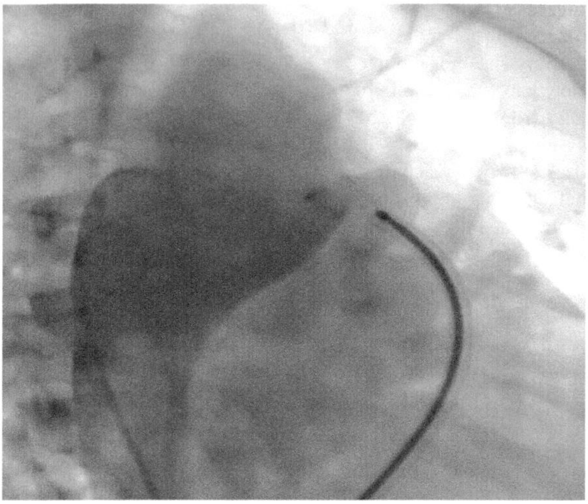

Fig. 65.11 Aortic injection, before releasing the device, showed the proper position of the device with mild residual shunt

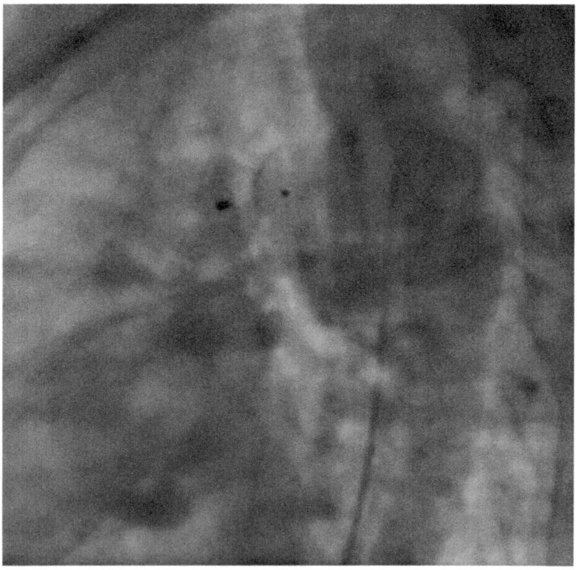

Fig. 65.12 Final angiography after releasing the device showed a moderate residual shunt

Conclusion

Results of transcatheter occlusion of PDA have been excellent. Complete closure rates at follow-up generally exceed 90–95% in most studies. As a result of device modifications, the evolution of new techniques, and increased operator skill, success rates for complete closure have improved significantly over time. Serious complications of transcatheter closure of the PDA are rare. The most common complications are device embolization, flow disturbance in the proximal left pulmonary artery or descending aorta from a protruding device, hemolysis from high-velocity residual shunting, femoral artery or vein thrombosis related to vascular access, and infection [3].

References

1. Carlgren LE. The incidence of congenital heart disease in children born in Gothenburg 1941–1950. Br Heart J. 1959;21:40–50.
2. 2018-AHA/ACC Guideline for the Management of Adults with Congenital Heart Disease. A Report of the American College of Cardiology/American Heart Association Task Force on Clinical Practice Guidelines. Circulation. 2019;139:e698–800. https://doi.org/10.1161/CIR.0000000000000603.
3. Rao PS. Summary and comparison of patent ductus arteriosus closure methods. In: Rao PS, Kern MJ, editors. Catheter based devices for the treatment of non-coronary cardiovascular disease in adults and children. Philadelphia, PA: Lippincott Williams & Wilkins; 2003. p. 219–28.

Chapter 66
Transcatheter Perimembranous VSD Device Closure

Ata Firouzi and Zahra Hosseini

Abstract The prevalence of VSD in adults is lower than the other defects with left to right shunts. When is detected in adulthood, it may cause LV volume overload or can be lead to Eisenmenger syndrome. It is off-label to close the perimembranous type (the most common type) percutaneously. But by recent advances in device types, it seems that trans-catheter closure of this type of VSD can be done safely with low complications.

History

The patient was a 32 years old man who was referred with complaints of exertional dyspnea and orthopnea since 2 years ago and recently with nocturnal palpitation. In TTE a large perimembranous VSD with mild AI was detected.

Isolated VSD accounts for 37% of all congenital heart disease in children. Because as many as 90% eventually closed spontaneously; the incidence is significantly lower in adults. Multiple synonyms have been classified and categorized VSDs into four major groups:

- Type 1: (Infundibular, outlet) This VSD is located below the semilunar valves (aortic and pulmonary) in the outlet septum of the right ventricle above the crista supraventricularis that is why sometimes also referred to as supra-cristal. It is the most uncommon type representing only 6% of all VSDs with the exception being in the Asian population where it accounts for approximately 30%. Aortic valve prolapse and regurgitation are common because of loss of support of the right and/or the noncoronary cusps of the aortic valve. It is unusual for these defects to close spontaneously.
- Type 2: (membranous) This VSD is, by far the most common type, accounting for 80% of all defects. It is located in the membranous septum inferior to the

A. Firouzi (✉) · Z. Hosseini
Interventional Cardiology, Cardiovascular Intervention Research Center, Rajaie Cardiovascular Medical and Research Center, Iran University of Medical Sciences, Tehran, Iran

M. Maleki, A. Alizadehasl (eds.), *Case-Based Clinical Cardiology*,
https://doi.org/10.1007/978-1-4471-7496-7_66

crista supraventricularis. It often involves the muscular septum when it is commonly known as perimembranous. The septal leaflet of the tricuspid valve sometimes forms a "pouch" that reduces the shunt and can result in spontaneous closure.

- Type 3: (Inlet or atrio-ventricular canal) This VSD is located just inferior to the inlet valves (tricuspid and mitral) within the inlet part of the right ventricular septum. It only represents 8% of all defects.
- Type 4: (muscular, trabecular) This VSD is located in the muscular septum, bordered by muscle usually in the apical, central, and outlet parts of the interventricular septum. They can be multiple, assuming a "Swiss cheese" appearance. They represent up to 20% of VSDs in infants. However, the incidence is lower in adults due to the tendency of spontaneous closure [1].

The presentation of unrepaired VSDs is dependent on the presence of hemodynamically significant shunt; that it is directly related to the size of the defect. Small VSDs only lead to minimal left-to-right shunt without hemodynamic effects; they are usually asymptomatic. Medium size VSDs result in a moderate LV volume overload and mild PAH; they present late in childhood with some congestive symptoms. Those with large defects develop CHF early in childhood due to severe LV overload and severe PAH and finally Eisenmenger syndrome which occurs in approximately 10–15% of patients. These patients present with dyspnea, cyanosis, syncope, palpitation, and sudden cardiac death.

Diagnostic Work-Up

In small size VSDs, a loud and harsh pansystolic murmur is heard in LSB, but it gets softer with increasing the size of the defects, and eventually, the typical murmur will be absent in the large ones with accentuated P2 sound. ECG shows LVH in moderate size defects. In those with Eisenmenger syndrome, right axis deviation and RVH is seen. TTE is the essential tool for the detection of VSDs (defect size, numbers, location, the relationship of the VSD with other structures, hemodynamic effects, LV and RV size and function, associated anomalies, and PAP).

Indications and Contraindications of VSD Closure (Table 66.1)

RHC

- Qp/Qs: 2.5
- PVR: 2 WU
- SVR: 120 WU
- PAP: 55/20 mm Hg

Table 66.1 AHA/ACC 2018 guideline

COR	LOE	Recommendations
Therapeutic		
I	B-NR	1. Adults with a VSD and evidence of left ventricular volume overload and hemodynamically significant shunts (Qp:Qs ≥ 1.5:1) should undergo VSD closure, if PA systolic pressure is less than 50% systemic and pulmonary vascular resistance is less than one third systemic.[54.1.3-1]
IIa	C-LD	2. Surgical closure of perimembranous or supracristal VSD is reasonable in adults when there is worsening aortic regurgitation (AR) caused by VSD.[54.1.3-1.54.1.3-2]
IIb	C-LD	3. Surgical closure of VSD may be reasonable in adults with a history of IE caused by VSD if not otherwise contraindicated.[54.1.3-3]
IIb	C-LD	4. Closure of a VSD may be considered in the presence of a net left-to-right shunt (Qp:Qs ≥ 1.5:1) when PA systolic pressure is 50% or more than systemic and/or pulmonary vascular resistance is greater than one third systemic.[54.1.3-4-54.1.3.6]
III: Harm	C-LD	5. VSD closure should not be performed in adults with severe PAH with PA systolic pressure greater than two third systemic, pulmonary vascular resistance greater than two thirds systemic and/or a net right-to-left shunt.[54.1.3-7-54.1.3.9]

- RVSP: 55/12 mm Hg
- mRAP: 12 mm Hg
- So2: 95%

Transcatheter PM-VSD Device Closure

Right femoral artery and vein sheaths (6F) were inserted then IV Heparin was completed to achieve ACT > 200 s. After LV injection in LAO 60-Cranial20 in order to profile the defect (Fig. 66.1a), Under general anesthesia, in retrograde approach, the VSD was crossed from LV via JR and 0.035 inch hydrophilic guide-wire (in some cases based on the location of the defects, another tip angled catheters like IMA or cutoff pigtail are used). After crossing the defect with the wire and the catheter that was being passed through it and inserted in the LPA, the wire was exchanged with long 260 cm Terumo wire. Through venous access,

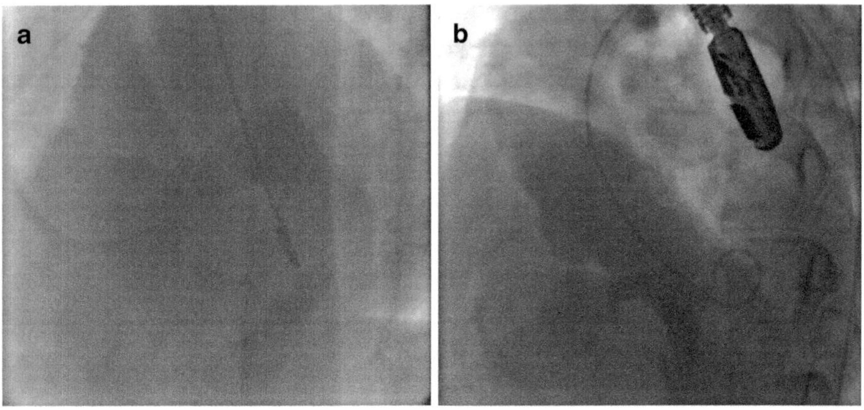

Fig. 66.1 (**a**, **b**) LV and aortic root angiography showed, a large perimembranous VSD with RV opacification

a pigtail catheter without guide-wire was inserted in the same pulmonary artery that the Terumo wire was passed (to reduce the interference with the Tricuspid valve chordae), then the pigtail was exchanged with JR guiding catheter. To make an arterio-venous loop, the guide-wire was then snared and exteriorized via venous access. A Delivery sheath (10F) was advanced carefully to RV, LV, and aortic arch with Kissing catheter technique (Fig. 66.1b). Then dilator was removed from the vein access and guide-wire and the end hole catheter were removed from the arterial line. Under TEE guiding and expert echo-man, according to the defect size (8 mm - largest diastolic phase on LV side) and acceptable distance between the defect and the aortic cusps, Membranous VSD Occluder (Cera Lifetech symmetric) device 10 mm was chosen. After the device was screwed to the delivery cable and de-aired, it passed through the long sheath and under TEE and fluoroscopy guidance, first Left disk was partially opened in ascending aorta and gently pulled back through the AV to the LV (Fig. 66.2a) and slowly, by retracting the delivery sheath and fully deploying distal disk at the LV side of VSD, the entire system was then pulled back into the defect (Fig. 66.2b) and the sheath was retracted to deploy the waist and finally after confirming the right position of the device by TEE and LV injection, the proximal (Right disk) was deployed (Fig. 66.2c). The operator must fully check the position and stability of the device without any compromising of the surrounding structures. If there is any doubt about the impingent of the valves or other structures, the device should be recaptured. If the device position is correctly confirmed by the TEE and angiography, it can be released by unscrewing it using pin vice (Fig. 66.3a, b). In this case, the AI severity or TR was not increased without any conduction abnormality.

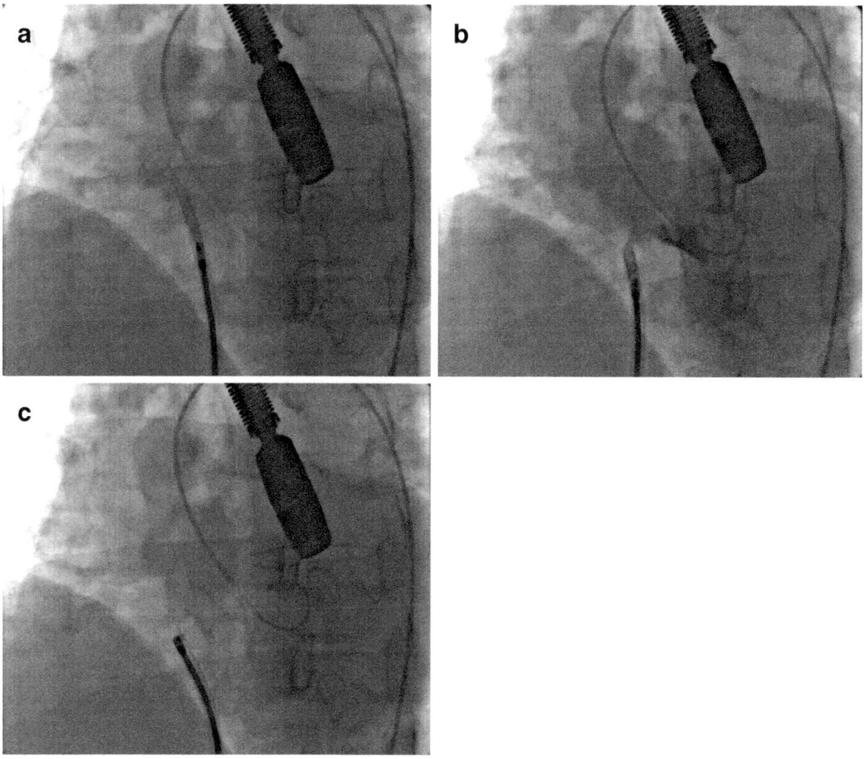

Fig. 66.2 (**a**, **b**, **c**) According to the defect size (8 mm - largest diastolic phase on LV side) and acceptable distance between the defect and the aortic cusps, Membranous VSD Occluder (Cera Lifetech symmetric) device 10 mm was chosen. first Left Disk was partially opened in the ascending aorta and gently pulled back through the AV to the LV and slowly, by retracting the delivery sheath and fully deploying distal disk at the LV side of VSD, the entire system was then pulled back into the defect and the sheath was retracted to deploy the waist and finally after confirming the right position of the device by TEE and LV injection, the proximal (Right Disk) was deployed

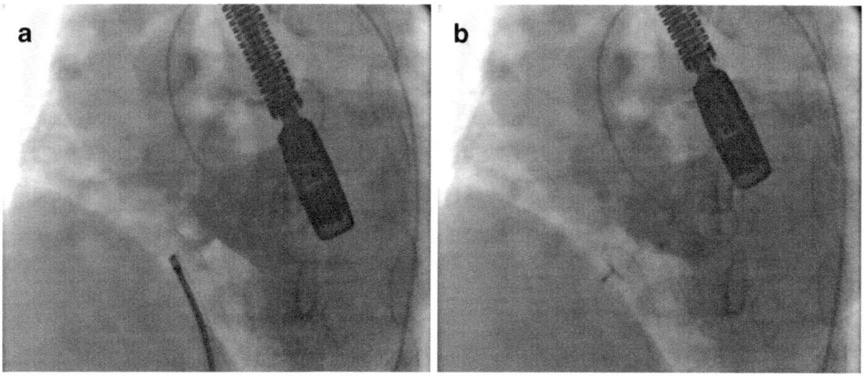

Fig. 66.3 (**a**, **b**) After confirming the right position of the device with no interaction with surrounding structures, the device was released and final LV angiography showed tiny residual shunt

Conclusion

Percutaneous closure of PM-VSD is a challenging procedure, owing to variable anatomical morphology, proximity to valves and conduction systems as well as complex manipulation process. The major key to improve the results of this treatment, while minimizing complications (such as: CHB, device embolization, valvular malfunction, and hemolysis) consists in the careful case and device selections as well as accurate defect sizing strategy [2].

References

1. Lopez L, Houyel L, Colan SD, Anderson RH, Béland MJ, Aiello VD, Bailliard F, Cohen MS, Jacobs JP, Kurosawa H, Sanders SP, Walters HL, Weinberg PM, Boris JR, Cook AC, Crucean A, Everett AD, Gaynor JW, Giroud J, Guleserian KJ, Hughes ML, Juraszek AL, Krogmann ON, Maruszewski BJ, St Louis JD, Seslar SP, Spicer DE, Srivastava S, Stellin G, Tchervenkov CI, Wang L, Franklin RCG. Classification of ventricular septal defects for the eleventh iteration of the international classification of diseases-striving for consensus: a report from the international society for nomenclature of paediatric and congenital heart disease. Ann Thorac Surg. 2018;106(5):1578–89.
2. Behzad Alizadeh. Transcatheter closure of congenital VSDs: tips and tricks, angiography. Burak Pamukçu, IntechOpen. 2019. https://doi.org/10.5772/intechopen.83641. https://www.intechopen.com/books/angiography/transcatheter-closure-of-congenital-vsds-tips-and-tricks

Chapter 67
Percutaneous Pulmonary Valve Commissurotomy (PTPC)

Ata Firouzi and Zahra Hosseini

Abstract Isolated valvular PS, is a commissural fusion with domed shape leaflets. Adults are usually asymptomatic and it progress gradually in these patients. In those with severe stenosis and RV pressure overload, if missed, it leads eventually to RV failure, although this event is rarely happened. The choice procedure is trans-catheter commissurotomy with appropriate balloons. The procedure is safe with minimal complications.

History

The patient was a 40 years old lady who was referred with complaints of exertional dyspnea for 6 months and one episode of syncope during an exercise last week. According to ECG and TTE, Isolated severe PS was diagnosed.

Isolated valvular Pulmonary Stenosis (PS) comprises approximately 10% of all congenital heart disease. Typically, the valve commissures are partially or completely fused and the three leaflets are thin and pliant, resulting in a dome-shaped structure and rarely dysplastic leaflets with a narrowed central orifice. Post-stenotic pulmonary artery dilatation may occur owing to "jet-effect" hemodynamics which is a good predictor of successful interventional treatment [1]. Most children and adults with mild-to-moderate RVOT obstruction are asymptomatic. Moderate valvular PS can progress in 20% of unoperated patients especially in adults. Those with severe PS may experience exertional dyspnea, chest pain (RV ischemia), fatigue, palpitation, syncope, cyanosis, or sudden cardiac death. Peripheral edema and other signs of RV failure may occur in advanced cases particularly in later life due to RV pressure overload, elevated RV End Diastolic Pressure (RVEDP), diminished RV

A. Firouzi (✉) · Z. Hosseini
Interventional Cardiology, Cardiovascular Intervention Research Center, Rajaie Cardiovascular Medical and Research Center, Iran University of Medical Sciences, Tehran, Iran

M. Maleki, A. Alizadehasl (eds.), *Case-Based Clinical Cardiology*,
https://doi.org/10.1007/978-1-4471-7496-7_67

compliance, elevated RA pressure and Tricuspid regurgitation. Cyanosis is present in those with significant right-to-left shunt via a patent foramen oval, atrial septal defect, or ventricular septal defect.

Diagnostic Work-Up

The diagnostic findings in physical exam are systolic ejection murmur in the second left intercostal space that its severity is correlated with duration, late systolic peaking murmur and diminished P2. ECG in severe cases demonstrates evidence of RVH and RA enlargement. TTE is the essential tool for diagnosis: in severe cases, RV and RA enlargement with D-shaped septum, moderate-to-severe TR which can estimate the RV systolic pressure (RVSP), fused and domed shape PV with narrowing orifice and post-stenotic PA dilatation is seen. Another anomalies like ASD, PFO, VSD, PDA, subvalvular or peripheral PS, Aortic Stenosis, and evaluation of all other valves should be considered. The key finding for selecting the appropriate size balloon is the hinge to hinge annulus diameter.

Indications for Valvular PS Intervention in Adults (Tables 67.1 and 67.2)

RHC (Right Heart Catheterization)

- RVSP: 130/15 mm Hg
- PAP: 25/10 mm Hg
- Trans-valvular gradient: 105 mm Hg
- mRAP: 18 mm Hg
- CI: 2.3 L/min
- So2: 95%

Table 67.1 Pulmonary valve stenosis severity

Mild	Peak gradient <36 mm Hg (peak velocity <3 m/s)
Moderate	Peak gradient 36–64 mm Hg (peak velocity 3–4 m/s)
Severe	Peak gradient 64 mm Hg (peak velocity >4 m/s); mean gradient >35 mm Hg

Table 67.2 Management of patients with pulmonary valve stenosis- ACC-AHA 2018 guideline

COR	LOE	Recommendations
I	B-NR	1. In adults with moderate or severe valvular pulmonary stenosis and otherwise unexplained symptoms of HF, cyanosis from interatrial right-to-left communication, and/or exercise intolerance, balloon valvuloplasty is recommended.[54.3.1.1-54.3.1-4]
I	B-NR	2. In adults with moderate or severe valvular pulmonary stenosis and otherwise unexplained symptoms of HF, cyanosis and/or exercise intolerance who are ineligible for or who failed balloon valvuloplasty, surgical repair is recommended.[54.3.1-1,54.3.1-5-54.3.1-8]
IIa	C-EO	3. In asymptomatic adults with severe valvular pulmonary stenosis, intervention is reasonable.

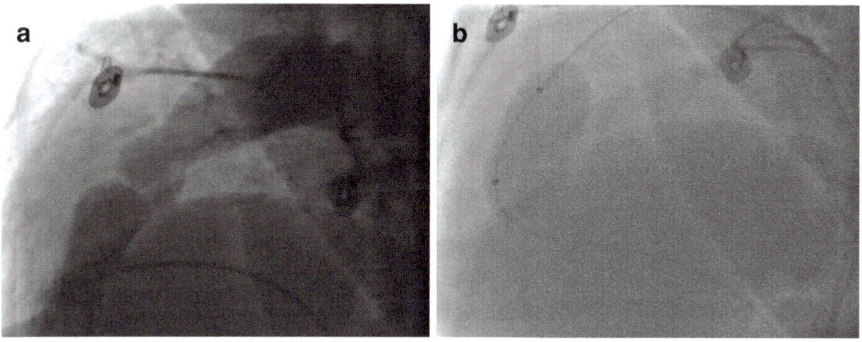

Fig. 67.1 (**a**, **b**) RV angiography in lateral projection showed thick and dome-shaped PV with post-stenotic PA dilatation. Commissurotomy was performed in lateral projection with Numed II 24*40 (Annulus diameter: 20 mm) successfully with complete disappearance of the waist

Procedural Technique

After insertion of two femoral arterial and venous sheaths (6F) and RHC during local anesthesia, RV injections in AP and lateral projections showed severe RVH and enlargement combined with thick, dome-shaped PV and post-stenotic PA dilatation (Fig. 67.1a). In fluoroscopy, the hinge to hinge annulus diameter was 20 mm (in TTE: 21 mm), so as we can choose the balloon size, 110–140% of annulus size, Numed II 24*40 balloon was chosen. After crossing the PV with 0.035 inch 260 cm long guide-wire with over which pigtail catheter was tracked, the wire was replaced with 0.035 inch Amplatzer Superstiff 260 long guide-wire in LPA, then after adjusting the site of the valve and the balloon in the lateral view, the balloon was inflated with diluted contrast by PTMC syringe until the waste disappeared (Fig. 67.1b), the most important issue in this step is stabilizing the balloon in its position (no slippage). Each inflation–deflation time should not take more than 10 s (with closed hemodynamic monitoring). After the procedure, via Multipurpose catheter the final transvalvular gradient was measured, the gradient was more than 30 mm Hg, again the procedure was repeated with higher pressure inflation (It can repeat up to eight times) or with larger balloons. Residual transvalvular gradient between 20 and 30 mm Hg is acceptable.

PTPC is currently the preferred therapeutic modality for valvular PS in children and adults. Current approaches of PTPC utilize various fixed size balloon catheters using a single or a double-balloon technique. Regardless of the type of balloons, long-term outcomes were good over the first 20 years and those with surgical approach seemed to have more reintervention 20–40 years after procedure, compared with those undergoing PTPC [2].

Anyway, PTPC is not without complications: annulus, RVOT or PA perforation, PI (mild-to-moderate in 10–40% of cases which rarely progress over time) or TR and transient subvalvular stenosis, although rare can happen.

Conclusion

Experience to date indicates that percutaneous balloon valvuloplasty is safe, effective, and can be performed at any age with good short- and long-term outcomes. Freedom of re-intervention (more often for restenosis as for insufficiency) is 95, 88, and 84% after 5, 10, and 20 years [3]. The limiting factor is the judgment of the balloon size to be used. We believe that our recent, more aggressive approach is achieving better results. Although hard and fast indications have not yet been established, it is currently our treatment of choice for congenital pulmonary valve stenosis [4].

References

1. Xiushui R, Lange R (ed.). Pulmonic stenosis, n.d.. Retrieved from http://emedicine.medscape.com/article/157737overview#showall
2. Voet A, Rega F, De Bruaene AV, et al. Long term outcome after treatment of isolated pulmonary valve stenosis. Int J Cardiol. 2012;156(1):11–5.
3. McCrindle BW. Independent predictors of long term results after balloon pulmonary valvuloplasty. Valvuloplasty and angioplasty of congenital anomalies (VACA) Registry investigators. Circulation. 1994;89:1759.
4. Rao PS. percutaneous ballon pulmonary valvuloplasty state of the art. Cath Cardiovasc Interv. 2007;69:747–63.

Chapter 68
Percutaneous Trans Mitral Valve Commissurotomy (PTMC)

Ata Firouzi and Zahra Hosseini

Abstract Rheumatic fever is the most common cause of Mitral Stenosis (MS). The pathologic finding in rheumatismal MS is commissural fusion with thickening and calcification of the leaflets and sub-valvular apparatus. The disaster sequelae of MS is systemic thromboembolism especially in cerebral vessels. TEE is the best tool which determine the treatment options. In the absence of absolute contraindications, PTMC is the first choice in symptomatic patients. In the long term outcome trials, is comparable to open commissurotomy.

History

The patient was a 40 years old lady, who was referred with complaints of exertional dyspnea and palpitation since one year ago. In TTE severe rheumatic MS was diagnosed.

The predominant cause of mitral stenosis is rheumatic fever, with rheumatic changes present in 99% of stenotic mitral valves excised at the time of mitral valve replacement. Approximately 25% of all patients with rheumatic heart disease have isolated MS, and approximately 40% have combined MS and mitral regurgitation (MR). Multivalve involvement is seen in 38% of patients with MS, with the aortic valve affected by approximately 35% and the tricuspid valve in approximately 6%. The pulmonic valve is rarely affected. Two-thirds of all patients with rheumatic MS are female. The interval between the initial episode of rheumatic fever and clinical evidence of mitral valve obstruction is variable, ranging from a few years to more than 20 years. Rheumatic fever results in characteristic changes of the mitral valve; diagnostic features are thickening at the leaflet edges, fusion of the commissures, and chordal shortening and fusion. The symmetric fusion of the commissures results in a small, central oval orifice in diastole that on pathologic specimens is shaped like

A. Firouzi (✉) · Z. Hosseini
Interventional Cardiology, Cardiovascular Intervention Research Center, Rajaie Cardiovascular Medical and Research Center, Iran University of Medical Sciences, Tehran, Iran

M. Maleki, A. Alizadehasl (eds.), *Case-Based Clinical Cardiology*,
https://doi.org/10.1007/978-1-4471-7496-7_68

a fish mouth or buttonhole because the anterior leaflet is not in the physiologic open position. The most useful descriptor of the severity of mitral valve obstruction is the degree of valve opening in diastole or the mitral valve orifice area. In normal adults, the cross-sectional area of the mitral valve orifice (MVA) is 4–6 cm^2. When the orifice is reduced to approximately 2 cm^2, which is considered to represent mild MS, blood can flow from the left atrium to the left ventricle only if propelled by a small, although abnormal, pressure gradient. When the mitral valve opening is reduced to 1 cm^2, which is considered to represent severe MS, a left atrio-ventricular (AV) pressure gradient of approximately 20 mm Hg (and therefore, with normal LV diastolic pressure, a mean LA pressure >25 mm Hg) is required to maintain normal cardiac output at rest [1] (Table 68.1).

In the early stage of the disease, the most common symptoms of these patients are exertional dyspnea, orthopnea, pulmonary edema, hemoptysis, palpitation (AF),

Table 68.1 MS severity

Stage	Definition	Valve anatomy	Valve hemodynamics	Hemodynamic consequences	Symptom
A	At rifle for MS	Mild valve doming during diastole	Normal transmittal flow velocity	None	None
B	Progressive MS	Rheumatic valve changes with commissural fusion and diastolic doming of mitral valve leaflets Planimetered MVA > 1.5 cm^2	Increased transmitral flow velocities MVA >1.5 cm^2 Diastolic pressure half-time <150 ms	Mild to moderate LA enlargement Normal pulmonary pressure at rest	None
C	Asymptomatic severe MS	Rheumatic valve changes with commissural fusion and diastolic doming of mitral valve leaflets Planimetered MVA $\leq$1.5 cm^2 (MVA $\leq$1 cm^1 with very severe MS)	MVA $\leq$1.5 cm^2 (MVA $\leq$1 cm^2 with very severe MS) Diastolic pressure half-time $\geq$150 ms (Diastolic pressure half-time $\geq$220 ms with very severe MS)	Severe LA enlargement Elevated RASP >30 mm Hg	None
D	Symptomatic severe MS	Rheumatic valve changes with commissural fusion and diastolic doming of mitral valve leaflets Planimetered MVA $\leq$1.5 cm^2	MVA $\leq$1.5 cm^2 (MVA $\leq$1 cm^2 with very severe MS) Diastolic pressure half-time $\geq$150 ms (Diastolic pressure half-time $\geq$225 ms with very severe MS)	Severe LA enlargement Elevated PASP >30 mm Hg	Decreased exercise tolerance Exertional dyspnea

and even systemic embolic events especially cerebral vessel emboli (may be as a first presenting symptom). With long-standing severe MS and elevated LA pressure, pulmonary hypertension (reactive or obliterative changes) will happen which consequently leads to RV failure and severe TR, in this stage, patients usually present with fatigue, peripheral edema, and low cardiac output states.

Diagnostic Work-Up

In physical exam, in the early stage of disease (pliable valve), S1 is audible but in severe and advanced cases with sinus rhythm when the leaflets are rigid and highly calcified, S1 sound and opening snap disappeared and the diastolic, rumbling murmur is audible in apex and persists until end diastole with presystolic accentuation. Systolic murmur of TR, diastolic murmur of PI and P2 accentuation may also be audible with RV heave in advanced cases. In ECG, AF rhythm, LA enlargement (90%) in sinus ones, and finally RA enlargement and RVH in PH patients are seen. TTE is the first diagnostic modality for evaluation of LV and RV size and functions, MS severity, Wilkins score (Table 68.2), other valvular disease, and PAP estimation. TEE is obligatory before PTMC for rule out LA-LAA clot, evaluation of MR severity, symmetric or asymmetric commissural fusion and the degree of leaflets and subvalvular apparatus calcification.

Table 68.2 Wilkins score

Grade	Mobility	Thickening	Calcification	Subvalvular thickening
1	Highly mobile valve with only one leaflet tips restricted	Leaflets near normal In thickness (4–5 mm)	A single area of increased echo brightness	Minimal thickening just below the mitral leaflets
2	Leaflet mid and base portions have normal mobility	Midleaflets normal considerable thickening of margins (5–8 mm)	Scattered areas of brightness confined to leaflet margins	Thickening of chordal structures extending to one-third of the chordal length
3	Valve continues to move forward in diastole, mainly from the base	Thickening extending through the entire leaflet (5–8 mm)	Brightness extending into the mid-portions of the leaflets	Thickening extended to distal third of the chords
4	No or minimal forward movement of the leaflets in diastole	Considerable thickening of all leaflet tissue (>8–10 mm)	Extensive brightness throughout much of the leaflet tissue	Extensive thickening and shortening of all chordal structures extending down to the papillary muscles

The total score is the sum of the four Items and ranges between 4 and 16

Management (Fig. 68.1)

Treatments

Diuretics, B-blockers, Calcium channel blockers (CCBs), and anticoagulants are the basic medical treatments of MS patients. According to the functional class, MS severity, PAP, and other echocardiographic findings, the final decision for the PTMC, surgical MV repair, or MVR (according to the above figure) is taken.

PTMC Procedure

The TEE should be done at least 48 h before the procedure to rule out any contraindications of PTMC (LA clot, moderate to severe MR, severe bi-commissural calcifications, absence commissural fusion, or any mass on IAS) and confirmed the suitability of the patient for PTMC. The INR should be less than 1.5 during the procedure.

Under local anesthesia, after the right femoral artery and vein sheaths (6F) insertion, LV injection in RAO was done to evaluate the mitral valve, subvalvular apparatus, and MR severity (Fig. 68.2a). The essential part of the procedure is septostomy. In the Angiographic method, in AP projection, one pigtail catheter is inserted in ascending aorta on the right coronary cusp and with another pigtail catheter, RA angiography with delayed phase is done to mark the lateral and inferior borders of

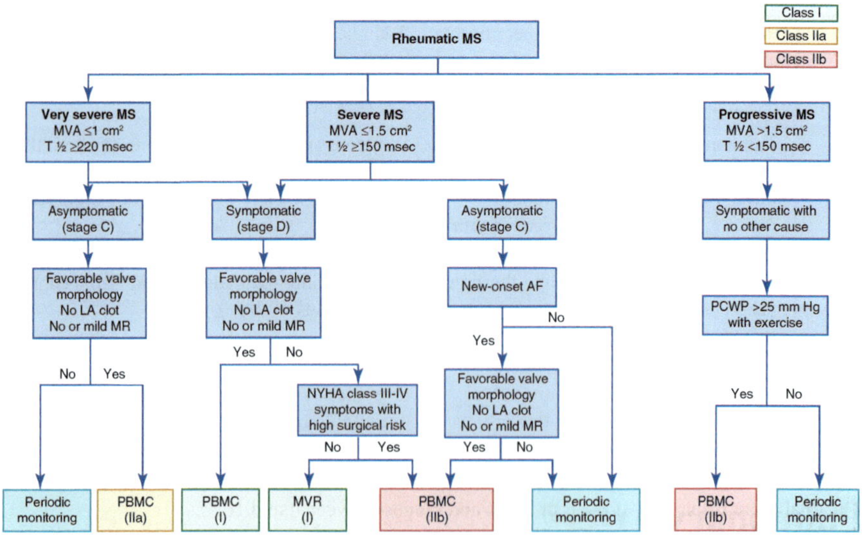

Fig. 68.1 Management of patients with mitral stenosis-AHA/ACC 2014

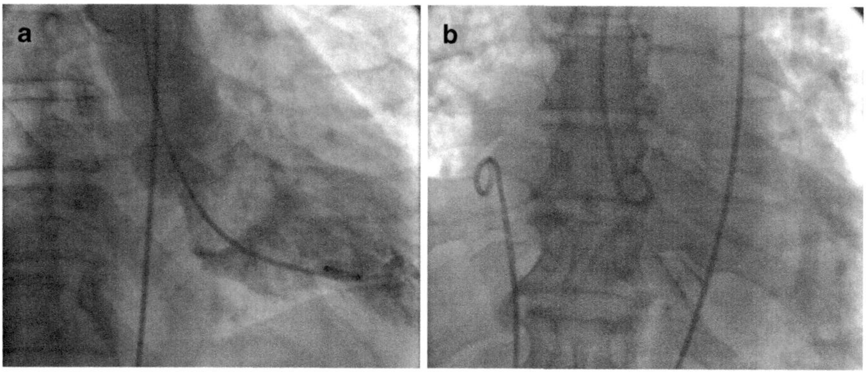

Fig. 68.2 (**a**, **b**) LV injection in RAO projection showed severe dome shape of the anterior mitral leaflet with no MR. In the Angiographic method, the LA border in levophase and the pigtail catheter in right coronary cusp as a marker of the lowest part of aorta and septal leaflet of the tricuspid valve. As previously described the catch point is localized

LA (Fig. 68.2b). The upper end of the tricuspid valve at systole (point T, marked as asterisk) is determined on a stop-frame frontal right atrial angiographic image (a) and translated to a stop-frame left atrial image (b). On the latter image, an imaginary horizontal line is drawn from point T to point L, where the line intersects the lateral border of the atrium encountered first (usually the left atrium). Point L is assumed to be the posterior limit of the septum. The dotted vertical line crossing at the midpoint between T and L is the "midline." In Fluoroscopic method (c), a horizontal line is drawn from the tip of the pigtail catheter (point A) to L, the left atrial silhouette (black arrows), to define the "midline." The dotted line indicates the right atrial silhouette [2] (Fig. 68.3).

The puncture site depends on the LA size, usually two-third above the lower border of LA (The best site is fossa ovalis) on the vertical line is chosen. The Mullins catheter is inserted via the right femoral vein over a 0.032 inch j tip guidewire into the SVC. The catheter is aspirated and flushed after the removal of the wire. Then, the Brockenbrough needle, which attached to the pressure connector, is inserted into the catheter and carefully advanced under fluoroscopic guidance until its tip reaches the predetermined position. The needle is allowed to rotate freely during its passage. The right hand stopper finger is now firmly kept between the catheter hub and the direction indicator of the needle to prevent the needle from moving forward. In AP view, the needle-fitted catheter with its direction indicator pointing at about 4 o'clock is slowly withdrawn downward (caudally) from the SVC. A clockwise rotation is applied to the direction indicator to align the catheter/needle on the "midline." The catheter/needle tip is further withdrawn until its tip reaches the target point (septal bounce is sense). Subsequently, the catheter-needle position is viewed in 30° RAO projection, to confirm optimal septal puncture site as well as to avoid puncture of the other structures. The catheter-needle tip is now seen usually just anterior to the vertebra, and inferior to ascending aorta. When the operator is satisfied with the intended puncture site, the catheter/

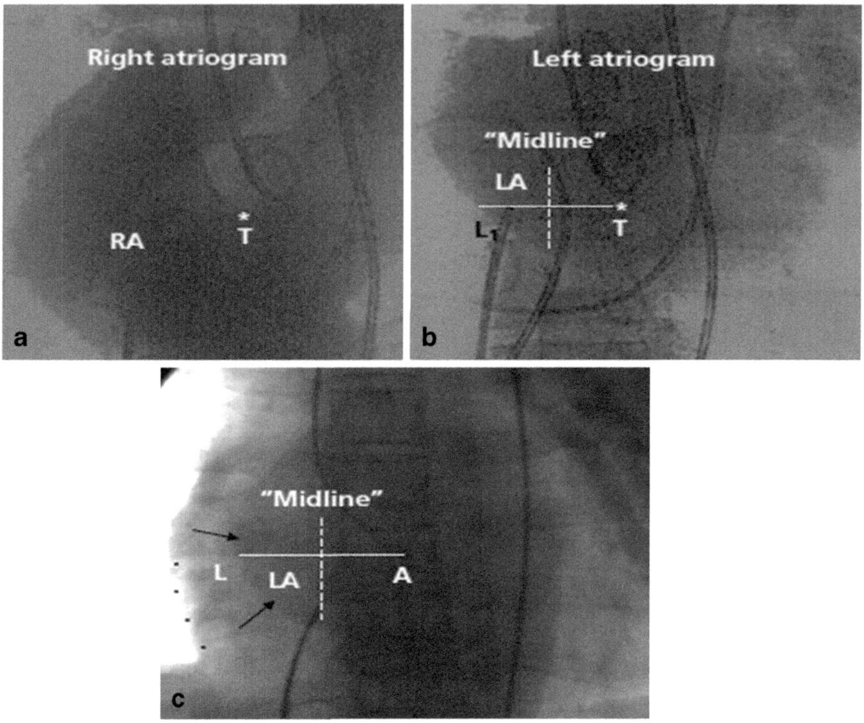

Fig. 68.3 The upper end of the tricuspid valve at systole (point T, marked as asterisk) is determined on a stop-frame frontal right atrial angiographic image (**a**) and translated to a stop-frame left atrial image (**b**). On the latter image, an imaginary horizontal line is drawn from point T to point L, where the line intersects the lateral border of the atrium encountered first (usually the left atrium). Point L is assumed to be the posterior limit of the septum. The dotted vertical line crossing at the midpoint between T and L is the "midline." In Fluoroscopic method (**c**), a horizontal line is drawn from the tip of the pigtail catheter (point A) to L, the left atrial silhouette (black arrows), to define the "midline." The dotted line indicates the right atrial silhouette

needle is pressed firmly against the septum. While keeping the catheter firmly against the septum to prevent it from slipping away from the puncture site, the operator releases the stopper finger and advances the needle forward. The needle is aspirated and the pressure curve is observed and contrast injected to confirm its entry into the LA (Fig. 68.4). After that, the Mullins catheter is advanced to mid LA and the needle removed. Spiral wire (0.025 inch-coiled tip) is advanced through the catheter to LA and after septal dilatation with a dedicated tapered dilator (14F), IV Heparin is completed.

The Inoue Balloon Catheter is manufactured of polyvinyl chloride with a balloon attached to the distal end. The balloon is two latex layers between which is polyester micromesh. The catheter is supplied in a 12F diameter with a length of 70 cm; the length of each balloon is 2.5 cm (unstretched). The balloon has three

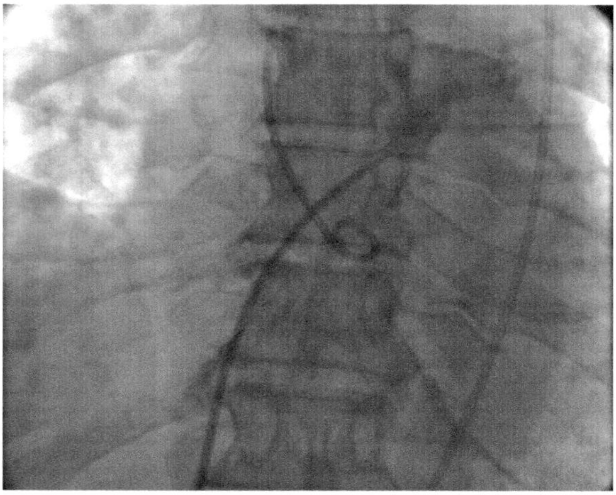

Fig. 68.4 Diluted contrast injection, confirmed the correct position of Brockenbrough needle

Table 68.3 Selection of Inoue Balloon Catheter

Reference size (RS) (mm)	
Height (cm) (rounded to nearest 0) × 1/10 + 10, e.g. height = 147 cm	
RS = 150 × 1/10 + 10 = 25 mm	
Catheter selection	
Valvular status	Balloon catheter
Pliable	RS matched (e.g. PTMC-26 for RS = 25 mm)
Calcified/SL	One-size < RS matched (e.g. PTMC-24 for RS = 25 mm)

distinct parts, enabling them to be inflated sequentially with stable positioning across the valve. There are four sizes of these balloons (24, 26, 28, and 30). Its diameter can be varied by up to 4 mm as required by circumstances (Table 68.3). Two proximally positioned stopcocks accomplish balloon inflation and catheter venting.

After pretesting for balloon-syringe matching and carefully de-airing the catheter, the stretching tube is advanced to the inner tube and fixed to the golden tube and both together advanced forward and tighten to slenderized the balloon (for this patient Inoue balloon 28 was chosen). The balloon gently was advanced through the subcutaneous tissue and crossed the septum with some clockwise rotation and forward pushing in AP view. At 12'o clock, simultaneously pulled back the stretching tube and pushed forward the balloon and at 3'o clock, pulled back the golden tube and the wire, while pushing the balloon forward, then the distal part of the balloon inflated. In RAO, with the stylet inserted to the catheter tip, the partially inflated distal balloon was directed toward the anteriorly located mitral orifice by applying a counterclockwise twist (usually 180°) to the stylet with the right hand. The catheter was then withdrawn slowly, using the left hand, until a horizontal bobbing motion of the balloon was noted, indicating close proximity of the

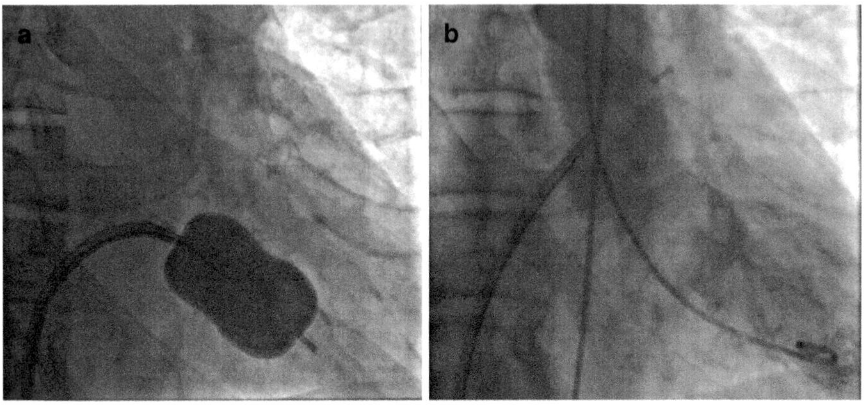

Fig. 68.5 (**a**, **b**) After septostomy and septal dilatation, the next step is crossing the Inoue balloon through the septum and with the guidance of stylet, pass the MV and enter the LV apex (good alignment of MV-Apex axis). Based on the size of the balloon and PTMC score and the degree of MR after each inflation, the procedure is completed. Finally, LV angiography is done for assessment the MR severity and any new wall motion abnormality

balloon to the mitral valve. Mitral valve crossing was then attempted by a combination of gently pulling the stylet with counterclockwise rotation while gently pushing the balloon catheter. After crossing the MV and good alignment of the balloon with MV-apex axis, the distal part of balloon was inflated (the syringe was filled with diluted contrast-26 mm) then by retracting the balloon catheter to the mitral orifice, the proximal and finally the central part inflated respectively with the disappearance of the central waist symmetrically at full inflation (total inflation and deflation time should be less than 6–8 s—Fig. 68.5a). If the residual waist is not satisfaction, stepwise dilation technique (according to the baseline Wilkins score, commissural and valvular calcification, subvalvular involvement and final MVA and MR by TTE-Fig. 68.6), the balloon size is increased up to the maximum size in 1 mm increments and inflated as the same way. Finally, the stylet was removed and after LVEDP measurement, the catheter was withdrawn into the LA and inflated the distal part to keep it in LA. After LV injection in RAO and evaluation of the final MR and any new wall motion abnormality (Fig. 68.5b), the balloon deflated and removed it just in a reverse manner (reintroduced the spiral wire and stretching tube to the inner catheter and fixed it to the golden tube in order to fully slenderized the balloon before withdrawal, then pulled back the catheter and the wire while only the soft part of the wire is left external in order to avoid a cutting effect which may occur if the stiff part of the wire is out of the tip of the balloon).

After 24–48 h, TTE is done for evaluation of MVA (by planimetry), commissural opening, MR severity, and mechanisms (commissural MR, leaflets tearing, or chordal rupture), residual ASD and any pericardial effusion.

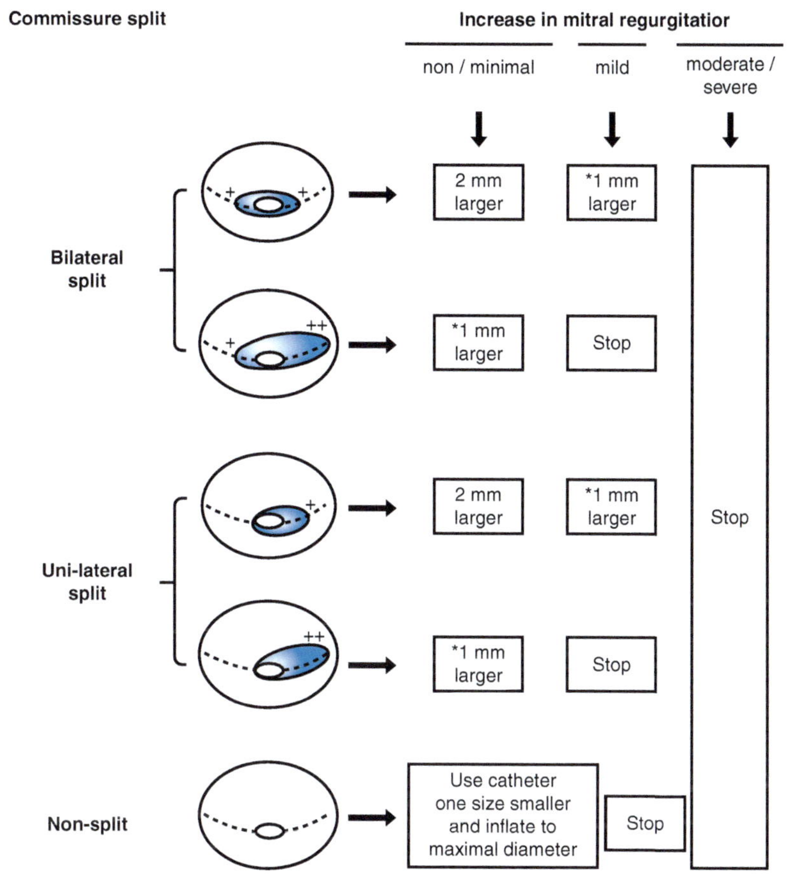

Fig. 68.6 Stepwise dilation technique

Successful Procedure

1. Final valve area larger than 1.5 cm^2 and an increase in valve area of at least 25%.
2. Final valve area larger than 1.5 cm^2 without MR greater than 2/4.

Failure Rate and Complications

The procedure is completely operator dependent, it ranges between 1 and 17% [3]. The most common causes are a failure in transseptal puncture and balloon crossing. The most complications are Tamponade (0.5–12%), severe MR (2–19%), embolism (coronary or cerebral), left-to-right shunt, and vascular site complications.

Conclusion

After more than 20 years, PTMC is now a mature technique as attested to by its use worldwide, based on a large number of series evaluating long-term results in a variety of patient subsets, PTMC has virtually replaced surgical commissurotomy. PTMC and surgery now appear as complementary techniques, which should be used appropriately in the different states and presentations of MS [4].

References

1. Tsang W, Freed BH, Lang RM. Three-dimensional anatomy of the aortic and mitral valves. In: Otto CM, Bonow RO, editors. Valvular heart disease: a companion to Braunwald's heart disease. Philadelphia: Saunders; 2013. p. 14–29.
2. Inoue K, Hung JS, Chen CR, et al. Mitral stenosis: Inoue balloon catheter technique. In: Cheng TO, editor. Percutaneous balloon valvuloplasty. New York: Igaku-Shoin Medical; 1992. p. 237–79.
3. Neumayer U, Schmidt HK, Fassabender D, et al. Early (three months) results of percutaneous mitral valvotomy with the Inoue balloon in 1,123 consecutive patients comparing various age groups. Am J Cardiol. 2009;90:190–3.
4. Palacios IF, Sanchez PL, Harrell LC, et al. Which patients benefit from percutanrous mitral balloon valvuplasty? Prevalvoplasty and postvalvoplasty variables that predict long term outcome. Circulation. 2002;105:1456–71.

Chapter 69
Transcatheter Coarctoplasty

Ata Firouzi and Zahra Hosseini

Abstract Isolated aortic coarctation is a kind of localized aortic stenosis (usually post-ductal), which usually being missed in adulthood and actually is detecting incidentally. In every new hypertensive cases, at least in first visit, both upper limbs pressure and Radial-Femoral pulses should be checked. If not treated, these patients usually don't survive more than 50 years. In the past, the gold standard of treatment was surgical repair but in the last 2 decades, balloon angioplasty and finally stenting have perceived their roles and long term outcome trials showed, the safety and effectiveness of trans-catheter coarctoplasty in adulthood.

History

The patient was a 30 years old man, a case of hypertension, who was referred with exertional dyspnea since one year ago. In TTE, he was diagnosed to have Bicuspid Aortic Valve (BAV), severe AI, and localized coarctation. He scheduled for percutaneous coarctoplasty and Bentall surgery.

Coarctation of Aorta (CoA) is a congenital abnormality of the heart producing obstruction to blood flow through the aorta; it consists of a constricted aortic segment comprising localized medial thickening with some infolding of the media and superimposed neo-intimal tissue. It may be a shelf-like structure in the posterolateral aortic wall or a membranous curtain-like structure with an eccentric or a central opening. Most commonly it is located at the junction of the ductus arteriosus with the aortic arch, just distal to the left subclavian artery. CoA accounts for 5–8% of children born with congenital heart disease, which is often associated with other congenital cardiac anomalies like: VSD, PDA, hypoplastic aortic arch, Shone complex, and BAV. BAV is commonly associated with CoA and is present in more than half of CoA patients which can lead to AI, AS, or aortic dilatation

A. Firouzi (✉) · Z. Hosseini
Interventional Cardiology, Cardiovascular Intervention Research Center, Rajaie Cardiovascular Medical and Research Center, Iran University of Medical Sciences, Tehran, Iran

M. Maleki, A. Alizadehasl (eds.), *Case-Based Clinical Cardiology*,
https://doi.org/10.1007/978-1-4471-7496-7_69

and dissection. Intracranial aneurysms may also occur (2–10%). Adequate and timely diagnosis of CoA is crucial for a good prognosis, as early treatment is associated with lower risks of long-term morbidity and mortality. The natural history of the condition is dismal, with death ensuring on average in the fourth decade of life and three-quarters of patients dying before their fiftieth birthday. The most common cause of death is CHF, dissection, and rupture of the aorta, endocarditis, premature coronary artery disease, and ICH. In adults, the most common presentation is systemic hypertension, accounts for 0.2% of all hypertension cases in adults [1].

Diagnostic Work-Up

In all new cases of hypertension, coarctation should be rule out by checking the upper and lower limb pulses and pressures. Radial-Femoral pulse delay is evident unless significant AI coexists, as well as a differential systolic blood pressure of at least 10 mm Hg between brachial and popliteal artery pressure is also suggestive. An inter-scapular systolic murmur may also reveal in auscultation. In ECG, various degree of LVH is seen. In CXR, 3 configuration and rib notching are diagnostic. TTE is an ideal modality for the detection of the stenotic segment, gradients, high-velocity jet with diastolic tail, and slow upstroke velocity flow in the abdominal aorta. CMR is the gold standard tool for detecting the type of the arch, coarctation types, collateral vessels, and the size of the aorta in arch and at the level of the diaphragm and any other vascular or cardiac anomalies.

Indications for Coarctoplasty

Significant native or recurrent aortic coarctation has been defined as follows: upper extremity/lower extremity resting peak-to-peak gradient >20 mm Hg or mean Doppler systolic gradient >20 mm Hg; upper extremity/lower extremity gradient >10 mm Hg or mean Doppler gradient >10 mm Hg plus either decreased LV systolic function or AR; upper extremity/lower extremity gradient >10 mm Hg or mean Doppler gradient >10 mm Hg with the collateral flow. This should be coupled with anatomic evidence for CoA, typically defined by advanced imaging (CMR, CTA) [2].

Coarctation of the Aorta

Recommendations for Coarctation of the Aorta		
COR	LOE	Recommendations
		Diagnostic
I	B-NR	Initial and follow-up aortic imaging using CMR or CTA is recommended in adults with coarctation of the aorta, including those who have had surgical or catheter intervention.
I	C-EO	Resting blood pressure should be measured in upper and lower extremities in all adults with coarctation of the aorta.
IIa	C-LD	Ambulatory blood pressure monitoring in adults with coarctation of the aorta can be useful for diagnosis and management of hypertension.
IIb	B-NR	Screening for intracranial aneurysms by magnetic resonance angiography or CTA may be reasonable in adults with coarctation of the aorta.
IIb	C-LD	Exercise testing to evaluate for exercise-induced hypertension may be reasonable in adults with coarctation of the aorta who exercise.
		Therapeutic
I	B-NR	Surgical repair or catheter-based stenting is recommended for adults with hypertension and significant native or recurrent coarctation of the aorta.
I	C-EO	GDMT is recommended for treatment of hypertension in patients with coarctation of the aorta.
IIb	B-NR	Balloon angioplasty for adults with native and recurrent coarctation of the aorta may be considered if stent placement is not feasible and surgical intervention is not an option.

Treatment

Surgery

The standard treatment in infants and children is surgical repair. Surgical repair progressed steadily with the development of several techniques (End to End anastomosis, patch aortoplasty (which has the highest risk of aneurysm formation), subclavian flap angioplasty and tubular bypass graft). The risk of recoarctation is about 10%, also there is rare reports of pseudoaneurysm at the site of surgical repair [3].

Balloon Angioplasty

The selected balloon angioplasty catheter is positioned across the aortic coarctation and the balloon is inflated with diluted contrast material to approximately three to five atmospheres of pressure or higher, depending upon the manufacture's recommendations. The balloon is inflated for a duration of about 5 s. A total of two to four balloon inflations are performed 5 min apart. Then repeat aortography and measurement of pressure gradients across the CoA are performed. Recording of heart rate, systemic pressure, and cardiac index prior to and fifteen minutes after balloon dilatation is made to assure that change in pressure gradient is not related to changes in patient status, but is, indeed related to balloon dilation. The size of the balloon chosen for angioplasty is two or more times the size of the coarcted segment, but no larger than the size of the descending aorta at the level of the diaphragm, as measured from a frozen frame of cineangiogram. Usually, a balloon that is midway between the size of the aortic isthmus (or transverse aortic arch) and the size of the descending aorta at the level of the diaphragm is chosen [4]. Aortic dissection, restenosis (15–25%) and aneurysm formation (10–15%) at the site of coarctation all have been documented.

Stenting

Primary stenting is the treatment of choice in native coarctation in older children and adults. It is superior to balloon angioplasty due to no elastic recoil and less aneurysm formation (By providing a scaffold for the weakened aortic wall, many believe that stent placement would decrease the likelihood of aneurysm formation). Nowadays, many balloon-expandable and self-expandable stents are available, which in multiple recent trials, there were no differences in midterm and long-term Major Adverse Cardiovascular Events (MACE) of patients based on the type of stent [5].

Procedural Technique

Under local anesthesia, after insertion of right femoral artery and vein sheaths (6F) (with fluoroscopic landmarks or ultrasonography guidance) and completed IV Heparin, (BP of the lower limb: 100/60). Femoral artery angiogram was done to evaluate the size of the Femoral and Iliac arteries and their capacity to pass large sheaths (Fig. 69.1). First, in AP and lateral projections descending aorta at the site of coarctation was injected with Pigtail catheter to characterize the residual segment, length, the distance to the left subclavian artery and the size of the aorta before and after the coarctation (Fig. 69.2). After crossing the stenotic segment with 0.035 inch wire and passing the Multipurpose catheter (BP of upper limb: 160/90, 60 mm Hg gradient), the wire exchanged with Amplatzer extra-stiff wire and positioned its tip in the ascending aorta. According to the size of the aortic arch (20 mm) and distal aortic size (24 mm), self-expandable stent 22*40 was chosen. After passing the delivery sheath (Cook 12) over the wire to the aortic arch, the delivery stent was passed through that to reach the tip of the sheath. In LAO view and angiography through the sheath, the correct position of the coarctation was confirmed. For optimal stent positioning, we covered the proximal stent with the delivery sheath and slowly expanded the distal stent to its full size, then by pulling the sheath off of the

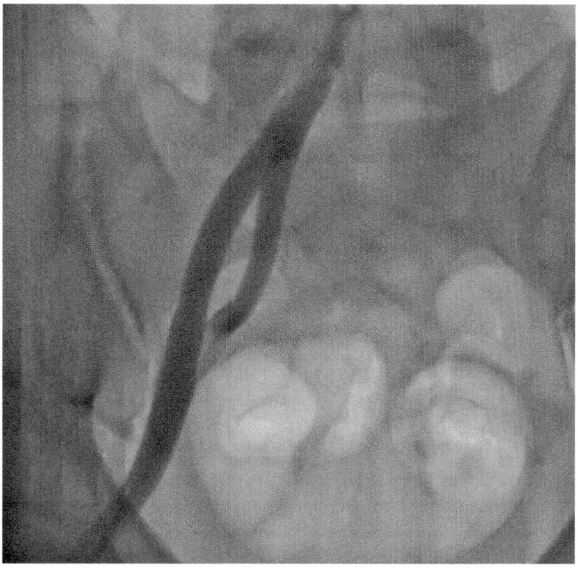

Fig. 69.1 Right CFA and CIA have an acceptable size

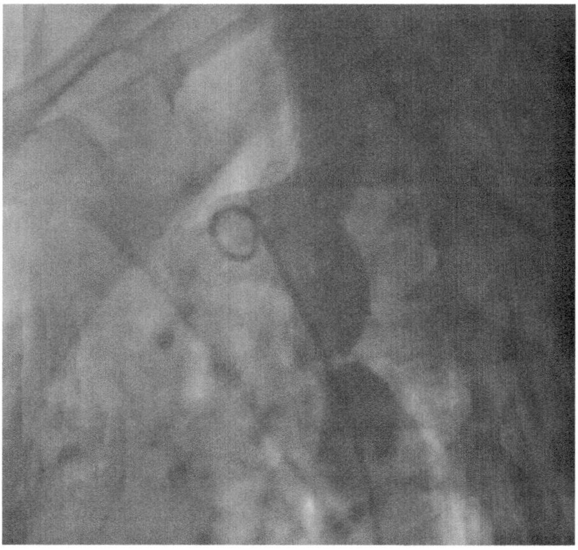

Fig. 69.2 Aortic arch injection showed significant narrowing after LSCA (50 mm Hg gradient) with post-stenotic dilatation

stent catheter, the remainder of the stent deployed across the coarctation segment (Fig. 69.3a, b). Following stent deployment, Pigtail catheter was passed to obtain simultaneous pressure measurements across the stent. Multiple angiograms was performed after stent deployment to rule out any complications (Fig. 69.4). Coarctoplasty is considered successful if the final gradient is less than 10 mm Hg and improvement in vessel caliber >80% of the normal adjacent aortic arch is achieved.

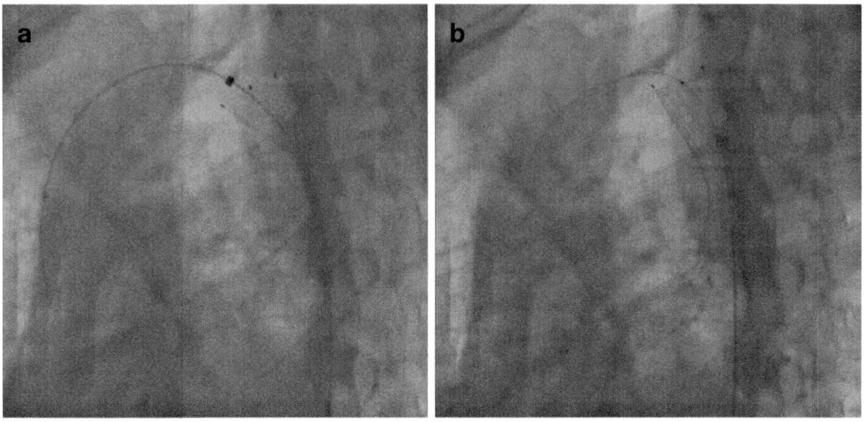

Fig. 69.3 (**a**, **b**) According to the size of the aortic arch (20 mm) and distal aortic size (24 mm), self-expandable stent 22*40 was chosen. The delivery stent was passed through the sheath to reach the tip of the sheath. In LAO projection and angiography through the sheath, the correct position of the coarctation was confirmed. For optimal stent positioning, we covered the proximal stent with the delivery sheath and slowly expanded the distal stent to its full size (**a**), then by pulling the sheath of the stent catheter back, the remainder of the stent deployed across, the coarctation segment (**b**)

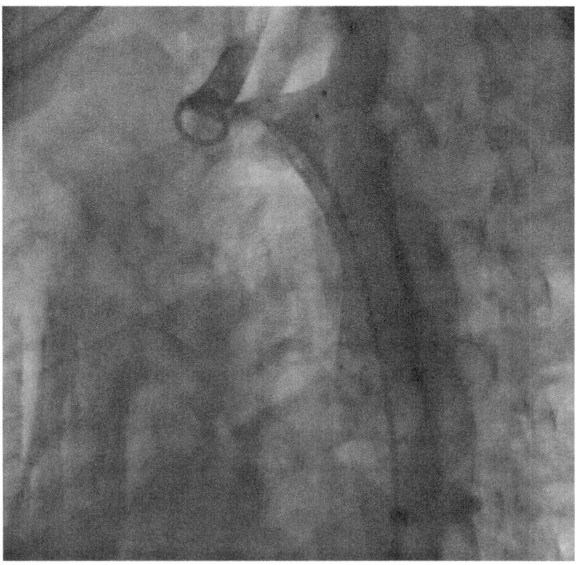

Fig. 69.4 Final aortic angiography showed, nice expansion of the device with residual gradient of 5 mm Hg without complications

Complications

During the procedure, major complications occur in approximately 15% of cases: Intimal tearing, dissection, perforation, stent migration, CVA, and the most important one, vascular complications. Late complications like: aneurysm and pseudoaneurysm formation, recoarct, and stent fracture are rare.

Conclusion

It is well established that stenting results in a marked improvement in aortic caliber. A successful procedure outcome is achieved in 98% of cases irrespective of whether it is native, recurrent, or its location. In one-third of patients, hypertension is ongoing, so lifetime follow-up of patients with coarctoplasty is mandatory for the evaluation of late complications and monitoring of blood pressure.

References

1. Hoimyr H, Christensen TD, Emmertsen K, et al. Surgical repair of coarctation of the aorta: up to 40 years follow up. Eur J Cardiothorac Surg. 2006;30:910–6.
2. Brown JW, Ruzmetov M, Hoyer MH, et al. Recurrent coarctation: is surgical repair of recurrent coarctation of the aorta safe and effective? Ann Thorac Surg. 2009;88:1923–30.
3. Matsui H, Adachi I, Uemura H, et al. Anatomy of coarctation, hypoplastic and interrupted aortic arch: relevance of intervention/surgical treatment. Expert Rev Cardiovasc Ther. 2007;5:871–80.
4. Rao PS, Galal O, Smith P. Five to nine year follow-up result of balloon angioplasty of native aortic coarctation in infants and children. JACC. 1996;27:462–70.
5. Firoozi A, Mohebbi B, Noohi F, et al. Self-expanding versus balloon- expandable stents in patients with isthmic coarctation of the aorta. Am J Cardiol. 2018;122(6):1062–7.

Chapter 70
Transcatheter Isolated Interrupted Aortic Arch Intervention

Ata Firouzi and Zahra Hosseini

Abstract Interrupted Aortic Arch (IAA), is a complex congenital heart disease which usually is associated with other anomalies. Actually it is luminal disruption between ascending and descending aorta. According to their types, the approach is different. Nowadays, with advances in interventional equipments and techniques, trans-catheter reconstruction of IAA with either antegrade or retrograde approach is growing up. Although, Surgical repair was the first option for those with associated other anomalies, but it seems that percutaneous reconstruction of IAA before surgical repair of other defects, help to the surgeon approach.

History

The patient was a 32 years old man, who was referred for more evaluation of refractory hypertension. In TTE and CMR Interrupted aortic arch was detected.

A rare type of congenital heart disease is an interrupted aortic arch (IAA), which affects approximately 1.5% of congenital heart disease patients. Interrupted aortic arch is an anomaly that can be considered the most severe form of aortic coarctation. In an IAA, there is an anatomical and luminal disruption between the ascending and descending aorta. IAA is a ductus dependent lesion since this is the only way the blood flow can travel to places distal to the disruption. There is posterior malalignment of the conal septum additional to the interrupted aortic arch, producing a ventricular septal defect as an associated lesion (80–90%). Due to this malalignment, there could be left ventricular outflow tract obstruction. Besides a ventricular septal defect, IAA can be associated with other more complicated cardiac anomalies; for example, transposition of the great arteries, truncus arteriosus, aortopulmonary window, single ventricle, aortic valve atresia, right-sided ductus,

A. Firouzi (✉) · Z. Hosseini
Interventional Cardiology, Cardiovascular Intervention Research Center, Rajaie Cardiovascular Medical and Research Center, Iran University of Medical Sciences, Tehran, Iran

M. Maleki, A. Alizadehasl (eds.), *Case-Based Clinical Cardiology*,
https://doi.org/10.1007/978-1-4471-7496-7_70

and double-outlet right ventricle. In the few cases reported in adults, the presentation varies from asymptomatic status to differential blood pressure recordings in the extremities and systemic arterial hypertension with its attendant complications. Survival into adulthood is dependent upon the development of substantial collateral circulation. These collateral vessels are subject to atrophy, atherosclerosis, and even spontaneous rupture, resulting in secondary complications [1].

According to the Celoria and Patton classification, interrupted aortic arch can be grouped into three types, depending on the site of the disruption [2]:

- Type A: The disruption is located distal to the left subclavian artery; this is the second most common disruption represents approximately 13% of the cases.
- Type B: The disruption is located between the left carotid artery and the left subclavian artery; this is the most common anomaly, representing approximately 84% of the cases.
- Type C: The disruption is located between the innominate artery and the left carotid artery; this is a rare type that represents approximately 3% of all cases.

Diagnostic Work-Up

In physical exam of isolated IAA patients, according to the type of interruption, different in pulses and pressures between left and right upper limbs or upper and lower limbs or even absent pulses is notable. Systemic HTN is usually present and sometimes systolic ejection murmur between inter-scapular areas is audible. Claudication and headache may also be the complaint of these patients. In ECG, evidence of LVH is frequently seen. TTE is the first modality for evaluation of LV and RV functions, Aortic valve evaluation (BAV, AS, AI), LVOTO, VSD, PDA, and any other concomitant anomalies also for detection of the stenotic segment of aorta (IAA type), gradients and collateral vessels (present of multiple collaterals in the absence of gradient in stenotic segment is infavor of the interrupted aorta). CMR is the gold standard tool for detecting the type of the arch, IAA types, collaterals, and the size of the aorta in arch and at the level of the diaphragm and any vascular (origin of subclavian arteries and their distance to IAA) and other cardiac anomalies. Cardiac CT Angiography is also another modality with good resolution in detecting the IAA and collateral vessels.

Management

The standard treatment of IAA is surgical repair especially in those with other anomalies. The objective of the surgery is to form unobstructed continuity between the ascending and descending aorta and to repair associated defects with the most common atrial and/or ventricular septum defect. The repair is done using either native arterial tissue, a homograph, or an autograph vascular patch. Advances in percutaneous interventions for congenital heart disease have included the percutaneous repair of coarctation of the aorta—from straightforward luminal narrowing through to full aortic interruption [3].

Transcatheter IAA (Type A) Reconstruction Technique [4]

Under local anesthesia, after insertion of right femoral artery and vein sheaths (6F) (with fluoroscopy guidance or ultrasonography) and completed IV Heparin, (BP of the lower limb: 90/60). Femoral artery angiogram was done to evaluate the size of the Femoral and Iliac arteries and their capacity to pass large sheaths (Fig. 70.1). According to the previous imaging data and the distance of the left subclavian artery to the interrupted segment (if less than 15 mm, left radial artery access is chosen and if it is more than 15 mm, right radial artery sheath is inserted). In this case left radial artery was chosen. (BP of the upper limb: 180/60). First, in AP and lateral projections, simultaneous descending aorta and aortic arch angiography was performed by Pigtail catheters to characterized the orientation and angulation of the ends and any visible nipple, residual luminal diameter, any micro-channels, length, collateral vessels and the size of the aorta before and after the interruption (Fig. 70.2a, b). The first operator was trying to pass the defect with 0.014 inch Conquest pro coronary guide-wire with end hole catheter from the femoral artery and the second operator was also tried to pass the Gaia second coronary guide-wire from the radial access (Fig. 70.3a). Under closed monitoring of patient's vital sign and sedation, after multiple trial and error, finally, in RAO-Caudal projection, the conquest guide-wire was passed retrogradely through the interruption with it tips in the left carotid artery (after confirming of being the wire in the true lumen by upper angiography Fig. 70.3a, b), the interrupted segment was dilated by coronary Tazuna balloon (2.5*15) and Multipurpose catheter was crossed through the defect. The wire was exchanged with Amplatzer Superstiff guide-wire with its tip in ascending aorta.

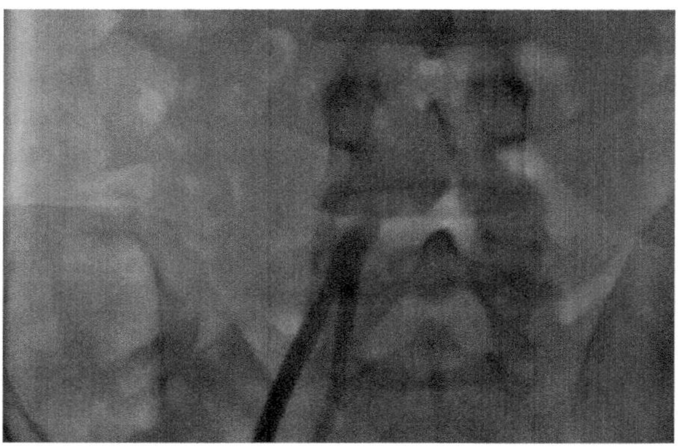

Fig. 70.1 Right CFA and CIA size

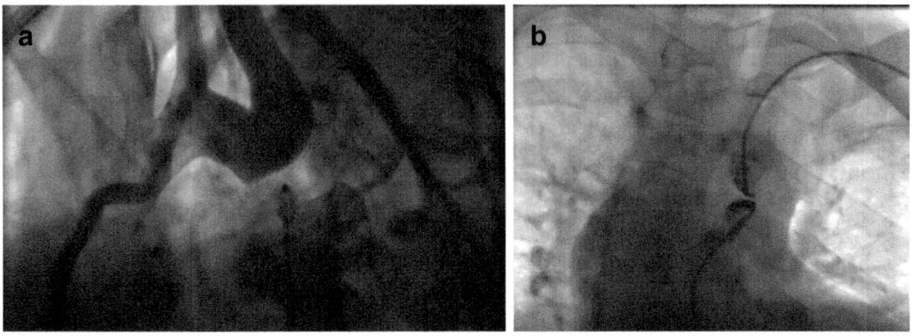

Fig. 70.2 (**a**, **b**) Descending aortic angiography showed a totally interrupted aorta with well-developed collateral vessels. Simultaneous injection of upper (left radial artery) and lower (descending aorta), showed the orientation of the ends

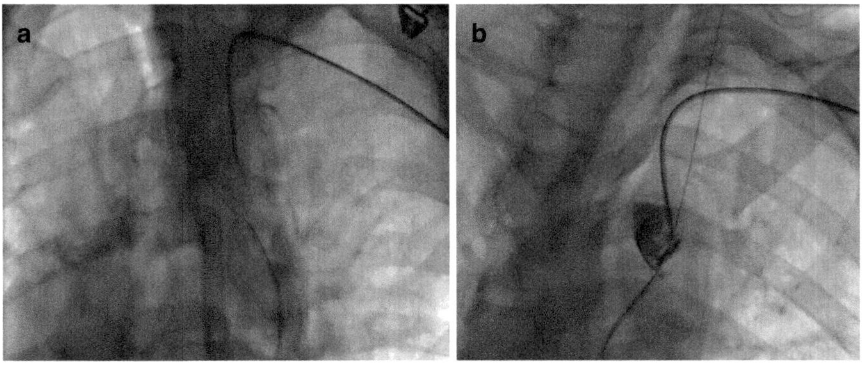

Fig. 70.3 (**a**, **b**) The first operator was trying to pass the defect with 0.014 inch Conquest pro coronary guide-wire with end hole catheter from the femoral artery and the second operator was trying to pass the Gaia second coronary guide-wire from the Radial access. After multiple trial and error, finally, in RAO-Caudal view, the conquest guide-wire was passed retrogradely through the interruption with its tips in the left carotid artery

According to the size of the aortic arch and descending aortic size, balloon-expandable stent (Covered CP8Z45 stent—premounted sheathed Covered Cheatham Platinum stent) and BiB 20*50 was chosen. After the passage of delivery sheath (Cook 14F) to the aortic arch, the delivery stent was passed gently through the sheath to reach the tip. Under fluoroscopy guidance and angiography from radial access in LAO and defining the correct position of the stent, the sheath was pulled back and the stent was deployed by inflating the inner and outer balloons (Fig. 70.4a). Finally, the delivery sheath was crossed again through the stent slowly to pull back the balloon to the sheath while keeping the wire in place. Following stent deployment, a Pigtail catheter was passed to obtain simultaneous pressure measurements across the stent. Multiple angiograms were performed after stent deployment to confirm the correct position and no dissection or perforation (Fig. 70.4b).

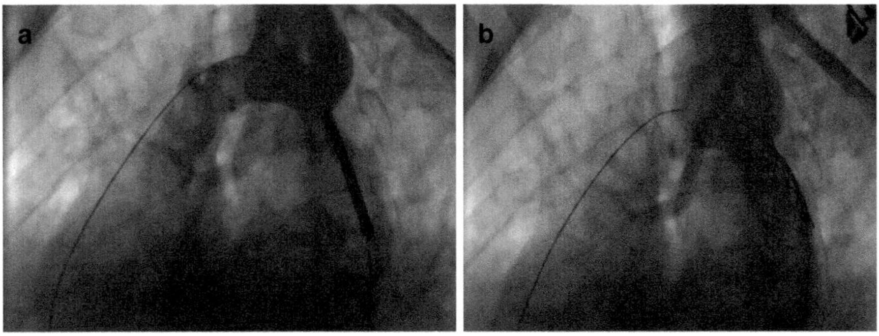

Fig. 70.4 (**a**, **b**) According to the size of the aortic arch and descending aortic size, balloon-expandable stent (Covered CP8Z45 stent- premounted sheathed Covered Cheatham Platinum stent) and BiB 20*50 was chosen. Under fluoroscopy guidance and angiography from radial access in LAO and defining the correct position of the stent, the sheath was pulled back and the stent was deployed by inflating the balloons

Conclusion

Although the gold standard treatment of IAA is surgical repair with acceptable long-term outcome, anyway, nowadays by improving in interventional technique and equipment, in isolated IAA, percutaneous intervention seems to be an alternative option with less complications by expert interventionist in the structural heart disease, although the long-term outcomes of these patients need more future studies.

References

1. Varghese R, Saheed SB, Omoregbee B, Ninan B, Pavithran S, Kothandam S. Surgical repair of interrupted aortic arch and interrupted pulmonary artery. Ann Thorac Surg. 2015;100(6):e139–40.
2. Schreiber C, Mazzitelli D, Haehnel JC, Lorenz HP, Meisner H. The interrupted aortic arch: an overview after 20 years of surgical treatment. Eur J Cardiothorac Surg. 1997;12(3):466–9. discussion 469–70.
3. Santoro G, Russo MG, Calabro R. Stent angioplasty in aortic arch interruption. Heart. 2006;92:1570.
4. Firouzi A, Hosseini Z, Sadeghipour P, et al. Paradigm shift in the management of isolated interrupted aortic arch in adulthood. cpcardiol.2020.100717. https://doi.org/10.1016/j.cpcardiol.2020.100717.

Chapter 71
Transcatheter Device Closure of Ruptured Sinus of Valsalva

Ata Firouzi and Zahra Hosseini

Abstract Aneurysmal sinus Valsalva (congenital or iatrogenic) is usually asymptomatic but when it ruptured, this catastrophic event lead to sudden onset chest chain, dyspnea, syncope or even sudden death. In this situation, right coronary cusp is the most one which frequently ruptured to the RVOT or RA with significant left to right shunt and eventually biventricular failure. It is obligatory to repair the ruptured cusp. Recently, trans-catheter device closure seems to be safe and effective strategy to close this shunt with minimal side effects.

History

A 35 years old man was referred to ER with complaints of sudden onset chest pain and dyspnea since 6 h ago who admitted with the impression of ACS. In TTE ruptured aneurysmal sinus Valsalva (NCC) was diagnosed.

Sinus of Valsalva aneurysm (SOVA) is an abnormal dilatation of the aortic root between the aortic annulus and ST junction. The estimated rate is about 0.09% of the general population. SOVA can be either congenital (connective tissue disease like Marfan syndrome) or acquired (bacterial endocarditis, Takayasu's arteritis, or trauma), the consequence of elastic lamina weakening and medial cystic necrosis. It can be an isolated anomaly or be associated with other CHD like: Bicuspid AV, Aortic regurgitation, VSD, PDA, and Coarctation of aorta. The most affected valve is RCC, followed by NCC (5–15%) and finally LCC. Non-ruptured ones are usually asymptomatic but can lead to sinus thrombosis or coronary artery compression and acute coronary syndrome. Ruptured sinus Valsalva aneurysm is a fatal event. In majority of cases, RCC or NCC ruptured results in communication between the aorta and RA or RVOT (significant left-to-right shunt with RV and LV overload and failure) who present with sudden onset chest pain, dyspnea, orthopnea, syncope,

A. Firouzi (✉) · Z. Hosseini
Interventional Cardiology, Cardiovascular Intervention Research Center, Rajaie Cardiovascular Medical and Research Center, Iran University of Medical Sciences, Tehran, Iran

M. Maleki, A. Alizadehasl (eds.), *Case-Based Clinical Cardiology*,
https://doi.org/10.1007/978-1-4471-7496-7_71

infective endocarditis, tamponade, hemodynamic instability or sudden cardiac death but ruptured LCC with communication to LVOT, is less clinically significant [1].

Diagnostic Work-Up

SOVA rupture diagnosis requires a low index of suspicion. In physical exam, a typical continues murmur with trill is sound in right and left LSB with bounding pulses and sometimes the murmur of AI is audible. In long-standing cases, the ECG shows LVH and RVH criteria. TTE is the first modality which shows LV and RV size and functions, aortic valve morphology and any aneurysmal or ruptured cusp with continues flow in systole and diastole into the communicated chambers, any vegetation and other anomalies and finally for more information, TEE is confirming tool for SOVA rupture and would differentiate it from a combination of VSD and AI. Cardiac CT is the test of choice for quantifying the size and morphology of SOVA.

Management

The ACC-AHA 2010 guideline-recommended surgical repair for those with non-ruptured sinus of Valsalva greater than 5.5 cm, greater than 5 cm in those with BAV and greater than 4.5 cm in those with connective tissue disease. But in SOVA rupture, the surgical or tans-catheter repair is urgent and mandatory as patients may quickly deteriorate. Medical treatment is just for stabilizing the patients before invasive procedures. Surgical intervention is recommended for a ruptured SOVA and/or a SOVA with associated intracardiac abnormalities such as VSD or significant AI. If ruptured SOVAs remain untreated, the prognosis is poor with a 1-year life expectancy [2].

Procedural Technique

The technique is similar to the TCC of perimembranous VSD, although the defect is located just above the aortic valve instead of below. Periprocedural TEE and color Doppler interrogation help us in sizing the defect, device selection (2–4 mm larger than the aortic end), delineating the SOVA anatomy in regards to its neighboring structures namely the aortic valve, tricuspid valve, and RVOT, ensuring proper seating of the aortic disk on the aortic side without slipping into the body of the aneurysm, and most importantly, monitoring AR and TR occurrence and residual shunting on color Doppler.

After loading ASA 325 mg and Plavix 600 mg and insertion of right femoral artery and vein sheaths (6F) and completed IV Heparin to achieved ACT > 200 s, Under general anesthesia, TEE guidance and re-evaluation of the defect (assessment of the maximum diameter of the aortic end of the RSOV, the minimum diameter and the length of the windsock, and the distance of the aortic end of the RSOV from the coronary ostium), aortic root and LV angiography was done for more evaluation (Fig. 71.1a, b). Then via retrograde approach, from the aortic side, after crossing the defect (Noncoronary cusp rupture to RA) via 0.035 inch, 260 cm long straight tipped Terumo wire and passing the JR catheter to the RA and manipulated to reach the IVC, the wire was snared from Femoral vein to create an arteriovenous loop (Fig. 71.2). After that, the delivery sheath (Occlutech 12F) was passed from the venous side over the wire across the RSOV. According to the defect size

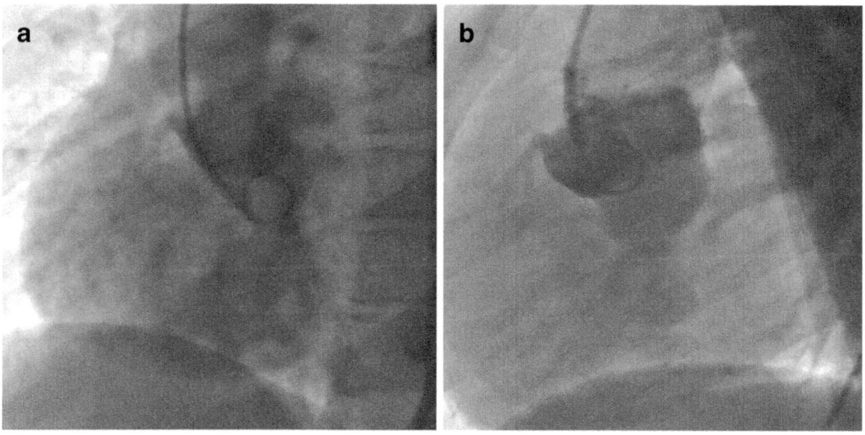

Fig. 71.1 (**a**, **b**) In both images the perforation of the aneurysmal noncoronary cusp to RA is noticeable

Fig. 71.2 Coarse of the catheter: CFA → Abdominal aorta → Aortic root → perforation defect → RA → IVC (arterio-venous loop)

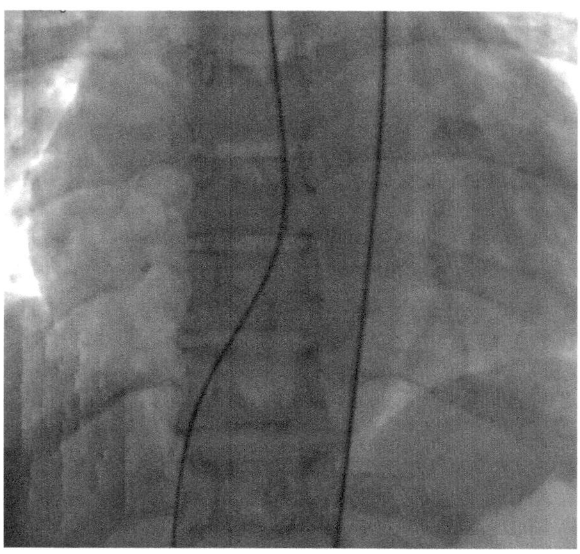

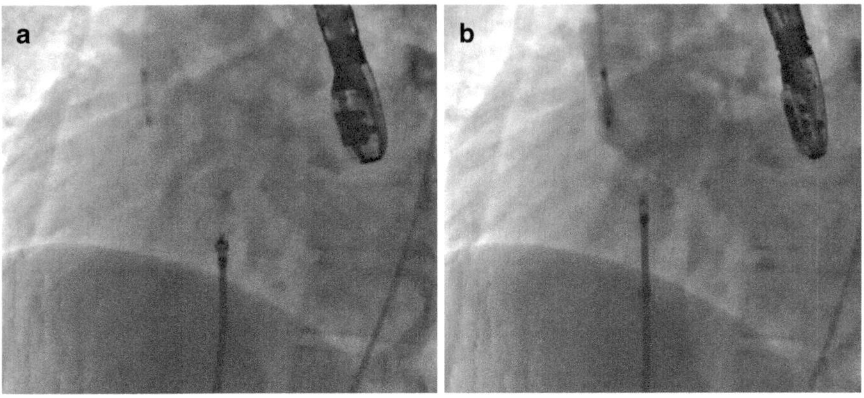

Fig. 71.3 (**a**, **b**) According to the defect size and length, Muscular VSD 8 mm (Occlutech) was chosen. Aortic disk was opened in the ascending aorta and the whole system was pulled back till it anchored at the aortic end of the RSOV and it was ensured that aortic valve leaflets were free as seen on TEE, then the proximal disk was deployed by retracting the sheath. After confirming the correct position of the device by aortic root injection and TEE (no interference with AV or occlusion of coronary ostia and the residual shunt), the device was released

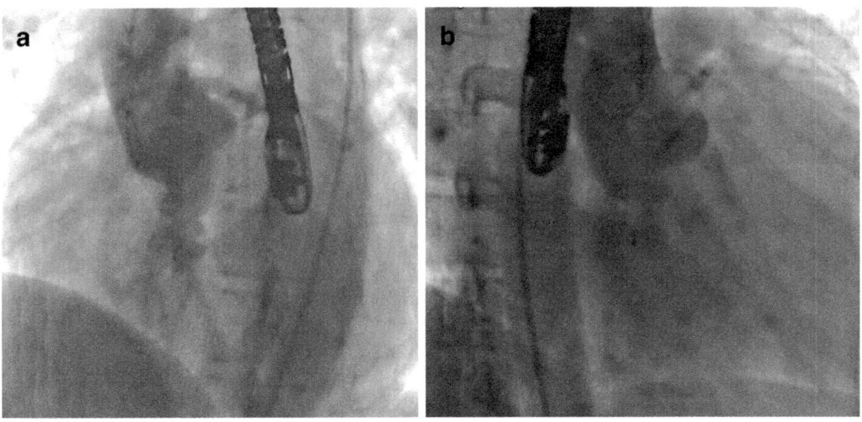

Fig. 71.4 (**a**, **b**) Selective aortic angiography in LAO and RAO projections showed, appropriate position of the device with minimal residual shunt

and length, Muscular VSD 8 mm (Occlutech) was chosen. After loading the device and connecting to the delivery cable and fully de-aired, the device was passed through the delivery sheath, under TEE guidance and fluoroscopy. Aortic disk was opened in the ascending aorta and the whole system was pulled back till it anchored at the aortic end of the RSOV and it was ensured that aortic valve leaflets were free as seen on TEE, then proximal disk was deployed by retracting the sheath (Fig. 71.3a). After confirming the correct position of the device by aortic root injection (Fig. 71.3b) and TEE (no interference with AV or occlusion of coronary ostia and the residual shunt), the device was released. Final angiography showed mild residual shunt, stable device position, and no AI (Fig. 71.4a, b).

Conclusion

Since the first report of device closure of RSOVA in 1994, it is increasingly being reported as either case reports or case series and is gradually replacing surgical correction with cardiopulmonary bypass, conventionally the mainstay of treatment. Transcatheter closure (TCC) had been performed using Amplatzer duct occluder (ADO), ventricular septal defect (VSD) occluder, atrial septal defect (ASD) occluder, Gianturco coils, and Rashkind umbrella. To conclude, transcatheter closure of RSOV is an effective and safe treatment modality for isolated RSOV. In patients where on-pump surgery is a high risk, due to poor general condition and comorbidities, transcatheter device closure can be lifesaving. An extended follow-up is required to assess the long-term outcome of these patients [3].

References

1. Serban AM, Batrana N, Cocoi M, et al. The role of echocardiography in the diagnosis and management of a giant unruptured sinus of Valsalva aneurysm. Med Ultrson. 2019;21(2):194–6.
2. Sakar M, Wehman B, Mukherjee R, et al. Left sinus of Valsalva aneurysm presenting as myocardial ischemia. J Thorac Cardiovasc Surg. 2018.
3. Supratim S, Amitabha C, Mily R, et al. Transcatheter device closure of ruptured sinus of Valsalva: immediate results and short term follow up. Ann Pediatr Cardiol. 2009;2(1):79–82.

Chapter 72
Pulmonary Hypertension (PH) and the Role of Transcatheter Atrial Flow Regulator (AFR) Device Implantation

Ata Firouzi and Zahra Hosseini

Abstract Pulmonary hypertension diagnosis is confirmed with RHC. Advanced cases of PH (mostly, group 1 and 4) who despite of optimized therapy (combination therapy), are being symptomatic (dyspnea functional class III/IV, recurrent syncope and clinical sign of RV failure), and eventually are candidate for lung transplant. In selected cases as bridge therapy, any strategy which can decrease the RV pressure and increase cardiac output, might improve RV function and patients symptoms. Atrial septostomy (which create a right to left shunt for increasing the cardiac output despite of desaturated the patients) has demonstrated to be effective in rare cases. But this procedure is very high risk and has the chance of reocclusion in short time. Recently in some pilot studies, the Occlutech AFR device which is a modified Figulla Flex II ASD Occluder that has been designed for using clinical conditions where creating the permanent inter-atrial communication which would lead to decompression of the right heart side. Further, it would increase cardiac output, blood pressure and organ perfusion and finally reduced the likelihood of syncope and acute right heart decompensation and death.

History

The patient was a 33 years old lady, a case of advanced Idiopathic PH who was referred with recurrent syncope attacks despite optimal medical therapy.

Pulmonary hypertension (PH) is defined as an increase in mean pulmonary arterial pressure (mPAP) of 20 mmHg or greater at rest, as assessed by right heart catheterization (RHC). Pre-capillary PH is defined as mPAP of 20 mmHg or more; a pulmonary capillary wedge pressure (PCWP) of 15 mm Hg or less; and a pulmonary vascular resistance (PVR) of more than 3 Wood units. Pre-capillary PH may

A. Firouzi (✉) · Z. Hosseini
Interventional Cardiology, Cardiovascular Intervention Research Center, Rajaie Cardiovascular Medical and Research Center, Iran University of Medical Sciences, Tehran, Iran

M. Maleki, A. Alizadehasl (eds.), *Case-Based Clinical Cardiology*,
https://doi.org/10.1007/978-1-4471-7496-7_72

being in group 1 pulmonary arterial hypertension (PAH), group 3 (PH due to lung disease), group 4 (CTEPH), or group 5 (PH due to unclear or multifactorial mechanisms) in origin. Post-capillary PH is present when the mPAP is 20 mmHg or more and the PCWP is 15 mm Hg or more [1]. Post-capillary PH is most common in group 2 patients or those with PH due to left heart disease. PH has multifactorial pathobiology in which an imbalance in vasoconstriction and vasodilation, thrombosis, and cell proliferation and remodeling of the walls of the pulmonary arteries contribute to increase PVR. Pulmonary vascular remodeling involves the intima, media, and adventitia of small pulmonary arteries (diameter <500 μm); all cell types (endothelial, smooth muscle, and fibroblastic), as well as inflammatory cells and platelets, may play a significant role in the condition. Pulmonary vasoconstriction has been regarded as an early component of the PH process, and excessive vasoconstriction has been related to abnormal function or expression of potassium channels and endothelial dysfunction. Endothelial dysfunction is characterized by impaired production of vasodilators such as a nitric oxide (NO) and prostacyclin, along with overexpression of vasoconstrictors such as endothelin-1. The most common initial symptoms of PH include exertional dyspnea or reduced exercise tolerance, chest pain, fatigue, and light-headedness. Manifestations of more advanced diseases include syncope, abdominal distention, lower extremity edema, and low cardiac output state attributable to right ventricular failure [2].

Diagnostic Work-Up

In physical exam, loud P2, RV heave, systolic murmur of TR, or diastolic murmur of PI and elevated JVP may be found. Central cyanosis, ascites, hepatomegaly, and peripheral edema is seen in advanced cases. In ECG, right axis deviation, RVH, and strain pattern are usually notable. TTE is the first noninvasive tool for evaluation the degree of LV, RV, RA, and LA size and dysfunctions, D-shaped septum, evaluation the causes of PH (left side valvular disease, HFPEF, congenital heart disease), TR and PI severity, estimation of PAP, stretched PFO and finally any pericardial effusion. Perfusion-ventilation lung scintigraphy is an essential tool for rule out of CTEPH. 6 MWT and CPET for evaluation of the functional capacity and finally, RHC is the gold standard modality for confirming the PH, hemodynamic assessment, treatment decision and predicting the prognosis of these patients (Fig. 72.1).

RHC

- So2: 92%
- Mixed venous saturation: 55%
- RVP: 100/20 mm Hg
- mRAP: 18 mm Hg

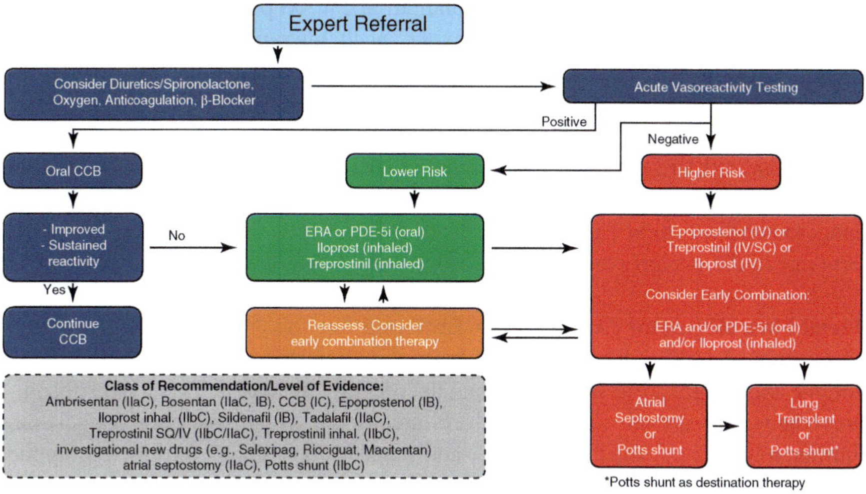

Fig. 72.1 Treatment approach

- mPAP: 70 mm Hg
- PVR: 22 WU
- SVR: 24 WU
- PCWP: 12 mm Hg
- CI: 1.8 L/min/m^2

Interventional Treatment

Balloon Atrial Septostomy (BAS) Atrial septostomy creates a right-to-left inter-atrial shunt, decreases the right-sided heart filling pressure, improves right ventricular function, and improves left-sided heart filling. Several case series have reported hemodynamic and clinical improvement following this procedure. Although the shunt created decreases systemic arterial oxygen saturation, the goal is an improvement in systemic oxygen delivery based on the improved CO. However, the procedural mortality rate is high, in the range of 9–22%, and it is driven by the severity of PAH and right-sided heart failure in patients undergoing this procedure. The recommended technique is graded balloon dilation of the fossa ovalis, which can be achieved in stages over a period of several weeks in unstable patients. It should not be performed in patients with impending death and severe right ventricular failure. Predictors of procedure-related failure or death include a mean right atrial pressure higher than 20 mm Hg, a PVR index higher than 55 units/m^2, or a predicted 1-year survival rate of less than 40%. Currently, atrial septostomy is recommended for patients with severe PAH and intractable right-sided heart failure despite maximal medical therapy. The goals of this procedure are palliation and restoration and maintenance of clinical stability until transplantation can be performed. Atrial septostomy should be performed only by experienced operators in centers with the resources to care for such critically ill patients. Expert-based consensus guidelines define the following as contraindications to atrial septostomy: mean right atrial pressure higher than 20 mm Hg, resting arterial oxygen saturation lower than 90% on room air, or LVEDP higher than 18 mm Hg [3]. The disadvantage of BAS is that the artificial shunt may be too large by inadvertent tear of the BAS, thus causing dangerous desaturation and potential death. Also, it may occlude within the short term due to the overgrowth of intimal cells.

Atrial Flow Regulator (AFR) Device Implantation An AFR device creates communication and allow blood to flow across the interatrial septum when the blood volume under right atrial side is high and the pressure increased. This would decompress the right heart side and reduce the clinically important right heart congestion. Further, it would give the left heart side additional blood volume, thus increasing the left-sided stroke volume, cardiac output, blood pressure, and organ perfusion and finally reduced the likelihood of syncope and acute right heart decompensation and death.

The Occlutech AFR device is a modified Figulla Flex II ASD Occluder that has been designed for using clinical conditions where creating permanent interatrial communication [4] (Fig. 72.2).

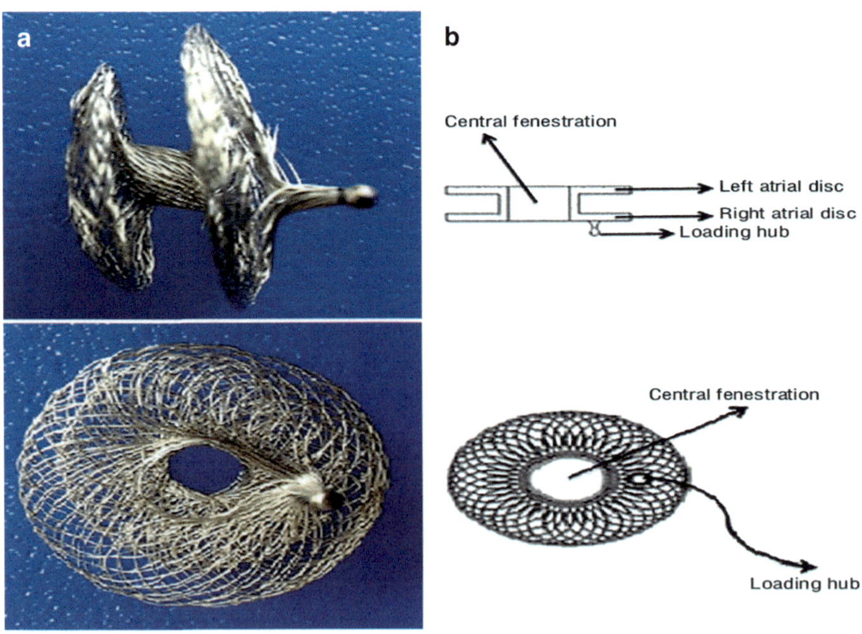

Fig. 72.2 AFR design

Procedural Technique

Under general anesthesia, and closed hemodynamic monitoring by heart failure team (Milrinone and Norepinephrine infusion), after insertion of femoral artery and vein sheaths (6F), under TEE guidance, septostomy was done by Brockenbrough needle with contrast injected to confirm of being in LA (Fig. 72.3) and spiral wire inserted in LA then IV Heparin completed to achieve ACT > 250 s. After septal dilatation by peripheral balloon 10*30 (OTW) (Fig. 72.4), the wire exchanged with Amplatzer Superstiff wire with its tip in LUPV, then the delivery sheath (Occlutech 10F) was crossed through the wire to mid LA and the dilator was removed to allow back bleed. After loading the device (AFR 8 mm) and connecting to the delivery cable, the device was passed over the sheath to reach the tip of the sheath. By retracting the sheath, the distal disk (DD) was deployed in LA then the whole system was pulled backed to the septum, after checking the orientation of the device by TEE, the proximal disk deployed (Fig. 72.5). Finally, after complete assessment of the device position and stability and the degree of right to left shunt, the device was released (Fig. 72.6). Final RHC showed the RAP decreased to 12 mm Hg and SO_2 was 90%. The patient referred to ICU for closed observation and hemodynamic monitoring.

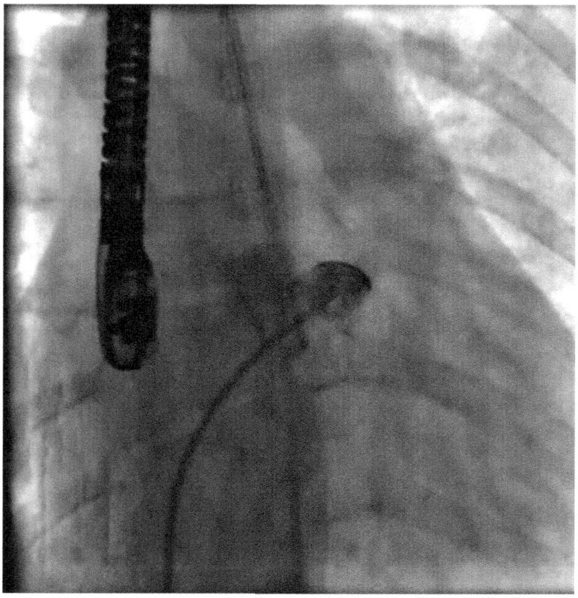

Fig. 72.3 After septostomy, diluted contrast showed the correct procedure

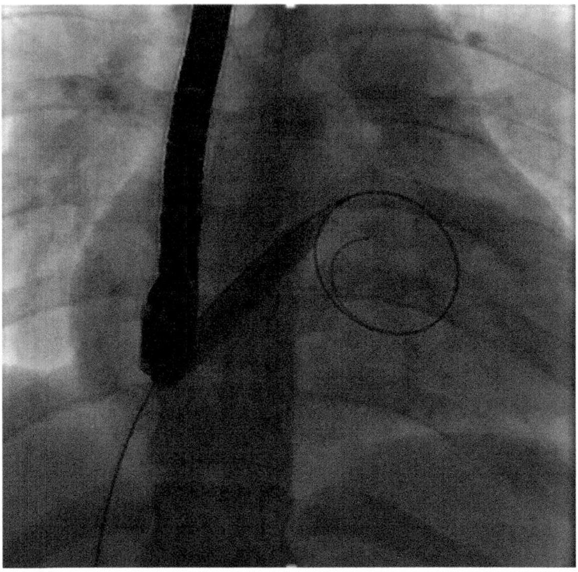

Fig. 72.4 Through the spiral wire, septal dilatation was performed with Powerflex (OTW) 10*30

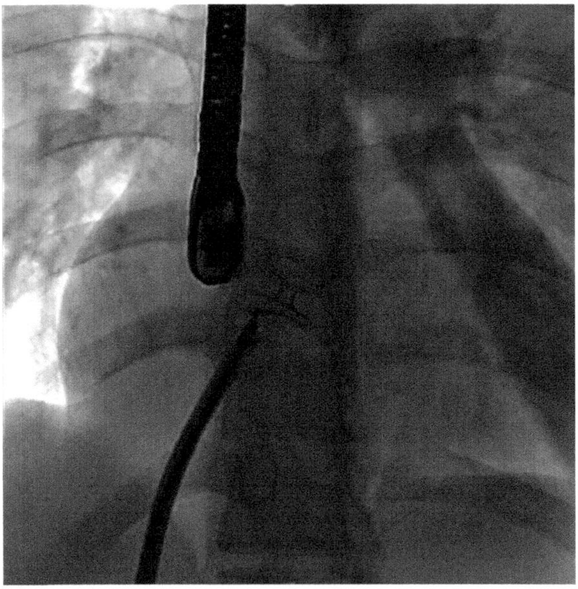

Fig. 72.5 By retracting the sheath, the distal disk (DD) was deployed in LA then the whole system was pulled back toward the septum, after checking the orientation of the device by TEE, the proximal disk deployed

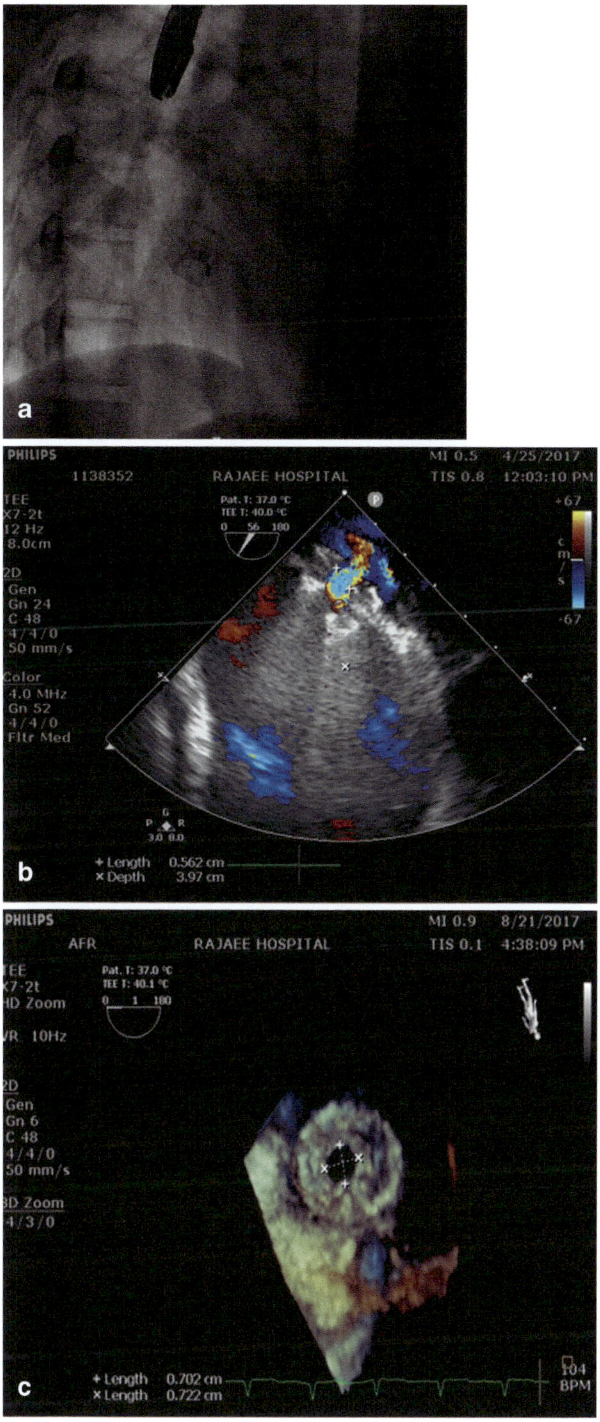

Fig. 72.6 (**a**–**c**) After complete assessment of the device position and stability and the degree of right-to-left shunt, the device was released

Conclusion

Although patients with advanced PH have a very poor prognosis, but any palliative interventions (bridge therapy) to buy the time for them to prepare these patients for lung transplant, is valuable. AFR implantation seems to be a safe procedure that needs more studies for determining the optimal time of intervention and long-term outcomes of these patients [5].

References

1. Galie N, Humbert M, Vachiery JL, et al. 2015 ESC/ERS guidelines for the diagnosis and treatment pulmonary hypertension: The joint task force for the diagnosis and treatment of pulmonary hypertension of the European Society of Cardiology (ESC) and the European Respiratory Society (ERS): Endorsed by: Association for European Paediatric and Congenital Cardiology (AEPC), International Society for Heart and Lung Transplantation (ISHLT). Eur Heart J. 2016;37:67–119.
2. Guignabert C, Tu L, Girerd B, et al. New molecular targets of pulmonary vascular remodeling in pulmonary arterial hypertension: importance of endothelial communication. Chest. 2015;147:529–37.
3. Braunwald Heart Disease, 11th edn.
4. Haas N, Schulze-Neick I, et al. Prospective, non-randomized, pilot study to assess safety and efficacy of a novel Atrial Flow Regulator in patients with Pulmonary Hypertension. The AFR-PROPHET Trial. 2016.
5. Vettukattil J, Rajeshkumar R, Dahdah N, Firouzi A, et al. Clinical impact of creating a predermined atrial communication in the management of severe pulmonary hypertention using the atrial flow regulator device. JACC. 2018;71(11). https://doi.org/10.1016/S0735-1097(18)32489-6.

Chapter 73
Transcatheter Post-MI VSR Device Closure

Ata Firouzi and Zahra Hosseini

Abstract Post MI VSR, is a catastrophic event with high mortality with and without treatment. Based on the patient's characteristic, LV and RV function, the location of the defect, it's size and the amount of shunt, the prognosis is individually different. Surgical repair is the first choice for treatment which there is some controversy about the time of surgery. Alternative approach in those with high surgical risk, is trans-catheter device closure, especially in apical VSR. The success rate again depends on patient's conditions.

History

The patient was a 50 years old lady who had presented with anterior STEMI one week ago and primary PCI on LAD was done for her. After 1 week, she referred with pulmonary edema and low cardiac output state which in TTE, post-MI apical VSR was diagnosed.

Post-MI VSR is the most catastrophic mechanical complication with high morbidity and mortality. The incidence of VSR has decreased from 1 to 3% following ST-segment elevation MI in the pre-reperfusion era to 0.17–0.31% following primary PCI. Depending on Becker classification (I–III), its presentation can occur within hours or within 3–5 days or even later of the index MI. Female gender, hypertension, no pervious MI, and delayed reperfusion are related risk factors. VSR is equally happened in both anterior and inferior MI. In anterior MI, the VSR is an apical segment, simple and slit like at the same level on both sides of septum with thinner rims while in inferior MI, the VSR is more complex, taking serpiginous routes through a hemorrhagic and necrotic basal inferoposterior septum [1].

Depending on the degree of left to right shunt, LV and RV volume overload and dysfunction and PAP, the patients may present with relatively hemodynamic stability to pulmonary edema and frank cardiogenic shock.

A. Firouzi (✉) · Z. Hosseini
Interventional Cardiology, Cardiovascular Intervention Research Center, Rajaie Cardiovascular Medical and Research Center, Iran University of Medical Sciences, Tehran, Iran

M. Maleki, A. Alizadehasl (eds.), *Case-Based Clinical Cardiology*,
https://doi.org/10.1007/978-1-4471-7496-7_73

Diagnostic Work-Up

In physical exam, a harsh, holo-systolic murmur with thrill is audible in LSB usually with S3 gallop. TTE should always be considered in patients with any murmur or hemodynamic instability after MI to rule out any mechanical complications including VSR. In RHC, a step-up of SO_2 in RV and large V wave in PCWP are confirming.

Management

Surgical closure is the definite treatment of these patients. After initial diuretic and vasodilators therapy and in selected cases, MCS (Mechanical Circulatory Support like IABP, Impella or pulsecath) implantation, the timing of surgery in the setting of VSR remains controversial and should be individualized. In hemodynamically stable patients with preserved end-organ function and favorable anatomy, early corrective surgery should be considered because sudden and unpredictable hemodynamic compromise is often noted. Delayed surgery in hemodynamically stable patients may be considered when surgical anatomy is complex and there is concern regarding tissue fragility and the ability to perform the definitive repair. Delay might facilitate successful repair by allowing friable tissue to organize, strengthen, and become well-differentiated from surrounding healthy tissue. In this scenario, close follow-up in the intensive care unit may be considered to enable tissue healing and promote chances of definitive repair. In recognition of the possible benefits of delayed repair, the 2017 European Society of Cardiology guidelines promotes delayed elective repair in patients initially responding to aggressive conservative management [2] (Fig. 73.1).

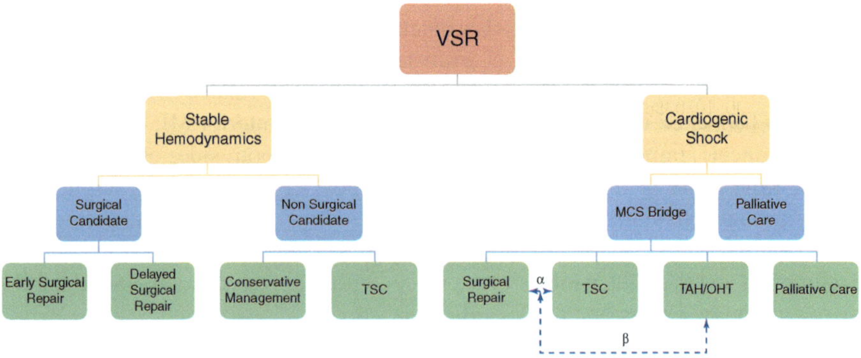

Fig. 73.1 (**α**) If deemed suitable for percutaneous repair, trans-catheter septal closure (TSC) may be used as primary repair, bridge to surgery, in conjunction with surgery, or as salvage of residual defect following surgical repair. (**β**) Candidacy for total artificial heart and/or cardiac transplantation should be considered for any unstable patient whether as an alternative to, in addition to, or following failure of repair. *MCS* mechanical circulatory support; *OHT* orthotopic heart transplant; *TAH* total artificial heart

Transcatheter Septal Closure (TSC)

Right femoral artery and jugular vein sheaths (6F) were inserted then IV Heparin was completed to achieve ACT > 200 s. Under general anesthesia, after complete assessment of VSR by TEE and LV angiography (Fig. 73.2), the apical VSR was crossed from LV via JR catheter and 0.035 inch hydrophilic guide-wire. After crossing the defect with the wire and the catheter and position the wire in the LPA, to make an arterio-venous circuit, the guide-wire was snared and exteriorized via venous access. A kink resistant delivery sheath (Lifetech12F) was advanced carefully to RV, LV, and aortic arch with the Kissing catheter technique. The dilator was removed from the vein access and guide-wire and the end hole catheter were removed from the arterial line. By TEE guidance and expert echo-man, according to the defect size (20 mm-largest diastolic phase on LV side), Atrial septal occluder (ASO-Figulla II Occlutech) device 33 mm was chosen. After the device was screwed to the delivery cable and de-aired, it passed through the long sheath and under TEE and fluoroscopy guidance, the whole system as a unit was pulled back gently through the AV to LV, and slowly by retracting the delivery sheath, distal disk (Left disk) at the LV side of VSR was deployed, then the entire system was pulled back into the defect and the sheath was retracted to deploy the waist and finally, after confirming the right position of the device by TEE and LV injection, the proximal disk (Right disk) was deployed (Figs. 73.3a, b and 73.4a). The operator must fully check the position and stability of the device without any compromising the surrounding structures. If the device position is correctly confirmed by the TEE and fluoroscopy, it can be released (Fig. 73.5). In this case, mild residual shunt at the end of the procedure was remained (Figs. 73.4b and 73.5).

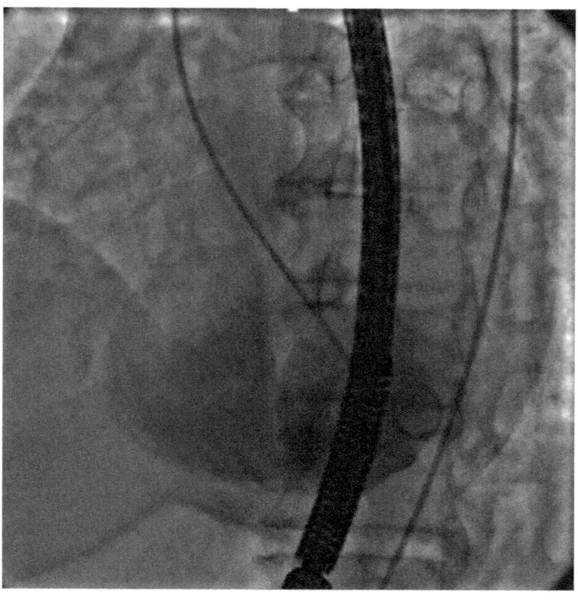

Fig. 73.2 LV injection showed a large post-MI VSR with significant shunt

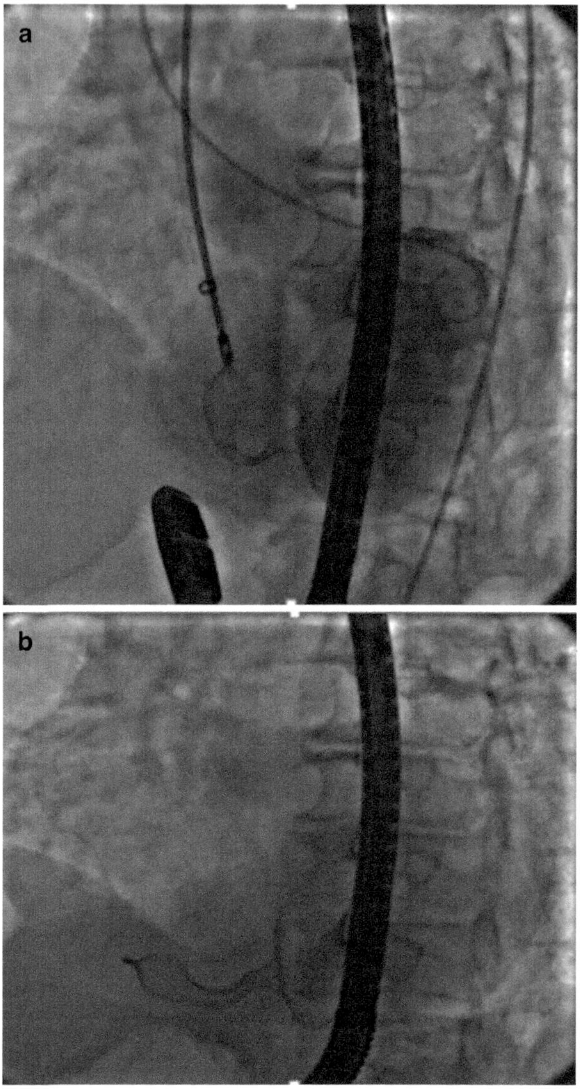

Fig. 73.3 (**a**, **b**) After wiring the defect and exteriorized via venous access, according to the size of the defect, Figulla II Occlutech device 33 mm was chosen, and by retracting the delivery sheath, the DD and PD were deployed. Initially, after deployment of the device, the Cobra configuration of RV disk is notable

Defects <15 mm are considered optimal for TSC, but successful closure has been reported with larger defects. Oversizing the disc may improve procedure success by accounting for defect enlargement due to tissue necrosis [3]. Challenges to TSC include inferior defects due to a lack of a circumferential septal rim, basal defects due to the proximity to the tricuspid valvular apparatus, serpiginous defects due to complicated morphology, and mitral soon following infarction due to tissue instability. Diligent defect characterization, device selection, and patient selection are perquisites to successful TSC.

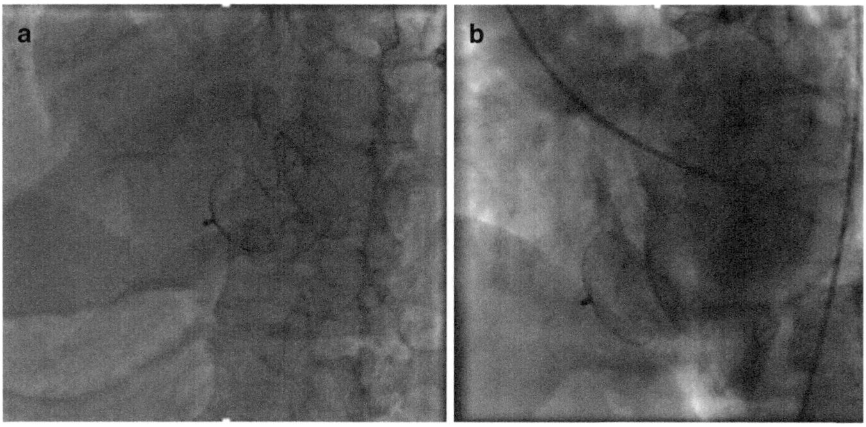

Fig. 73.4 (**a**, **b**) Under TEE guidance, after releasing the device, 5 min later the final configuration of the device is seen. Final LV angiography showed, well position of the device with mild residual shunt

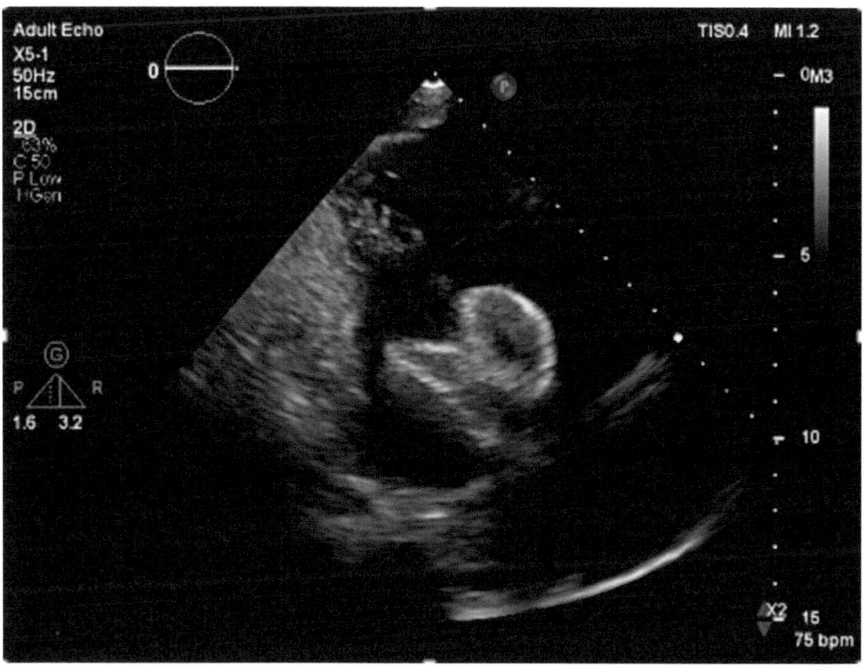

Fig. 73.5 Final assessment by TEE of the device position, which demonstrated nice position without impingement on the surrounding structures

Conclusion

Although surgical repair is the definite treatment for post-MI VSR patients, in stable but inoperable patients, percutaneous TSC may be considered. Successful device implantation rate is about 89% and overall in-hospital/30-day mortality is 32% in one systematic review [4]. Reported procedure complications include arrhythmias, device embolization, ventricular rupture, device-related hemolysis, and death. The post VSR closure course in the CCU is often stormy and requires careful monitoring to detect complications early and manage them appropriately. Coronary lesions should be addressed on a later date for better results and the primary focus should be on correction of mechanical complication.

References

1. Singh V, Rodriguez AP, Bhatt P, et al. Ventricular septal defect complicating ST-elevation myocardial infarctions: a call for action. Am J Med. 2017;130:863.e1–863.e12.
2. Ibanez B, James S, Agewall S, et al. 2017 ESC Guidelines for the management of acute myocardial infarction in patients presenting with ST-segment elevation: the task force for the management of acute myocardial infarction in patients presenting with ST-segment elevation of the European Society of Cardiology (ESC). Eur Heart J. 2018;39:119–77.
3. Schlotter F, de Waha S, Eitel I, Desch S, Fuernau G, Thiele H. Interventional post-myocardial infarction ventricular septal defect closure: a systematic review of current evidence. EuroIntervention. 2016;12:94–102.
4. Calvert PA, Cockburn J, Wynne D, et al. Percutaneous closure of postinfarction ventricular septal defect: in-hospital outcomes and long-term follow-up of UK experience. Circulation. 2014;129:2395–402.

Chapter 74
Transcatheter Coronary Arterio-Venous Fistulae (CAVF) Closure

Ata Firouzi and Zahra Hosseini

Abstract Coronary AVF, is account of 48.7% of all congenital coronary anomalies. It can be coronary- cameral or coronary to great vessels fistulae. The most common involved artery and entry sites are RCA and RV, RA, coronary sinus, pulmonary artery and left circulation. According to the feeding vessel and entry site, the left to right shunt is dissimilar. Steal phenomena, aneurysmal dilatation of feeding vessel and subsequently, thrombosis, rupture and endarteritis are reported complications. For all symptomatic patients or LV overload and rarely pulmonary hypertension, closure is recommended. Either surgical ligation or trans-catheter closure are effective. With advances in interventional equipments and devices, either retrogradely or antegradely can close the fistulae tract with minimal complication and high success rate.

History

The patient was a 40 years old lady, without any traditional cardiovascular risk factors, was referred with exertional chest pain and dyspnea functional class II–III since 6 months ago. In Gated Thallium myocardial perfusion scan, moderate ischemia in inferior and inferoseptal segments was reported. In selective coronary angiography, left and right coronary arteries were normal, but a large fistulous connection was seen between RCA and pulmonary artery.

An AVF is an abnormal connection between an artery and a vein bypassing interposed arterioles, capillaries, and venules. It usually causes venous dilatation due to exposure to arterial pressure. CAVF can be congenital (0.4% of all cardiac malformations, comprise 48.7% of all congenital coronary anomalies), associated congenital cardiovascular anomalies have been seen in 5–30% of these cases such as ASD, Tetralogy Of Fallot, VSD, and PDA or acquired (followed by trauma, cardiac

A. Firouzi (✉) · Z. Hosseini
Interventional Cardiology, Cardiovascular Intervention Research Center, Rajaie Cardiovascular Medical and Research Center, Iran University of Medical Sciences, Tehran, Iran

M. Maleki, A. Alizadehasl (eds.), *Case-Based Clinical Cardiology*,
https://doi.org/10.1007/978-1-4471-7496-7_74

transplant, CABG, myocardial infarction, PCI, and endomyocardial biopsy) [1, 2]. The fistulous tract may occur between any coronary arteries or their branches and any cardiac chambers (coronary cameral fistulae) or great vessels, either with the right side of the circulation (right atrium and its tributaries, coronary sinus, right ventricle, pulmonary artery) causing a left-to-right shunt, RV volume overload, and pulmonary hypertension or with the left atrium or left ventricle causing LV volume overload and LVH. The former is more frequent. According to Sakakibara et al, there are two types of angiographic classification: Type A: proximal type, where the proximal coronary segment is dilated to the origin of the fistula and the distal end is normal; and Type B: distal type, where the coronary artery is dilated over its entire length terminating as a fistula mainly into the right side of the heart (end-artery type) and the proximal coronary segment can or might have regular branches [3].

In congenital types, the most common feeding vessel is RCA (52%), followed by LAD (30%) and rarely LCX (18%). The most common entry sites are RV, RA, coronary sinus, LV, and pulmonary artery respectively [4] (Table 74.1).

The tract tends to be more tortuous if it originates from proximal RCA especially when enters the coronary sinus, or distal LAD to the LV chamber. Rarely some of CAVFs close spontaneously (1–2%), many are asymptomatic and incidentally detected by a continuous murmur in physical exam which frequently is mistaken for a PDA. Coronary "steal phenomenon" is believed to be the primary pathophysiological problem seen in CAVF without outflow obstruction. The mechanism is related to the runoff from the high-pressure coronary vasculature to a low-resistance receiving cavity (e.g., pulmonary vasculature) due to a diastolic pressure gradient. Eventually, there is a high risk of ischemia in the myocardium beyond the site of the origin of the fistula, which is most frequently evident in association with increased myocardial oxygen demand during exercise or activity [5]. Complications of CAVF are coronary artery dilatation, aneurysm formation, intimal ulceration, atherosclerotic change, calcification, side-branch obstruction, mural thrombosis, rupture, and even tamponade. A left-to-right shunt exists in over 90% of cases, the symptoms develop depending on the amount of the left-to-right shunt or the presence of coronary steal phenomenon of the fistulae, which usually present in young adults with angina (3–7%), exertional dyspnea (60%), CHF, endocarditis in the fistula (20%), syncope, arrhythmia, myocardial ischemia and infarction, and manifest in older adults with congestive heart failure (19%—Congestive heart failure is seen more

Table 74.1 Origin and drainage of fistulae

Origin	Prevalence (%)	Drainage	Prevalence (%)
LAD	25–42	RA	19–26
RCA	50–60	RV	14–40
Both	5	LA	5–6
Diagonal	1.9	LV	2–19
Marginal	0.7	PA	15–20.2
Circumflex	18.3	CS	7
Single coronary	3	SCV	1

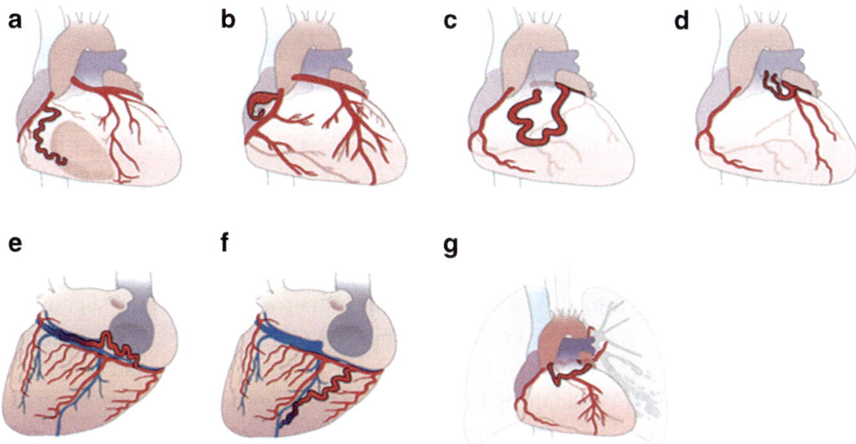

Fig. 74.1 Classification of CAFs based on drainage site. The following fistula types are illustrated: (**a**) Coronary cameral fistula involving the right ventricle chamber. (**b**) coronary cameral fistula involving the right atrium chamber. (**c**) coronary artery to pulmonary artery fistula involving a single large fistulous tract. (**d**) coronary artery to pulmonary artery fistula involving multiple small fistulous tracts. (**e**) coronary artery to coronary sinus fistula. (**f**) coronary artery to cardiac vein fistula, and (**g**) coronary artery to bronchial artery fistula

frequently in cases of a coronary artery-to-coronary sinus fistula than with other CAVF), atherosclerosis, cardiac arrhythmias and even sudden cardiac death [6] (Fig. 74.1).

Diagnostic Work-Up

In physical exam, usually a loud, soft continuous murmur is audible on the chest wall depending on the entry site, often lower than the PDA murmur site and peak at mid to late diastole. Depending on the amount of left-to-right shunt, any sign of LV volume overload or PH can be detected. In ECG, again depending on the severity and the entry site of the shunt, LVH or RVH pattern or any ischemic changes are seen. TTE can evaluate LV, LA and RV size and functions, any regional wall motion abnormality, coronary sinus dilatation, or concomitant anomalies. TEE can demonstrate the origin and the draining points of the fistulae. The gold standard tool is coronary angiography, which provides the hemodynamic effect and most detailed anatomy of the fistula giving information about the size, the course, the origin, the presence of any stenosis, and the drainage site. However, it yields two-dimensional projection images, which are often limited in the delineation of the complex anatomy of abnormal communications, with reported correct diagnosis rates of 35%–50% [7].

Another modality is coronary CT Angiography, which is useful for the evaluation of CAFs because it involves a shorter acquisition time and yields higher temporal and spatial resolution. Multi-planar reconstruction with 3D volume-rendered imaging yields excellent anatomic information, including the origin, course, and drainage site of CAFs, even in cases of complex anomalies and thus has the potential to serve as a basic guide for treatment planning. At cardiac CT angiography, a coronary-to-pulmonary artery fistula appears as an abnormal contrast blush, which is also referred to as the contrast shunt sign, in a relatively less opacified pulmonary trunk or as a well-visualized fistulous tract between the coronary artery and pulmonary trunk. In this type of CAVF, it has been shown that the LCA to be the most common origin site (84%), followed by the RCA (38%). The majority (89%) of CAFs drain into the pulmonary trunk rather than into other segmental pulmonary arteries. According to recent findings, two types of coronary-to-pulmonary artery fistulas occur: The first type is a single prominent fistulous connection between the LAD or RCA and the main pulmonary trunk and the other type involves multiple small-caliber fistulous connections from the LAD or RCA, which drains into the main pulmonary trunk [8]. CMR is another modality for anatomic assessment of the fistulae and finally, MPI is the functional test for evaluating the severity of myocardial ischemia related to the CAVF.

Management

There is general agreement that symptomatic patients should be treated. According to the ACC/AHA guidelines, a percutaneous or surgical closure is a Class I recommendation for large fistulae regardless of symptoms and for small- to moderate size fistulae with evidence of myocardial ischemia, arrhythmia, ventricular dysfunction, ventricular enlargement, or endarteritis [9]. In addition, closure of fistulae that arise in the proximal segment of the coronary vessel is highly recommended as this type of fistulae is more likely to become aneurysmal with a high possibility of rupture. Traditionally, asymptomatic patients with small shunts are managed conservatively owing to the benign course and the possibility of spontaneous closure.

Surgical Treatment Surgical ligation is generally recommended for treatment of large symptomatic fistulas with multiple communications, tortuous and aneurysmal arteries and for patients who require surgical management of other clinically important cardiac anomalies (Table 74.2).

Transcatheter CAVF Closure Percutaneous transcatheter closure is a noninvasive alternative for the treatment of CAFs. It is indicated in patients whose anatomy is favorable for the procedure, including those with a single narrow drainage site, a proximal fistula origin, an absence of multiple fistulas or large branch vessels, and/or an absence of concomitant cardiac disorders. It is preferred for older patients who are at risk for perioperative complications. Various devices are being used to perform percutaneous transcatheter procedures. These devices include coils, umbrella devices, vascular plugs, covered stents, and ductal occluders (Table 74.3). Addressing

Table 74.2 Indications for surgical ligation and percutaneous trans-catheter closure

Surgical ligation
Large symptomatic fistula with high fistula blood flow
Multiple communications and drainage sites
Tortuous and aneurysmal fistulous arteries
Need for simultaneous distal bypass
Large vascular branches that can be accidentally embolized
Percutaneous transcatheter closure
Proximal fistula origin
Single drain site
Nontortuous vessel with distal portion of fistula accessible with the closure device
Extra-anatomic termination of fistula away from normal coronary arteries
Older patients with high risk of perioperative complications
Absence of concomitant cardiac disorders

Table 74.3 Comparison of devices used in percutaneous coronary artery fistula closure

	Amplatzer® Vascular Plug	AMPLATZER Duct Occluder	Detachable balloon	Coils	Covered stent	Chemicals
Selected fistula size	Medium–large	Medium–large	Medium–large	Small–medium	Small–medium	Small–medium
Retraction before deployment	Yes	Yes	Yes	Yes/no	No	No
Clinical experience	High	High	Low	High	Moderate	Low
Delivery approach	Antegrade or retrograde	Antegrade	Retrograde	Antegrade or retrograde	Retrograde	Retrograde

the distal vessel entry site before performing the transcatheter embolization is clinically important. When the distal vessel is wide, the chance of distal coil migration increases. On the other hand, if the coil is placed proximal to a branching vessel, it may be difficult to completely occlude the shunt. Therefore, the focus of the pre-procedural radiologic report should be delineation of the distal entry site.

Procedural Technique

Under local anesthesia, after the right femoral artery and vein sheaths (6F) insertion, IV Heparin completed to achieve ACT > 200 s. After RHC and selective coronary angiography, precisely localized the entry and the distal end of the fistulae (the entry was at the proximal part of RCA after the Conus branch with a very tortuous tract which ended to the pulmonary trunk) (Fig. 74.2a, b). Retrogradely, through JR guiding catheter (6F), in LAO projection, gently, wiring of the tract was done under

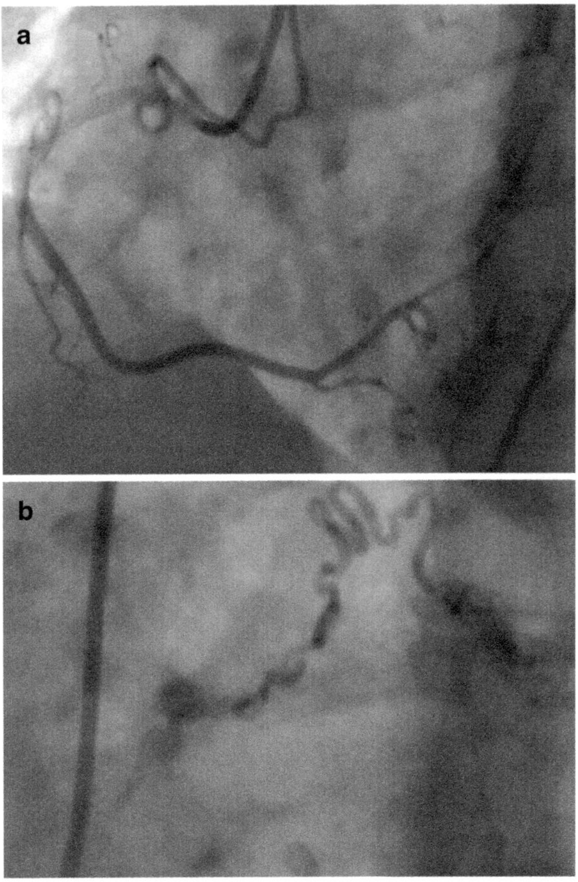

Fig. 74.2 (**a**, **b**) Selective RCA injection showed that an entry was at the proximal part of RCA after the Conus branch with a very tortuous tract which ended to the pulmonary trunk

support of micro-catheter (Caravel-135) with 0.014 inch coronary guide-wire (Sion black) to reach as distal as possible, then the Caravel was pushed forward over the wire with clock and counterclockwise rotation and positioned at distal end. According to the size of the fistulae, the detachable coil 6*30 (ev3) was chosen. After withdrawing the guide-wire, the coil was passed to reach the distal tip of the micro-catheter then after being sure about the size of the coil by angiography, the micro-catheter was retracted gently and the coil was deployed completely and detached (Fig. 74.3a). Final angiography showed no residual shunt or any RCA injury (Fig. 74.3b).

Complications

The success rate in multiple literatures have been reported between 87 and 97% [10]. Early complications related to occlusion procedures are transient myocardial ischemia or dysrhythmias, myocardial infarction, distal coronary spasm, fistula

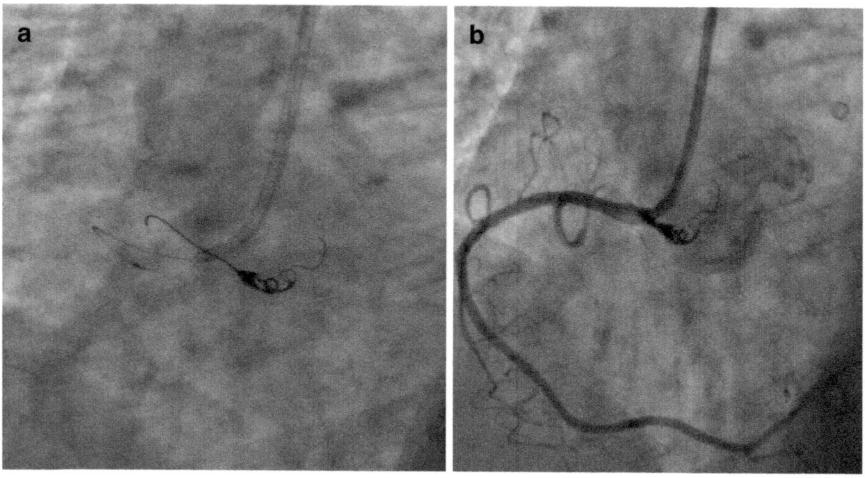

Fig. 74.3 (**a**, **b**) According to the size of the fistulae, the detachable coil 6*30 (ev3) was chosen. the coil was deployed completely and detached. Final angiography showed no residual shunt or any RCA injury

dissection, and device embolization [11]. Residual shunt (25%) and recurrence (9–19%) is reported [12]. Coronary artery dilatation may persist after the intervention, either with percutaneous closure or surgical ligation, in intermediate to long-term follow-up. Rupture of CAFs may occur in patients, independent of preceding dilation. Therefore, close follow-up is warranted, especially for thin-walled ectatic arteries. Although there is not a consensus regarding the antithrombotic or anticoagulant therapy for dilated coronary arteries after closure, some authors advocate antiplatelet therapy for dilated coronary arteries and anticoagulation with warfarin in severe coronary artery dilatation (>10 mm), especially in patients with the sluggish coronary flow [13]. The prognosis depends on the severity of the shunt and on certain complications that sometimes occur, such as heart failure, pulmonary hypertension, and bacterial endocarditis.

Conclusion

Currently, percutaneous management of CAFs provides a high degree of procedural success with a very low risk of serious complications. Device selection and delivery technique should be based on the anatomic and morphologic characteristics of the fistula. Although surgical ligation has previously been the standard treatment for CAF, specialized techniques, equipment, and newer devices have made the percutaneous approach a safe and effective first-line treatment modality in most patients with suitable anatomy, with good follow-up results. Long-term follow-up is essential owing to the possibility of post-procedural recanalization or residual flow, persistent dilation of the coronary artery, late thrombosis, and myocardial ischemia.

Therefore, even though most patients become asymptomatic after the intervention, they should not be dismissed from follow-up [14].

References

1. Fernandes ED, Kadivar H, Hallman GL, Reul GJ, Ott DA, Cooley DA. Congenital malformations of the coronary arteries: the Texas Heart Institute experience. Ann Thorac Surg. 1992;54(4):732–40.
2. Said SA, Lam J, van der Werf T. Solitary coronary artery fistulas: a congenital anomaly in children and adults. A contemporary review. Congenit Heart Dis. 2006;1(3):63–76.
3. Dodge-Khatami A, Mavroudis C, Backer CL. Congenital heart surgery nomenclature and database project: anomalies of the coronary arteries. Ann Thorac Surg. 2000;69(Suppl 4):S270–97.
4. Ata Y, Turk T, Bicer M, Yalcin M, Ata F, Yavuz S. Coronary arteriovenous fistulas in the adults: natural history and management strategies. J Cardiothorac Surg. 2009;4:62.
5. Dimitrakakis G, Von Oppell U, Luckraz H, Groves P. Surgical repair of triple coronary-pulmonary artery fistulae with associated atrial septal defect and aortic valve regurgitation. Interact Cardiovasc Thorac Surg. 2008;7(5):933–4.
6. Shiga Y, Tsuchiya Y, Yahiro E, et al. Left main coronary trunk connecting into right atrium with an aneurysmal coronary artery fistula. Int J Cardiol. 2008;123(2):e28–30.
7. Shabestari AA, Akhlaghpoor S, Fatehi M. Findings of bilateral coronary to pulmonary artery fistula in 64-multislice computed tomographic angiography: correlation with catheter angiography. J Comput Assist Tomogr. 2008;32(2):271–3.
8. Verdini D, Vargas D, Kuo A, et al. Coronary-pulmonary artery fistulas: a systematic review. J Thorac Imaging. 2016;31(6):380–90.
9. Warnes CA, Williams RG, Bashore TM, et al. ACC/AHA 2008 guidelines for the management of adults with congenital heart disease: executive summary—a report of the American College of Cardiology/American Heart Association Task Force on Practice Guidelines (Writing Committee to Develop Guidelines for the Management of Adults with Congenital Heart Disease). Circulation. 2008;118(23):2395–451.
10. Said SA, Nijhuis RL, Op den Akker JW, et al. Diagnostic and therapeutic approach of congenital solitary coronary artery fistulas in adults: Dutch case series and review of literature. Neth Heart J. 2011;19(4):183–91.
11. Armsby LR, Keane JF, Sherwood MC, Forbess JM, Perry SB, Lock JE. Management of coronary artery fistulae. Patient selection and results of transcatheter closure. J Am Coll Cardiol. 2002;39(6):1026–32.
12. Zhu XY, Zhang DZ, Han XM, et al. Transcatheter closure of congenital coronary artery fistulae: immediate and long-term follow-up results. Clin Cardiol. 2009;32(9):506–12.
13. Mcmahon CJ, Nihill MR, Kovalchin JP, Mullins CE, Grifka RG. Coronary artery fistula. Management and intermediate-term outcome after transcatheter coil occlusion. Tex Heart Inst J. 2001;28(1):21–5.
14. Oto MA, Yorgun H, Aytemir K, et al. Percutaneous approaches to closure of coronary artery fistulas. Interv Cardiol. 2011;3(1):79–89.

Chapter 75
Transcatheter Pulmonary Vein Stenosis (PVS) Venoplasty

Ata Firouzi and Zahra Hosseini

Abstract In adults, the most common cause of pulmonary vein stenosis (PVS), is iatrogenic (the most cause is radiofrequency AF ablation). Left side veins are more involved. Frequently patients with one vein stenosis are asymptomatic, but sometimes even in these patients symptoms have been shown 3-6 months after the ablation. Treatment indications are controversy, in those who are symptomatic with severe stenosis or those ones with lung perfusion defect>20-25% are candidate for repair. Some believe that even asymptomatic patients with more than 75% stenosis are better to undergo intervention. Both surgical and trans-catheter interventions are available. In adult patient the preferred strategy is trans-catheter balloon venoplasty, although the rate of restenosis is high and stenting seems to be more durable.

History

The patient was a 45 years old lady, a case of post AF (lone AF) ablation 6 months ago who was referred with exertional dyspnea and occasional palpitation which in TTE, turbulent flow in LUPV-LA junction with high gradient was detected.

Pulmonary vein stenosis (PVS) can be congenital (o.4% of all CHD), the syndrome of primary endo-luminal pulmonary vein stenosis with no preceding surgery or catheter intervention has been postulated to result from abnormal incorporation of the common pulmonary vein into the left atrium in the later stages of cardiac development. Affected patients most often become symptomatic in the first few months to years of life, frequently have one or more additional cardiac anomalies, and have no active inflammation in or around the involved segments of vein. Estimates of the incidence of associated cardiac defects have ranged from 30 to 80% [1]. The most commonly associated congenital heart defects are septal defects, but pulmonary vein stenosis has been seen in conjunction with all major types of congenital cardiac malformations, the timing and severity of symptoms in pediatric

A. Firouzi (✉) · Z. Hosseini
Interventional Cardiology, Cardiovascular Intervention Research Center, Rajaie Cardiovascular Medical and Research Center, Iran University of Medical Sciences, Tehran, Iran

M. Maleki, A. Alizadehasl (eds.), *Case-Based Clinical Cardiology*,
https://doi.org/10.1007/978-1-4471-7496-7_75

patients with pulmonary vein stenosis appear to depend largely on the number of pulmonary veins involved and the obstruction severity of individual pulmonary veins. Most patients present with a history of significant respiratory symptoms. Patients are often tachypneic and have recurrent pneumonias. As the disease progresses, signs of PH become increasingly prominent. In acquired ones, after surgical repair of a total or partial anomalous pulmonary venous connection (10%), myxoma resection, Lung transplant, AF radiofrequency ablation (the most common cause (60%) of PVS which usually missed), sarcoidosis, neoplasm, and mediastinal fibrosis (Fig. 75.1) [2], patients most often present with dyspnea, orthopnea and sometimes have a radiographic appearance of a localized infiltrate or localized edema. Hemoptysis is not uncommon. In both the congenital and acquired forms of PVS, histological findings show a variable manifestation of neo-intimal proliferation leading to occlusion of the lumen of one or more of the pulmonary veins. It is estimated that approximately 60% of patients have unilateral disease, of which most stenosis involves the left pulmonary veins. Approximately 40% of patients have bilateral pulmonary vein disease [3]. Three patterns of PVS have been described: bilateral tubular hypoplasia extending from the veno-atrial junction for a variable length, discrete hourglass constriction at the veno-atrial junctions, and bilateral multiple short pulmonary veins that are hypoplastic for their entire extra-pulmonary course [4]. The prognosis is often poor. The disease tends to be progressive and is associated with high mortality (30–50%) in the first 2 years after diagnosis (the development of progressive pulmonary venous congestion followed by pulmonary arterial hypertension (PH) and eventual death). At the present time PV ablation for AF has become the principal cause of PVS. Incidence derived from recent studies reaches a mean and median of 2% and 3.1%, respectively [5]. These figures represent a significant reduction in comparison with those reported in pioneer series. The main factors contributing to this finding are operator experience and improvements in the procedure (changing of ablation site from the PVs antra to ostia, reduction of temperature applied to tissue, cryoablation, and ICE guidance). However real occurrence of PVS is probably underestimated as screening is only performed within the

Fig. 75.1 The most common Causes of pulmonary vein stenosis (Congenital or Acquired etiologies)

Causes of pulmonary vein stenosis
Congenital
Cardiac defects associated:
Total anomalous pulmonary venous return
Septal defects
Transposition of the great vessels
Acquired
Pulmonary vein ablation
Sarcoidosis
Neoplasm
Fibrosing mediastinitis
Post cardiovascular surgery

first 3 months in some centers (it has been demonstrated that PVS can occur over this time period) and asymptomatic patients are not always imaged. Therefore screening with available imaging modalities in patients with PV ablation who develop respiratory symptoms is warranted.

Clinically, almost all patients with mild (<50%) or moderate stenosis (50–70%) of the PV do not have symptoms. The occurrence of respiratory symptoms (coughing, hemoptysis, and dyspnea) which usually appear 3–6 months after the procedure is associated with severe stenosis of a single PV (>70%), lung perfusion reduction by >20–25% or the involvement of multiple PV [6]. However, it is also known that patients with severe stenosis or occlusion of a single PV can remain asymptomatic. In this context, although still controversial, the strategy of systematically screening for PV stenosis with CT scan or CMR for all patients undergoing PV isolation, regardless of symptom manifestation, can be considered [7]. In asymptomatic patients, the failure or delay in recognizing PV stenosis, with the consequent interruption of the anticoagulation after the procedure can result in thrombotic occlusion of the PV, with adverse effects on pulmonary perfusion and the risk of the development of pulmonary infarction, respiratory infections, and even long-term pulmonary hypertension.

Diagnostic Work-Up

CXR may demonstrate signs of congestion either diffuse or localized, depending on the PVs involve. TTE and TEE are useful tools for PV investigation. Studies have shown high diagnosis accuracy for the detection of PVS after PV ablation (sensitivity: 82–100%, specificity: 95–100%) compared to other techniques. There is no standard definition of PVS, nevertheless, it seems that an increased maximum PV Doppler flow velocity (>1.1 m/s) combined with color Doppler turbulence may be a reliable index [8]. Cardiac CT Angiography, allows assessment of the extension of mediastinal neoplastic and non-tumoral diseases infiltrating or compressing the PVs and enables the diagnosis of PVS after PV ablation by directly depicting vessel ostia and distal part diameter (significant stenosis >50%). The main benefits of CT are short examination time, multi-planar views, and high spatial resolution (Fig. 75.2). PVs (typically the left inferior) can be compressed between the LA and the descending aorta appearing stenotic (pseudostenosis).

CMR is also an accurate modality for the evaluation of PVs and flow dynamic. This allows for anatomic measurements in any desired plane, including determination of the perimeter and cross-sectional area that may be more meaningful measures of pulmonary vein size. The maximal diameter, perimeter, and cross-sectional area are measured at the location in the sagittal plane at which the pulmonary veins separate from the LA and each other (Fig. 75.3).

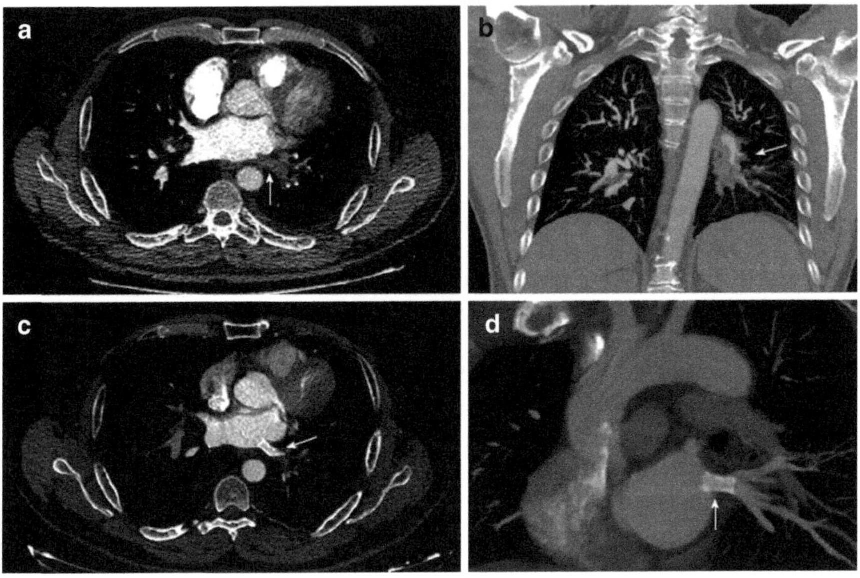

Fig. 75.2 CT of a patient who had AF radiofrequency ablation two months before and recent onset of dyspnea on exertion. (**a**) Absent of contrast (arrow) in the left lower pulmonary vein (complete occlusion); (**b**) Extensive infiltrate within the left lung (arrow) caused by localized edema; (**c** and **d**) After stent implantation (arrows) flow was successfully restored

Fig. 75.3 Advantages of imaging modalities (TEE, CT, MRI, and VQ) used for pulmonary vein stenosis evaluation

Advantages of imaging modalities used for pulmonary vein stenosis evaluation

	TEE	CT	MRI	VQ
Availability	Yes	Yes	No	No
Non-invasive	No[1]	Yes	Yes	Yes
Caliber assessment	No	Yes	Yes	No
Functional assessment	Yes	No	Yes	Yes
Evaluation of surrounding tissues	No	Yes	Yes	No
Radiation avoidance	Yes	No	Yes	No

Management

PVS in Pediatric Population

Surgery is the preferred approach in most congenital or acquired significant symptomatic PVS. The conventional interventions include: (1) endarterectomy (excision of the stenotic ring and direct anastomosis of the PV to the LA endocardium), and (2) pericardial patch venoplasty (resection of the stenotic tissue and patch anastomosis to enlarge the tightened segment). The newer sutureless marsupialization technique can help to prevent deformation of the suture line and reduce tissue growth stimulus decreasing therefore restenosis risk. Overall, published surgical outcomes are modest, only half of the cases are free from re-intervention or death at 5 years [9].

PVS in Adult Population

Transcatheter therapy is the most commonly chosen approach. The degree of PVS after PV ablation is classified as severe with luminal narrowing more than 70%, moderate for 50–70% narrowing, and mild for <50% narrowing. There is a general agreement that patients with symptomatic severe stenosis of one or multiple PVs should be treated with PV angioplasty with or without stenting. For asymptomatic patients with severe stenosis of a single PV, there is no consensus on whether intervention is warranted, although the available evidence suggests that early intervention in such patients leads to clinical benefit [6]. Despite most authors recommend clinical and imaging monitoring every 3–6 months in asymptomatic patients with 50–85% stenosis, some promote angioplasty if a single stenosis >75% and others in cases of a cumulative stenosis index (average stenosis of the PVs of one site) >75% [10]. The main arguments for early intervention are: Inadequate recovery of lung perfusion at advanced stages caused by fixed venoconstriction leading to permanent PH and fast progression to PV occlusion in some cases which may be difficult to amend. Regarding the technique itself, stenting appears better than isolated balloon venoplasty in terms of vessel restenosis (60 vs. 36% for PV over 8 mm). Mid- to long-term patency is directly related to vessel size with higher rates of restenosis observed in PV < 1 cm.

Procedural Technique

Under general anesthesia, after the insertion of right femoral artery and vein sheaths (6F), RHC was done (mPAP: 30 mm Hg, PCWP: 18 mm Hg). Through venous access, after septostomy with Brockenbrough needle and contrast injection to confirm of being in LA and insertion of Spiral wire (coiled tip, 0.025 inch) in LA for more support and LA border illustration (Fig. 75.4a), IV Heparin completed to achieve ACT > 250 s. Through a 125-cm 6F multipurpose diagnostic catheter telescoped through a steerable transseptal sheath (Agilis sheath), a 0.035 inch straight hydrophilic wire was manipulated to cross the origin of LUPV under TEE and fluoroscopic guidance, after some minutes, the wire was crossed and advanced as distal as possible, then gently the Multipurpose catheter passed over the wire with its tip at the most distal part. After exchanging the wire with Amplatzer Superstiff guidewire, the catheter slowly pulled back to measure the mean gradient between LA and LUPV (MPG: 10 mm Hg) (Fig. 75.5b). Contrast-enhanced venography was

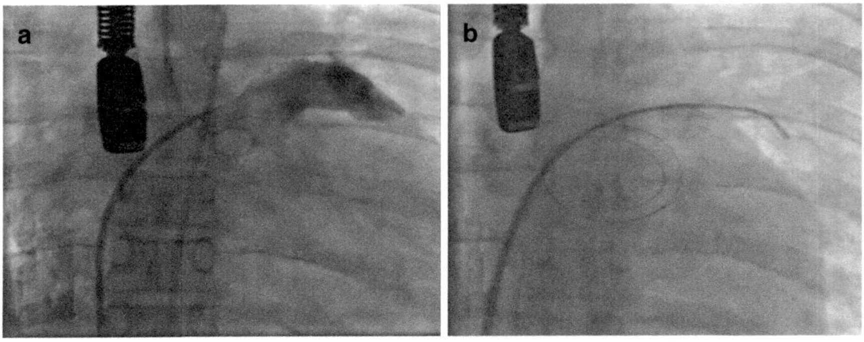

Fig. 75.4 (**a**, **b**) After successful septostomy, via Multipurpose catheter, the gradient between LA and LUPV was measured (10 mm Hg)

Fig. 75.5 (**a**, **b**) Selective LUPV-L angiography showed significant narrowing at the origin of LUPV-LA junction. Through long sheath, sequential dilatation of LUPV ostia at site of maximal stenosis was performed with peripheral balloons (OTW) 10*30 and 12*30 under TEE guidance

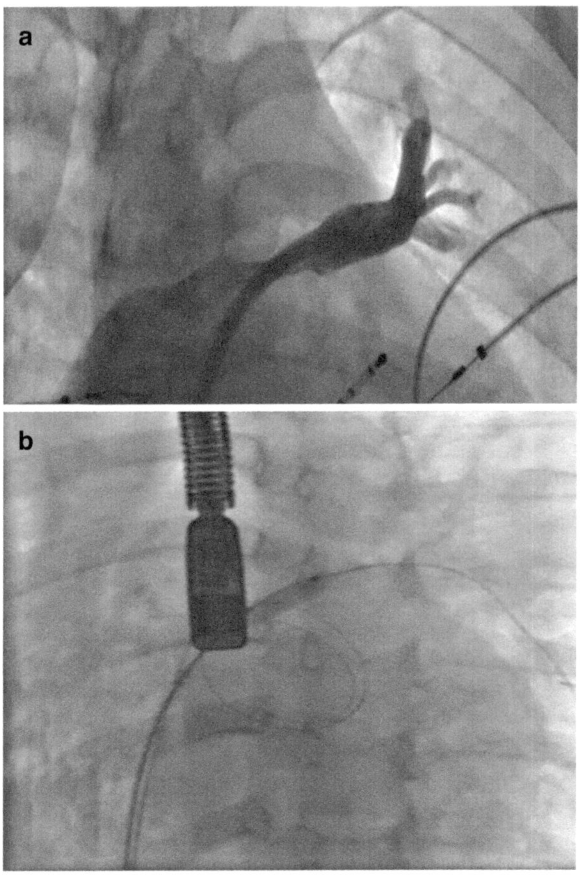

performed for confirmation and characterization of the stenosis (Fig. 75.5a). After withdrawing the Agilis sheath, a long delivery sheath (Cook 12F) was advanced through the septum and the end tip was passed over the guide-wire to cross the ostium of LUPV. According to the CT data (distal LUPV diameter was 12 mm), sequential dilatation of LUPV ostia at the site of maximal stenosis was performed with peripheral balloons (OTW) 10*30 and 12*30 under TEE guidance with closed hemodynamic monitoring (Figs. 75.5b and 75.6). Despite of full inflation of the balloons for long duration (30–60 s) and disappearance of the waist, in TEE, the recoil of the ostium occurred with no decrease in mean gradient. So, in this situation, a BiB balloon 14*30 was maximally inflated for a long duration (Fig. 75.7a).

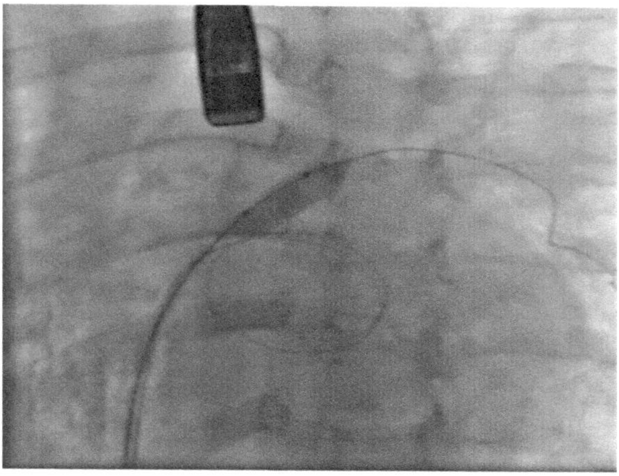

Fig. 75.6 Balloon dilatation with peripheral balloon 12*30

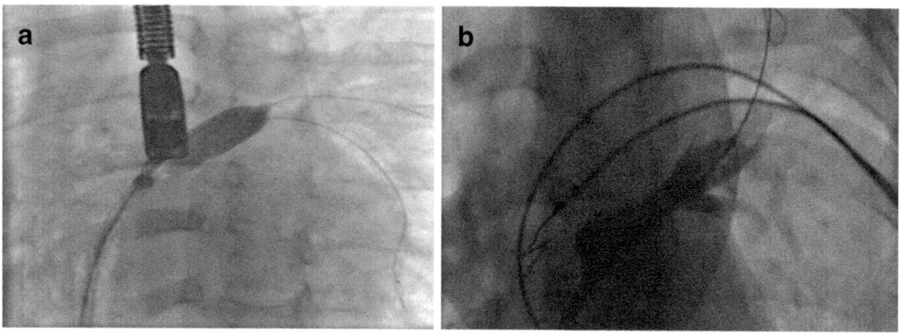

Fig. 75.7 (**a**, **b**) Despite full inflation of the balloons for a long duration (30–60 s) and disappearance of the waist, in TEE, the recoil of the ostium occurred with no decrease in mean gradient. So, in this situation, a BiB balloon 14*30 (**a**) was maximally inflated for a long duration. At the end, final LUPV angiography showed the disappearance of the ostial narrowing with the final gradient of 3 mm Hg and no complications

Finally, TEE showed no any residual recoil and decreasing the mean gradient to 2 mm Hg. The LA angiography also showed acceptable ostial opening (residual narrowing less than 20%) and well LUPV branches contrast opacification with no oozing (Fig. 75.7b), residual gradient was 3 mm Hg.

Complications

Complication rates in transcatheter PVS venoplasty or stenting is about 10–13%. The most are, wire induced PV perforation or injury, balloon induced PV perforation and tamponade, stent migration to LA, acute stent thrombosis and CVA or restenosis, and recoil after balloon venoplasty. The pathophysiological effect of restenosis after balloon venoplasty is an elastic recoil and happens typically at an early stage after the procedure. In comparison, restenosis after stent implantation occurs at a later stage because of neo-intimal hyperplasia [11].

Conclusion

In general, pulmonary vein stenosis has a high rate of restenosis (defined as narrowing more than 70%) and a high rate of mortality regardless of surgical or transcatheter therapy (angioplasty, stenting). In one study, it reported that angioplasty success and restenosis rates of 42% and 72%, respectively. In contrast, stenting resulted in success and restenosis rates of 95% and 33%, respectively [12]. After angioplasty, 90% of patients reported that their symptoms have improved, despite restenosis. This may be due to collateralization or other beneficial physiological adaptations [13]. The long-term risk of developing pulmonary hypertension in patients with pulmonary venous stenosis remains unknown, and it remains unclear whether intervention is needed in asymptomatic patients with severe stenosis. In spite of reasonable immediate results, restenosis is not uncommon, and repeat dilations following stenting may be needed. A few reports indicate that the stented diameter of 7–10 mm or greater may play a role in minimizing the risk of restenosis. It is not uncommon to re-intervene as a bridge to lung transplant. Despite the lack of randomized studies, currently available published research seem to indicate that stent implantation should be the first-line therapy in patients with RFA-induced severe PVS. To minimize the restenosis rate, stents with diameters $\geq$8 mm should be preferred [14]. In our experience, surgical repair can be considered in selected patients with three or more severe PVS or complex cases with prior failed PTA. There is a strong need for a prospectively randomized comparison of these two interventional treatment options for PVS following AF ablation procedures and for adequate products meeting the needs for PV stenting with short-length, large-diameter stents [15].

References

1. Edwards JE. Congenital stenosis of pulmonary veins. Pathologic and developmental considerations. Lab Invest. 1960;9:46–66.
2. Albers EL, Pugh ME, Hill KD, Wang L, Loyd JE, Doyle TP. Percutaneous vascular stent implantation as treatment for central vascular obstruction due to fibrosing mediastinitis. Circulation. 2011;123:1391–9.
3. King W, Kenneth O, Schowengerdt, et al. Pulmonary disease associated with congenital heart disease. Kedig's disorders of respiratory tract in children. Elsevier; 2019, p. 615–25.e2
4. Ward KE, Mullins CE. Anomalous pulmonary venous connections, vein stenosis, and atresia of the common vein. In: Garson A, Bricker JT, Fisher DJ, Neish SR, editors. The science and practice of pediatric cardiology. Baltimore, MD: Williams and Wilkins; 1998. p. 1431–61.
5. Calkins H, Hindricks G, Cappato R, et al. 2017 HRS/EHRA/ECAS/APHRS/SOLAECE expert consensus statement on catheter and surgical ablation of atrial fibrillation: executive summary. Europace. 2018;20:e1–e160.
6. Di Biase L, Fahmy TS, Wazni OM, Bai R, Patel D, Lakkireddy D, et al. Pulmonary vein total occlusion following catheter ablation for atrial fibrillation: clinical implications after long-term follow-up. J Am Coll Cardiol. 2006;48:2493–9.
7. Saad EB, Rosillo A, Saad CP, Martin DO, Bhargava M, Erciyes D, et al. Pulmonary vein stenosis after radiofrequency ablation of atrial fibrillation: functional characterization, evolution, and influence of the ablation strategy. Circulation. 2003;108:3102–7.
8. Yu WC, Hsu TL, Tai CT, Tsai CF, Hsieh MH, Lin WS, Lin YK, Tsao HM, Ding YA, Chang MS, Chen SA. Acquired pulmonary vein stenosis after radiofrequency catheter ablation of paroxysmal atrial fibrillation. J Cardiovasc Electrophysiol. 2001;12:887–92.
9. Shi G, Zhu Z, Chen H, Zhang H, Zheng J, Liu J. Surgical repair for primary pulmonary vein stenosis: single-institution, midterm follow-up. J Thorac Cardiovasc Surg. 2015;150:181–8.
10. Holmes DR, Monahan KH, Packer D. Pulmonary vein stenosis complicating ablation for atrial fibrillation: clinical spectrum and interventional considerations. JACC Cardiovasc Interv. 2009;2:267–76.
11. Schoene K, Arya A, Jahnke C, Paetsch I, et al. Acquired pulmonary vein stenosis after radiofrequency ablation for atrial fibrillation. Single-center experience in catheter interventional treatment. JACC. 2018;11(16). https://doi.org/10.1016/j.jcin.2018.05.016
12. Prieto LR, Schoenhagen P, Arruda MJ, et al. Comparison of stent versus balloon angioplasty for pulmonary vein stenosis complicating pulmonary vein isolation. J Cardiovasc Electrophysiol. 2008;19:673–8.
13. Mahapatra S, Peterson LA, Monihan KM, Munger TM, Packer DL. Long-term symptom improvement in patients with pulmonary vein stenosis from atrial fibrillation ablation despite restenosis. Heart Rhythm. 2004;1:S88.
14. Buiatti A, von Olshausen G, Martens E, et al. Balloon angioplasty versus stenting for pulmonary vein stenosis after pulmonary vein isolation for atrial fibrillation: a meta-analysis. Int J Cardiol. 2018;254:146–50.
15. Neumann T, Kuniss M, Conradi G, et al. Pulmonary vein stenting for the treatment of acquired severe pulmonary vein stenosis after pulmonary vein isolation: clinical implications after long-term follow-up of 4 years. J Cardiovasc Electrophysiol. 2009;20:251–7.

Chapter 76
Percutaneous Closure of Aortic Paravalvular Leakage

Ata Firouzi and Zahra Hosseini

Abstract Aortic para-valvular leakage, is a regurgitation jet between swing ring and native valve tissue. The etiology of this side effect depends on the time of surgery (technical issues, endocarditis, severe calcification of the surrounding tissue). Depends on the size of the defects, patient's symptoms range between asymptomatic to pulmonary edema. The standard treatment in severe leakage is surgical repair, but in those with high surgical mortality, trans-catheter device closure (if anatomically being suitable) is an alternative approach by expert interventionist. Dedicated device is not available, but according the shape and location of the defect in 3-D TEE, various device can be used.

History

The patient was a 65 years old man, a case of coronary bypass surgery, Aortic Valve Replacement (AVR) and Mitral Valve Replacement (MVR) 15 years ago who was admitted with refractory CHF (Five times admissions within recent 6 months). In TEE, he had severe paravalvular leakage of aortic mechanical valve.

Paravalvular leak (PVL) is a regurgitant jet that originates between the outer margin of the prosthetic ring and the native tissue around the valve. It is a common complication of aortic valve replacement that has been found to occur in about 10% of cases. The majority of patients remain asymptomatic, however, 1–5% Of them present with congestive symptoms [1], hemolytic complications, or both. The congestive heart failure symptoms are related to the defect size, numbers, and LV volume overload degree, whereas hemolytic complications have no correlation with defect size and even occur in small defects. Surgery is the gold standard treatment for operable patients with intractable symptoms and severe PVL (Class I), while in those with high-risk surgery, intractable symptoms and anatomically suitable for catheter-based closure in hands of expert operators is reasonable.

A. Firouzi (✉) · Z. Hosseini
Interventional Cardiology, Cardiovascular Intervention Research Center, Rajaie Cardiovascular Medical and Research Center, Iran University of Medical Sciences, Tehran, Iran

M. Maleki, A. Alizadehasl (eds.), *Case-Based Clinical Cardiology*,
https://doi.org/10.1007/978-1-4471-7496-7_76

For the aortic valve, the LCC is located between 11 and 3 o'clock, the RCC between 3 and 7 o'clock and the NCC between 7 and 11 o'clock. The aortic PLVs are most often between 7 and 11 o'clock (46%) and also between 11 and 3 o'clock (36%) [2] (Figs. 76.1 and 76.2).

Diagnostic Work-Up

TTE is the first modality for evaluation of LV, RV size and functions, mechanical valve evaluation, the severity of trans-valvular or paravalvular leaks, any clots, pannus formation, or vegetation. The 3-D TEE can precisely demonstrate the location,

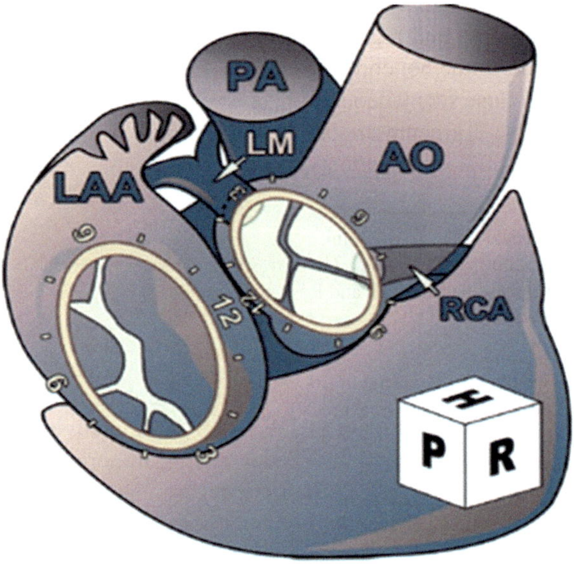

Fig. 76.1 Paravalvular leaks locations diagram

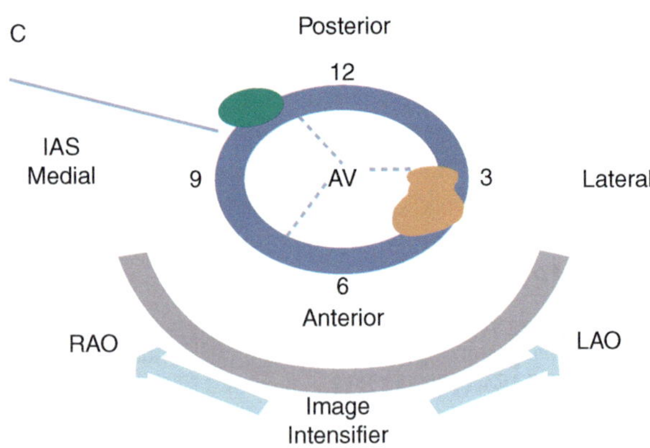

Fig. 76.2

shape, size, depth, and number of the defects, dehiscence, surrounding structures, and differentiated PVL from trans-valvular regurgitations. Another modalities like CT Angiography and CMR can also give more information for better evaluation of the defects.

Procedural Technique

Under general anesthesia, after insertion of right femoral arterial sheath (6F), aortic root injections was done in LAO and RAO projections to localized the site, size, and severity of the paravalvular leakage (Fig. 76.3a). Then under TEE guidance and fluoroscopy, by retrograde approach, in LAO view, the defect (at 10 o'clock) crossed with straight hydrophilic wire and the JR catheter was passed over it (Fig. 76.3b). After that, the wire was exchanged with Extra-support wire (Lunderquist) over that, a hydrophilic delivery sheath (Epsylar 7F) was advanced to the LV. Based on the TEE defect size (6 mm) and shape, the Muscular VSD 8 mm (Occlutech) device was chosen. After loading the device and connecting to the delivery cable, the device was passed over the delivery sheath. First distal disk (DD) was partially extruded in the LV then by retracting the whole system toward the defect, the DD was totally deployed in the ventricular side and anchored within the defect (Fig. 76.4a), then after rechecking by TEE and angiography, the waist and the proximal disk (PD) was deployed (Fig. 76.4b). Prior to the release the device, the most attention (by TEE and fluoroscopy) must be paid to the prosthetic valve to be sure that there is no interference with valve function (free moving leaflets) and no coverage of coronary ostia (Fig. 76.5). Final injection showed mild residual leakage, no interference with leaflets, and stable position of the device. In case of device implantation in the area of NCC, anterior mitral valve leaflet should be check.

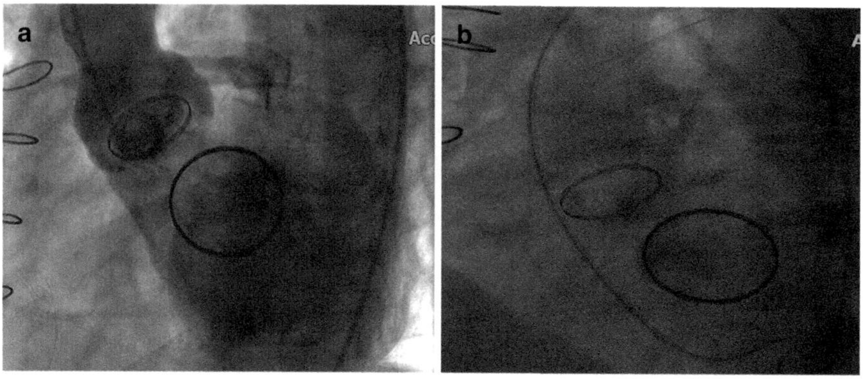

Fig. 76.3 (**a**, **b**) Aortic root injection showed severe paravalvular leakage from the medial side of the swing ring. Under TEE guidance, the wiring of the defect was done

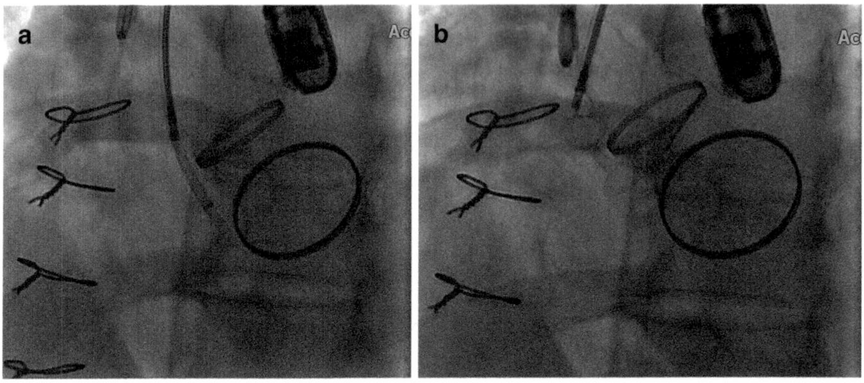

Fig. 76.4 (**a**, **b**) Based on the TEE defect size (6 mm) and defect shape, Muscular VSD 8 mm (Occlutech) device was chosen. First distal disk (DD) was partially extruded in the LV then by retracting the whole system toward the defect, the DD was totally deployed in the ventricular side and anchored within the defect, then after rechecking by TEE and angiography, the waist and the proximal disk (PD) was deployed

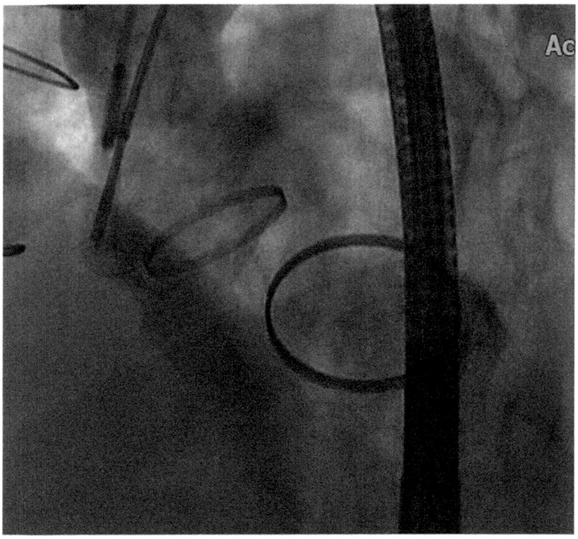

Fig. 76.5 Prior to release of the device, the most attention (by TEE and fluoroscopy) must be paid to the prosthetic valve to be sure that there is no interference with valve function (free moving leaflets) and no coverage of coronary ostia

Conclusion

Experience with percutaneous PVL closure is still limited. The procedural success rate varies from 63–95% based on the location of PVL and available devices. After successful closure, the congestive symptoms improve within the weeks, on the other hand, the hemolysis may continue or even worsen for the first few months until device endothelialization [3].

References

1. Ionescu A, Fraser AG, Butchart EG. Prevalence and clinical significance of incidental paraprosthetic valvular regurgitation: a prospective study using transoesophageal echocardiography. Heart. 2003;89:1316–21.
2. Hammermeister K, Sethi GK, Henderson WG, et al. Outcomes 15 years after valve replacement with a mechanical versus a bioprosthetic valve: final report of the Veterans Affairs randomized trial. J Am Coll Cardiol. 2000;36:1152–8.
3. Pate GE, Al Zubaidi A, Chandavimol M, et al. Percutaneous closure of prosthetic paravalvular leaks: case series and review. Catheter Cardiovasc Interv. 2006;68:528–33.

Chapter 77
Transcatheter Closure of Mitral Paravalvular Leakage (PVL)

Ata Firouzi and Zahra Hosseini

Abstract Mitral paravalvular leakage is more frequent than aortic valve. Patient's symptoms are dependent of the size of the defect and the severity of regurgitation. In severe type, they usually are symptomatic and finally leads to biventricular failure. The recommended treatment is surgical repair but in those with prohibited surgical risk, trans-catheter closure is an option. This intervention is very complex and should be evaluated completely by experience team for defining the anatomical feature of the defect. Various devices are available for closure (off-label), depending on the defect shape and size.

History

The patient was a 70 years old man, the known case of Mechanical Mitral Valve Replacement (MVR) 16 years ago, who was referred with refractory dyspnea F/C III–IV since 3 months ago despite high dose diuretic therapy. In TEE severe paravalvular leakage in the medial side of the swing ring was detected.

Percutaneous paravalvular closure is a complex procedure that requires multiple imaging modalities to visualize the 3D relationship of intracardiac structures and the operator' ability. Three approaches can be employed to cross the defect and the delivery device: transseptal, retrograde trans-aortic, and direct trans-apical. There is no dedicated device for this procedure. Paravalvular leakage in the Mitral prosthetic valve has occurred more than Aortic valve (17 vs. 10%) [1]. PVL can affect any valve in any position but is more common with mitral mechanical prostheses, supra-annular aortic prostheses and use of sutures without pledgets or continuous sutures in the mitral position [2]. Although surgical repair is the gold standard treatment for severe paravalvular regurgitation in those with intractable symptoms (right and left

A. Firouzi (✉) · Z. Hosseini
Interventional Cardiology, Cardiovascular Intervention Research Center, Rajaie Cardiovascular Medical and Research Center, Iran University of Medical Sciences, Tehran, Iran

M. Maleki, A. Alizadehasl (eds.), *Case-Based Clinical Cardiology*,
https://doi.org/10.1007/978-1-4471-7496-7_77

side congestive symptoms, hemolytic anemia), but in high-risk patients (STS risk score >8% or at a >15% risk of mortality at 30 days) with refractory symptoms and anatomically suitable for percutaneous closure at a center with expertise in this field, this is a better option (Class IIa) which has been appeared to have superior outcomes and less complications in compared with open surgery.

For the description of paravalvular leaks an adaptation of the accepted surgical nomenclature can be used. Each valve can be compared to a clock, so there are two clocks horizontally inverted one to another: one is in the aortic valve position and the other in the mitral valve position as seen from a cephalad position. The 12 o'clock in both clocks corresponds to the mitral-aortic fibrous continuity, and from there each location is named in a clockwise fashion (Fig. 77.1).

For the mitral valve, the 3 o'clock corresponds to the area of the interatrial septum, the 6 o'clock corresponds to the posterolateral free wall and the 9 o'clock corresponds to the LAA. Mitral PVL is most located between 10 and 2 o'clock (mitro-aortic fibrous continuity) and between 6 and 10 o'clock (posterior wall) [3] (Fig. 77.1 and 77.2).

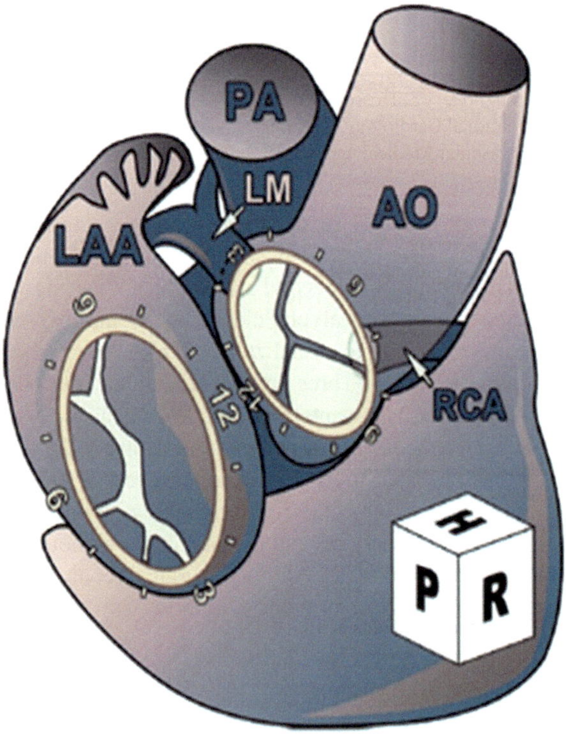

Fig. 77.1 Paravalvular leaks locations diagram

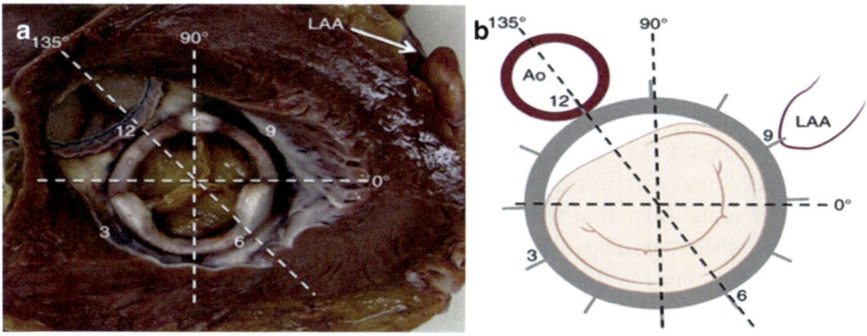

Fig. 77.2 Mitral valve (MV) as viewed from the left ventricle. The angles shown refer to the cuts made by a transesophageal echocardiography imaging crystal. The numbers correspond to the clock face perspective of the MV (numbering is as viewed from the left atrium). *Ao* Aorta; *LAA* left atrial appendage

Diagnostic Work-Up

TTE is the first modality for evaluation of LV, RV size and functions, mechanical valve evaluation, the severity of the valvular or paravalvular leak, any thrombus, or vegetation. The 3D TEE can accurately demonstrate the location, shape, size, number of the defects, dehiscence, any rocking motion and surrounding structures and differentiated PVL from valvular regurgitations. Another modalities like CT Angiography and CMR can also give more information for better evaluations of the defects.

Closure Strategy

It is clear that PVLs of the MVR are more challenging to treat. This procedure should only be undertaken by a team of structural and imaging cardiologists with experience in advanced structural interventions.

After insertion of right femoral artery and vein sheaths (6F) and IV Heparin injection to achieve ACT > 250 s, LV injections were done in LAO and RAO projections to localize the defect site and paravalvular leakage severity. Under general anesthesia and 3D TEE guidance, after complete assessment of the mechanical valve, the degree of trans-valvular and paravalvular regurgitation, defect numbers, shape, location, and rule outing any thrombus, vegetation or dehiscence, according to the defect location (clock number), transseptal or trans-apical approach is utilized. In this patient, the largest defect was crescent-shaped, 6 mm and at 2 o'clock corresponds to mitro-aortic fibrous continuity. Because of the absent hybrid room in our center, the transseptal approach was chosen.

Transseptal Approach: This approach is usually used for mitral PVL between 6 and 11 o'clock. For defects away from the septum, the location of the puncture is less critical. However, for medial defects near the IAS, a posterior and slightly superior puncture provides the appropriate working height within the LA. After septostomy by Brockenbrough needle and contrast injection to be sure of being in LA (Fig. 77.3a), Spiral wire was inserted in LA for more support and LA borders localization and septal dilatation was performed. Through a 125-cm 6F multipurpose diagnostic catheter telescoped through a steerable transseptal sheath (Agilis sheath), after several attempts, a 0.035 inch straight hydrophilic wire was manipulated by TEE and fluoroscopy guidance to cross the defect and advanced to the ascending aorta, then the catheter was passed over the wire (Fig. 77.3b). After that, the wire was exchanged with Amplatzer Superstiff guidewire and hydrophilic kink resistance delivery sheath (Epsylar 7F) was advanced gently over the wire in to the LV. (In case of significant difficulty in crossing the delivery sheath, more support can be obtained by building an arterio-venous rail). In this case, based on the defect characteristics, Muscular VSD 8 mm (Occlutech) was chosen. After loading the

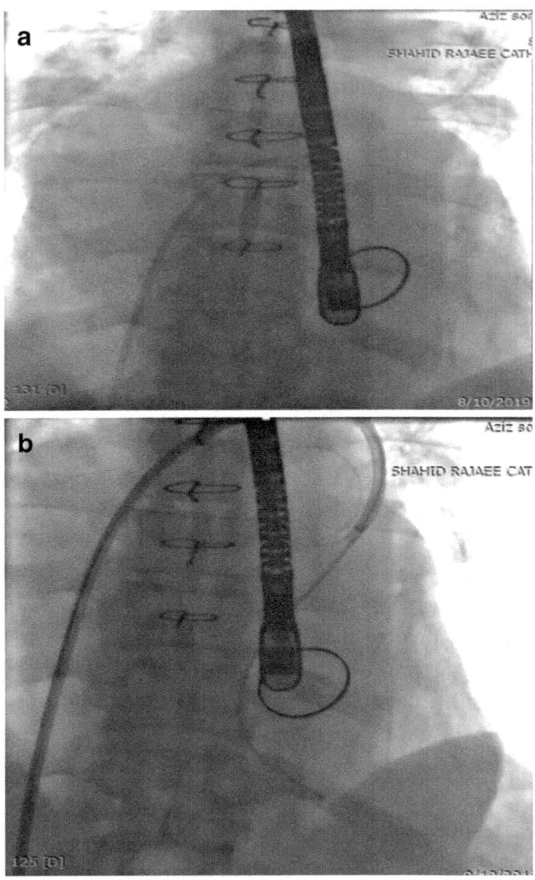

Fig. 77.3 (**a**, **b**) After septostomy, through Agilis sheath, wiring of the defect at 6 o'clock was performed

device and connected to the delivery cable, the device passed over the delivery sheath and under TEE and fluoroscopy guidance, after partially exposed the Distal Disk (DD), the whole system was pulled back, then the DD fully deployed in the LV, after reassurance about the correct position of the DD by TEE and LV injection, the waist, and proximal disk was deployed in LA (Fig. 77.4a). Before releasing the device, TEE should show mobile mitral leaflets, open pulmonary veins, the residual leakage, and the stability of the device. After final angiography and TEE evaluation, the stability of the device was confirmed and the device was released (Fig. 77.4b). The residual leakage was minimal.

Trans-Apical Approach: This approach can be a good alternative for mitral PLV between 11 and 6 o'clock (posterior or septal defects) to avoid complications associated with excessive forces on the septal wall from the delivery catheter. The advantage is less difficult wiring of the PVL.

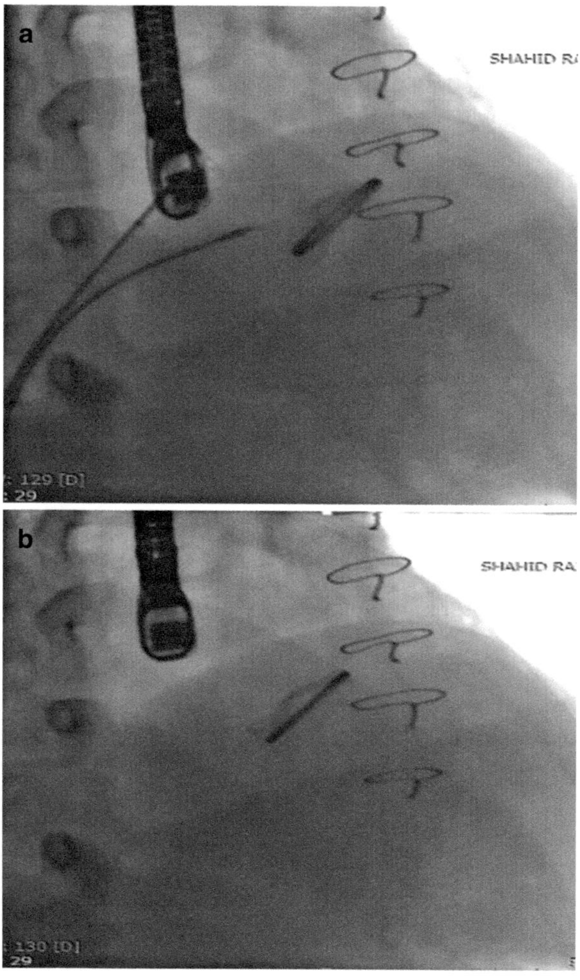

Fig. 77.4 (**a**, **b**) In this case, based on the defect characteristics, Muscular VSD 8 mm (Occlutech) was chosen. Under TEE and fluoroscopy guidance, after partially exposed the Distal Disk (DD), the whole system was pulled back, then the DD fully deployed in the LV, after reassurance about the correct position of the DD by TEE and LV injection, the waist and proximal disk was deployed in LA. Before releasing the device, TEE should show mobile mitral leaflets, open pulmonary veins, the residual leakage, and the stability of the device

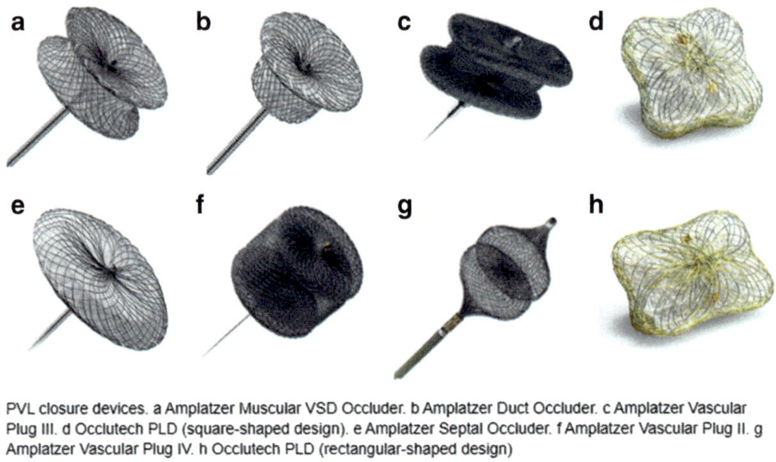

Fig. 77.5 Most of the devices are used off-label for this procedure. PVLs are variable in size, shape (crescentic, oval, serpiginous, or cylindrical), so, one device is not fit in all PVLs. Usually, for a small cylindrical PVL, AVP II or PDA Occluders are used, for oval types AVP III and for small and angulated ones AVP IV Occluders can be considered

Device Selection

Most of the devices are used off-label for this procedure. PVLs are variable in size, shape (crescentic, oval, serpiginous, or cylindrical), so, one device is not fit in all PVLs.

Usually, for a small cylindrical PVL, AVP II or PDA Occluders are used, for oval types AVP III and for small and angulated ones AVP IV Occluders can be considered [4] (Fig. 77.5).

Conclusion

TPVL closure in symptomatic patients is a less invasive option than surgery (most complications are: device embolization, cardiac perforation, vascular complications, prosthetic valve impingement, and stroke), with lower morbidity and mortality. To continue to improve procedural success and outcome, new advancements in device design are necessary.

References

1. Ionescu A, Fraser AG, Butchart EG. Prevalence and clinical significance of incidental paraprosthetic valvular regurgitation: a prospective study using transoesophageal echocardiography. Heart. 2003;89:1316–21.
2. Meloni L, Aru G, Abbruzzese PA, Cardu G, Ricchi A, Cattolica FS, Martelli V, Cherchi A. Regurgitant flow of mitral valve prostheses: an intraoperative transesophageal echocardiographic study. J Am Soc Echocardiogr. 1994;7:36–46.
3. Ruiz CE, Jelnin V, Kronzon I, et al. Clinical outcomes in patients undergoing percutaneous closure of periprosthetic paravalvular leaks. J Am Coll Cardiol. 2011;58:2210–7.
4. Shapira Y, Hirscg R, Kornowski R, et al. Percutaneous closure of perivalvular leaks with Amplatzer occluders: feasibility, safety, and shortterm results. J Heart Valve Dis. 2007;16:305–13.

Index

M. Maleki, A. Alizadehasl (eds.), *Case-Based Clinical Cardiology*,
https://doi.org/10.1007/978-1-4471-7496-7

GPSR Compliance

The European Union's (EU) General Product Safety Regulation (GPSR) is a set of rules that requires consumer products to be safe and our obligations to ensure this.

If you have any concerns about our products, you can contact us on ProductSafety@springernature.com

In case Publisher is established outside the EU, the EU authorized representative is:

Springer Nature Customer Service Center GmbH
Europaplatz 3
69115 Heidelberg, Germany

Batch number: 10703867

Printed by Printforce, the Netherlands